Genetics - Research and Issues

nova
Medicine & Health
New York

Genetics - Research and Issues

Genetic Instability and Some Unusual Radiobiological Effects
Ekaterina S. Evstratova, Vladislav G. Petin,
Andrey D. Kaprin and Petr V. Shegai (Editors)
2022. ISBN: 978-1-68507-886-7 (Hardcover)
2022. ISBN: 979-8-88697-007-4 (eBook)

Fragile X Syndrome: From Diagnosis to Treatment
Fabrizio Stasolla, PhD (Editor)
2022. ISBN: 978-1-68507-572-9 (Softcover)
2022. ISBN: 978-1-68507-593-4 (eBook)

Recurrence Risk in Autism Spectrum Disorders
Michael Beenstock
2021. ISBN: 978-1-68507-129-5 (Hardcover)
2021. ISBN: 978-1-68507-244-5 (eBook)

p53: Structure, Functions and Role in Disease
Monte Stevens (Editor)
2020. ISBN: 978-1-53618-771-7 (Softcover)
2020. ISBN: 978-1-53618-808-0 (eBook)

A Comprehensive Guide to Genetic Counseling
Benjamin A. Kepert (Editor)
2020. ISBN: 978-1-53616-975-1 (Softcover)
2020. ISBN: 978-1-53616-976-8 (eBook)

Living with Huntington's Disease: Challenges, Perspectives and Quality of Life
Sherman Howell (Editor)
2019. ISBN: 978-1-53616-729-0 (Softcover)
2019. ISBN: 978-1-53616-730-6 (eBook)

More information about this series can be found at https://novapublishers.com/product-category/series/genetics-research-and-issues/

Sevgi Durna Daştan
and Nazan Yurtcu
Editors

Epigenetics

Beyond the Genetics and Medicine

nova
Medicine & Health
New York

DOI: 10.52305/IVZP1313.

Library of Congress Cataloging-in-Publication Data

ISBN: 979-8-88697-228-3

Published by Nova Science Publishers, Inc. † New York

Contents

Preface

Epigenetics refers to the study of changes in organisms that are caused by modifications of gene expression instead of alteration of the genetic code itself. This volume includes 30 chapters that explore epigenetics from a variety of perspectives, including the role of epigenetics in aging, cancers, fetal brain development, epilepsy, and more.

Chapter 1 - Epigenetics is termed as non-sequence deoxyribonucleic acid (DNA) alterations in the gene expression profile that is heritable. With these, cellular identity is preserved, and gene function is transferred from one cell to another. Epigenetic changes occur with the effect of DNA methylation, chromatin structure changes, and non-coding ribonucleic acids, histone modifications. Even though cells in different tissues have the same DNA, differences may occur between the steps that take place during protein synthesis from DNA, and this can be explained by epigenetic regulation. In addition to the genetic basis, it is known that epigenetic differences are also effective in the development of many diseases, especially cancer. Changes in gene expression should be investigated with epigenomics rather than gene analysis in a particular region. In the investigation of diseases of unknown etiology, such as obesity, insulin resistance, neurodegenerative, cardiovascular, and immune system diseases, it has been determined that many internal and external environmental factors directly affect gene expression. Understanding the differences that cause diseases with epigenetic mechanisms makes it possible to develop molecular diagnostic tests and targeted treatment strategies. In this chapter, basic information about epigenetics will be given and the situations where disruptions in epigenetic mechanisms may lead to related gene expression, and the importance of epigenetics in these situations will be emphasized.

Chapter 2 - Epigenetic changes occur in the phenotype due to differences in the expression of genes while remaining the same in the existing DNA sequence. Disruptions in the promoter methylation pattern, histone modifications, and non-coding RNA irregularities can be given as examples of epigenetic changes. The positive or negative effects of lifestyle changes lead to epigenetic mechanisms and these mechanisms often work together to cause changes that affect all organ systems. These changes can result in autoimmune diseases or syndromes. Therefore, further research on epigenetic mechanisms can significantly contribute to the diagnosis, follow-up, and the treatment of many organ systems diseases.

Chapter 3 - Epigenetic modifications include DNA methylation and covalent modifications of histones. In spite of the fact that they are reversible, these alterations have an unavoidable effect on gene expression and are very stable. Cytosines are more frequently methylated than guanine nucleotides or CpG sites in DNA. In addition to regulating tissue-specific gene expression, DNA methylation also affects genomic imprinting and the inactivation of X chromosomes. It is possible that DNA methylation in different genomic regions may influence gene activity differently depending on the genetic sequence.

Methylation changes in the promoter or first exon can mimic the effects of mutations in various tumor suppressor genes (TSGs) or protooncogenes. Cancer may also develop from abnormal DNA methylation, such as hyper- or hypomethylation of cancer-related genes' promoters or first exons. The transcriptional silencing of a variety of TSGs is caused by hypermethylation of their promoters. Activating the transcription of protooncogenes, retrotransposons, and genes that encode proteins that have a role in genome instability and malignant cell metastasis is accomplished by hypomethylating regulatory DNA sequences.

In carcinogenesis, DNA methylation has a critical role in gene expression. In this chapter, hypo- and hyper-DNA methylation on cancer as well as recurrence risk of human cancers are discussed along with the mechanisms and cell-regulating effects of both hypo- and hyper-methylation.

Chapter 4 - Epigenetics refers to changes that do not affect the DNA sequence but can affect gene expression. Healthy cells transform into malignant cells through some complex mechanisms. The simultaneous evaluation of tumor suppressor genes and oncogenesis with epigenetics makes it easier for us to understand this complex process. Among epigenetic mechanisms, there are two mechanisms that directly control gene expression, which are DNA methylation and histone modification. DNA methylation is involved in cellular control, while histone modifications have functions in transcriptional activity and modifications at the chromatin structure level. It has been determined that epigenetic mechanisms such as DNA methylation and histone modifications also regulate the expression of miRNAs. miRNAs are non-coding RNA molecules composed of twenty-two nucleotide sequences that are short and involved in the development of both physiological and important diseases such as malignancies. Tumor-associated abnormalities in miRNA or epigenetic mechanisms are commonly found in human cancers. Abnormal proliferation, apoptosis, and genetics are involved in the development of malignant cells. miRNAs are considered to be actively involved in the regulation of these processes. Available data reveal that miRNAs, which can be used as biomarkers, are biomarkers that can be used in early diagnosis, tumor subtyping, early treatment, prognosis prediction, and treatment resistance. Thus, it is considered that they can increase the disease-free lifetime and quality of life of cancer patients. In this paper, it was attempted to describe the relationship between dysregulated miRNA and epigenetic mechanisms in cancer.

Chapter 5 - Genetics cannot solely explain genetic variations in humans and disease developments. We see varying differences in phenotypes and disease susceptibility in organisms that have the same genetic make-up, e.g., monozygotic twins and cloned animals. The information carried by the genomic sequence is the blueprint, but the final product requires environmental determinants. Here comes the concept of epigenetics, as it is the framework where biochemical interactions between the genome and the environment blend. We can describe epigenetics as mechanisms that are beyond genetics, as such mechanisms alter the result of the genomic blueprint without altering the information itself, i.e., the sequence. Both epigenetics and epigenomics are trending research fields to better evaluate the genotype and the phenotype. The methylation of genetic material is a well-studied and well-known epigenetic marker. The epigenome, as a term, describes the inheritable changes in both the DNA and histone molecular structures, where the methylation and acetylation mechanisms are studied extensively. As the building blocks of the chromatin structure, nucleosomes depend on epigenetic changes, which lead to becoming either tight or loose, based on the particular mechanisms. Chromatin structure changes directly affect the gene expression, e.g., particular gene expression becomes silenced if the gene position has DNA hypermethylation and histone hypoacetylation that leads to the condensed form of the chromatin. Inversely, if the said changes were removed, genes in that position would express themselves again. Therefore, epigenetics provides a vigorous and remarkably malleable means for gene expression regulations. Epigenomics includes both the epigenetic mechanisms on the DNA and histones and complicated interactions between the genotype and the phenotype. There are well-known epigenomic changes in DNA, RNA, and protein levels. DNA base changes in somatic cells and chromosome positioning are among the aspects determining the epigenomic scene. Alternative splicing mechanism, RNA processing (editing, capping, Poly-A tailing, etc.), RNA methylation, and regulations conferred by the non-coding RNAs (ncRNAs) are RNA level epigenomic changes. Epigenomic changes at the protein level include various mechanisms of the post-translational modification. Epigenomics research includes total hypomethylation profile of the genome, identification of hypermethylated genes, microRNA-driven gene silencing with DNA methylation, epigenome projects, and DNA-based clinical therapies for different biomedical conditions. This chapter will detail fundamental concepts and basic approaches to both epigenomics and epigenomes.

Chapter 6 - Epigenetic changes are important mechanisms that have a role in the etiology and/or progression of cancer by causing the activation of oncogenes or the silencing of tumor suppressor genes. Epigenetic mechanisms that alter chromatin structure can be separated into four categories: histone modifications, DNA methylation, nucleosome remodeling, and non-coding RNAs (e.g., miRNAs). These mechanisms work together to organise the functioning of the genome by regulating the accessibility of chromatin and altering the structural dynamics of chromatin. These epigenetic mechanisms are necessary for normal mammalian development and regulation of gene expression. Disorders in epigenetic regulators have been determined in both blood and solid cancers, and the significance of epigenetic changes in cancer cells has been emphasized by several groups in different types of cancer.

Chapter 7 - The human is a superorganism called the holobiont, which consists of human cells and a larger proportion of microbial cells. Microbiota is the ecological communities of microorganisms that live in a particular environment. It is known that the human microbiota, especially the gut microbiota, is known to affect the physiology and pathology of the host through various mechanisms. For example, the intestinal microflora regulates many epigenetic pathways, such as modifications to DNA or histones, their metabolites, and noncoding RNAs. Epigenetic factors are also known to regulate the gut microbiota within the host by various mechanisms.

Chapter 8 - The study of epigenetics examines how genetic changes in gene expression are transmitted from one generation to another and are not caused by changes in the DNA sequence. A key role played by epigenetic mechanisms is thought to be in cellular growth, differentiation, and autoimmune diseases. There are several epigenetic mechanisms, including DNA methylation, histone modifications, and non-coding RNA regulation.

Transcripts that do not have protein-coding capacity in our genome are defined as non-coding RNA (ncRNA). The post-transcriptional regulation of genes is greatly influenced by non-coding RNAs. These ncRNAs are composed of small non-coding RNAs (sncRNA) and long non-coding RNAs (lncRNA) according to their length. Epigenetic mechanisms (genetic imprinting and dosage compensation) have been found to regulate the expression of lncRNAs. The function of centromeres is regulated by sncRNAs, which are involved in gene expression, chromatin organization, and modification.

In this chapter, the potential epigenetic mechanisms of ncRNAs and their associated cellular processes are presented. The importance of non-coding RNAs in the etiology of diseases has been revealed in recent genetic studies. Non-coding RNAs have been shown to have functions ranging from control of gene expression, epigenetic mechanisms, and signal transduction. In particular, it has been determined that some piRNAs, miRNAs, and siRNAs function in common pathways and are involved in regulatory mechanisms.

Chapter 9 - Epigenetics generally describes inherited DNA methylation, histone modifications, and chromatin-based events including chromatin structure that regulate gene expression. In the field of epigenetics, microRNAs have also been shown to have a role in epigenetic regulation. While DNA methylation and histone modifications add a new dimension to gene regulation at the transcriptional level, miRNAs are involved in the regulation at the post-transcriptional level. Analysis of histone modifications is done by chromatin immunoprecipitation (ChIP) and 3C Chromosome conformation capture. There are many methods used for DNA methylation analysis. These methods are hybridization (Southern blot and microarray), restriction enzyme PCR, methylation-sensitive single-nucleotide primer extension, cutting with methylation-sensitive restriction enzymes, bisulfite genomic DNA sequence analysis techniques and epigenetic MR. This chapter offers a reference of various techniques for epigenetic analysis.

Chapter 10 - Epigenetics is a new critical field that has arisen to investigate the effect of elements apart from genes on the character and on the role of an organism. Using computational tools constitutes the core of this new research area and has critical roles because controlling the choice of basic tests, developing recent provable theories from precise examination of complicated genomic knowledge, which is not attainable utilizing classical methods, only possible with computational tools. Epigenomics connects conventional genomics with computer science, biochemistry, mathematics, chemistry, proteomics for the extensive investigation of hereditary diversities in phenotype, and gene activity or gene interpretation, which are not dependent on gene array. Moreover, it helps us to better understand transcriptional adjustment, nuclear arrangement, improvement, and illness. Here, current computational approaches to investigate epigenetic factors are explored. Essential data sources and bioinformatic apparatus in this fast-developing area have been evaluated.

Chapter 11 - Aging is a multifactorial process happening with many biological, biochemical, and physiological changes. There are a lot of theories to explain the nature of aging. There are also many data supporting the relationships between epigenetic modifications and the aging process. Nucleosomal remodeling is frequently stressed by numerous research due to its critical nature in cellular senescence and aging. Different mechanisms are postulated for nucleosomal remodeling, which include (1) modification of nucleosome residency by histone loss, (2) alteration of nucleosome affinity to either DNA or histones induced by histone protein variants, and (3) ATP-dependent nucleosome relocation to modify recruitment of transcriptional factors and other modifiers. Recent advances have revealed aging-related genes that have modifying properties for histone repositioning, which supports the fact that both aging and senescence are directly related to the disruption of heterochromatin and euchromatin ratios in the chromatin landscape. Thus, leading to the dissolution of the clear distinctions between chromatin regions in cellular senescence, which is more pronounced in the aging process. This dissolution correlates with the downregulation of genes in the senescence that are normally in an active state before the senescence period. However, conflicting results are present in terms of the genome-wide heterochromatin association with the aging and senescence processes.

Therefore, specific analyses are necessary of which genomic regions, related loci, and gene expressions are affected. This review will try to describe the intricate associations between cellular senescence and known epigenetic mechanisms, e.g., chromatin remodeling and restructuring. Also, the currently established properties of the aging process with epigenetic mechanisms are described using different models for the aging phenomenon.

Chapter 12 - FMF represents an autosomal recessive hereditary disease, which may have recurrent episodes of fever, serositis, and arthritis/arthralgia and accompanying skin findings. Its prevalence varies from society to society and changes in the range of 1/200-1/1000 on average. The gene responsible for FMF is the MEFV (Mediterranean Fever) gene on chromosome 16, which encodes the pyrin protein. The problem in FMF is the change in pyrin protein due to the MEFV gene mutation. Mutation in pyrin reduces the activation threshold of the inflammasome, which excessively increases IL-1 secretion and initiates the inflammatory process. Mutations of M694V, V726A, M680I, and M694I are observed most frequently worldwide, and these are known as pathological mutations. The most feared complication is secondary AA-type amyloidosis. With the use of colchicine in the treatment, attacks are prevented, subclinical inflammation between attacks is taken under control, and the risk of amyloidosis is eliminated. Alternative treatments should be considered in the presence of partial remission with colchicine therapy, in cases of unresponsiveness to colchicine, or in cases of colchicine intolerance. TNF-a inhibitors, IL-1 inhibitors (anakinra, rilonacept, and canakinumab), and Janus kinase inhibitors are among alternative treatments.

It has been recently revealed that changes in DNA cannot be explained only by genetics, and the role of epigenetic mechanisms is also quite significant. In epigenetics, the DNA sequence does not change; however, since the promoter region of the gene changes, quantitative and qualitative changes emerge in gene transcription. As a result of transcriptional changes, the transcription of the relevant gene can be silenced or activated. These quantitative and qualitative changes are not permanent and can be regulated when needed. Furthermore, these alterations in gene transcription can be transferred to the following generations. When epigenetic mechanisms are mentioned, DNA methylation, histone acetylation, histone methylation, histone ubiquitination, histone phosphorylation, histone citrullination, histone ribosylation, non-coding RNA, and chromatin re-modeling come to mind.

Epigenetics tries to explain different phenotypes of FMF patients with the same genotype (patients with the same mutation and individuals from the same family), the absence of the clinical presentation of a patient with the mutation or the FMF clinical presentation of patients without the mutation, drug response or drug resistance. Histone modification, DNA methylation, and microRNA (miRNA) represent the epigenetic mechanisms that are accused the most of the correlation between FMF and epigenetics.

Chapter 13 - Genetic and environmental interactions have a significant role in the evolution, development, and functioning of the central nervous system. Epigenetic mechanisms including, DNA methylation, non-coding RNAs, and histone modifications are important to clarify how genetic and environmental interactions alter neurobiology and behavior. Alterations in epigenetic mechanisms induce remarkable changes in cognitive and behavioral phenotypes. It is becoming apparent that the epigenetic machinery is involved in the pathogenesis of neurobehavioral and neurobiological disorders. A better understanding of the altered epigenetics mechanism underlying these disorders is important to inventing new therapies for neurobiological disorders.

Chapter 14 - The physiological and behavioral development of an individual is a dynamic event that includes the interaction between genes and the environment. The brain and nerve development period of the baby in the womb is between the 4th and 10th weeks of pregnancy. Although the early stages of the brain development are affected by genetic factors, the decision of where and how genes are utilized is determined by environmental factors. This situation solely depends on the pregnancy period of the mother, meaning it is tightly related to the level of food intake and stress exposure which affects the early phases of brain architecture. Environmental factors and experience leave traces on certain parts of genes, and these epigenetic changes can change the activity or expression of the genes.

Chapter 15 - Epilepsy is a common neurological disorder manifested by recurrent seizures, and its underlying causes could be significantly associated with genetic. Epigenetic hereditary changes in gene expression that are not caused by changes in the DNA sequence.

DNA methylation, post-transcriptional changes of histones, and the action of non-coding RNA molecules are currently the most well-researched epigenetic mechanisms. These processes control gene expression, and interruption of these molecular pathways can lead to disease development. Investigating the epigenetic processes involved in epilepsy is a potential avenue of search that will lead to a better understanding of the etiology and treatments of epilepsy.

Chapter 16 - Epigenetic mechanisms occurring in DNA methylation, histone modification, and RNA-based mechanisms may generate heritable phenotypic changes without a change in DNA sequence. The disruption of gene expression patterns governed by epigenetics may lead to various diseases such as cardiovascular diseases, autoimmune diseases, and cancers. Genetic studies guide for preventive measures, appropriate treatment selection, drug interactions, drug efficacy, and patient compliance. Cardiovascular diseases (CVDs) are the most common cause of mortality worldwide. The increase in risk factors is predictive of the fact that the frequency of CVDs will further increase. Thus, detailed genetic data screening will become important in the diagnosis and prevention of CVD in the near future.

Chapter 17 - Obesity is an important health problem that has reached the level of pandemic today, has important effects on high prevalence diseases such as cardiovascular, diabetes, and cancer, and even leads to deaths. Obesity occurs from multifactorial effects, primarily genetic and environmental factors. Studies have identified a large number of genes that cause obesity, but the rapid increase in obesity in a short time cannot be explained only by genetic factors alone. Epigenetic changes that occur through environmental factors such as nutrition and physical activity also have an important role in the current increase in the incidence of obesity. Gene-environment interaction causes different phenotypic variations to occur in organisms. These different phenotypes, which occur without any changes in the DNA sequence, are explained by epigenetics. Therefore, the view that interindividual differences in susceptibility to obesity are due to epigenetic factors has recently gained considerable importance. Many studies have shown that epigenetic mechanisms such as DNA methylation, histone modifications, and non-coding RNAs are closely related to obesity.

The aim of this review is to present the relationship between epigenetics and obesity and the effects of epigenetic mechanisms on obesity.

Chapter 18 - Diabetes mellitus (DM) is a metabolic disease characterized by hyperglycemia resulting from a partial or absolute decrease in insulin secretion, with varying degrees of peripheral resistance to the impact of insulin. The prevalence of type 2 diabetes mellitus increases exponentially every day, along with an increase in obesity and bad eating habits.

Prolonged hyperglycemia causes microvascular (retinopathy, nephropathy, neuropathy, and cardiovascular diseases) and macrovascular (cardiovascular diseases) complications and major morbidity and mortality in patients. The causes of disease in DM, which is such an important public health problem, are largely based on the interaction of genetic and environmental factors. Nevertheless, the etiopathogenesis of the disease has not been completely elucidated. Since epigenetics can provide a molecular link between genetic, environmental factors and diabetes and can be transmitted over generations, it is promising in elucidating the etiopathogenesis of diabetes and identifying new treatment options for its etiology. Even if hyperglycemia is corrected, epigenetic mechanisms are included in metabolic memory, and in the long term, complications secondary to DM persist. Furthermore, studies on epigenetics and metabolic memory demonstrate that diabetes and its complications can be prevented by changing environmental factors such as calorie control.

Chapter 19 - Osteoporosis is a disease that is more common in old age nowadays, significantly reduces bone quality and causes severe morbidity with fractures and in the development of which many factors have a role. It has extensive etiopathogenesis, and it has been investigated for many years. Along with the increasing knowledge of genes, the evolving technological developments open new windows, and the adventure that starts with this small window turns into a large world. New approaches, new possible drugs, and new etiopathogenesis for osteoporosis are present in this new world of epigenetic science. Determining this cycle of bone tissue, which starts with gene sequences and turns into the most robust tissue of people, through genetic, epigenetic, and molecular mechanisms has still been discussed in studies. The fact that epigenetic factors are modifiable, editable, and recyclable causes this world to be much more interesting.

Chapter 20 - Osteoarthritis (OA) is a common degenerative joint disease worldwide. Considering the large number of people it affects, it creates serious limitations on patients and creates a serious burden on the healthcare system. Obesity, gender, genetic predisposition, trauma, and some systemic diseases can be listed as the most common causes of OA. However, in recent years, with the research on the concept of epigenetics and its relationship with various diseases, there have been serious changes in the view of the etiology of OA. The imbalance of anabolic and catabolic events that have a role in cartilage physiology is the most important element in the pathogenesis of OA. Epigenetic factors are also blamed for the disruption of this balance. DNA methylation, Histone modification, and non-coding RNAs are the most widely accepted epigenetic mechanisms in OA. Many published studies have revealed the relationship of each of these mechanisms with the pathogenesis of OA. New doors will likely be opened in the prevention and treatment of OA with the studies that have been conducted and will be conducted in this regard.

Chapter 21 - Degenerative disc disease (DDD) is one of the most common spine-related diseases. Its etiology is not exactly known, but recent studies have elucidated that this disease is a complex and multifactorial disease resulting from the interaction of genetic and environmental factors. In general terms, these studies focus on changes in genes encoding the structural components of the intervertebral disc.

Chapter 22 - Spinal deformity in neuromuscular scoliosis is the result of various neurological or muscular pathologies. Loss of muscle tone and weakness, which are often the main symptoms. Sometimes in addition to the clinical picture of muscle retraction, sensitivity disorder, accompanied by mental retardation, and digestive, heart, or respiratory problems. DNA modifications are thought to have a role in epigenetic deterioration and disease formation in congenital scoliosis (CS) that occurs with congenital deformity of the vertebrae. When DNA is extracted from the hemivertebra and spinal process during surgical correction operations, aberrant DNA methylation has been found to be associated with the development of hemivertebrae and congenital scoliosis. In studies conducted in recent years, TGFR1, EGFR, IGF1R, and GHR are in spinal growth stages; Chondrogenic alteration of the SOX9, PAX1, PAX9, and IHH genes and during differentiation; In the cartilage matrix structure of the ACAN, LUM, VCAN, COL1A1, COL2A1, and HAPLN1 genes; It has been shown that the SLC26A2, CHST1, and CHST3 genes are involved in the formation of the extracellular matrix in vivo. In a different study, it has been observed that there is a predisposition to spinal pathologies in the CALM1 gene polymorphism, which is involved in muscle contraction and bone synthesis. Statistical differences were found in the polymorphic distribution of the rs2234693 region of the ER1 gene in patients with double curve, Cobb angle $\geq 40°$, and thoracic curve. In addition, it was determined that there was a difference in the polymorphic distribution of the rs12885713 region in the CALM1 gene in patients with double curves and in the polymorphic distribution of the same gene in patients with thoracic curves.

Chapter 23 - The endometrium is a functional tissue under the control of ovarian steroid hormones. The endometrium shows cyclic changes including biochemical and morphological. These cyclic changes occur with the growth, proliferation, and death of endometrial stromal and glandular cells. Cyclic changes of endometrial tissue are regulated by levels and nuclear receptors of ovarian steroid hormones. During the normal menstrual cycle, epigenetic mechanisms, especially DNA methylation, have important roles in gene expression regulation and influence functional changes.

Epigenetic mechanisms affect gene expression with transcriptional regulation and control endometrial cell proliferation, angiogenesis, desidualization, and embryo implantation. DNA methylation is an essential modification for the normal cell cycle. Abnormal DNA methylation can be associated with abortus and other endometrial pathologies. Recent studies focus also on the combination of epigenetic changes with genetic changes in the development of endometrial pathologies such as endometriosis and endometrial cancer.

The most known epigenetic mechanisms are DNA methylation, post-translational modifications, and non-coding RNAs. Understanding the epigenetic mechanisms and identifying the methylation profile can help create personalized treatment for each patient.

Chapter 24 - Polycystic ovary syndrome (PCOS) is a common disease in women of reproductive age. Recently, research has shown that the interaction of genomic and environmental factors can modify the clinical condition through epigenetic modifications in the pathophysiology of this disease.

Chapter 25 - Preeclampsia (PE) is a disease that affects pregnant women at rates ranging from 2% to 10%, causing perinatal and maternal morbidity as well as maternal and perinatal mortality. PE is typically characterized by the onset of new hypertension with proteinuria at and after the 20th week of pregnancy; It may be associated with various causes such as inflammatory cytokines and poor trophoblast invasion. Several epigenetic changes can be associated with PE, such as histone modifications, environmental factors, microRNAs (miRNAs), and DNA methylation. In this perspective, the most important epigenetic factor associated with PE; is abnormal DNA methylation during placentation. In addition, acetylation-like histone modifications and low regulation of miRNAs or the effect of ovarian regulation and long non-coding RNAs in various signaling pathways may be involved in the etiology of PE and its epigenetics. PE is associated with low birth weight (LBW) and intrauterine growth restriction (IUGR). When children born as a result of pregnancies with a diagnosis of PE were followed, it was determined that these children were at risk of cardiovascular disease. The cause of PE, which carries serious risks for the mother and the child, is unfortunately not known precisely, and there is no effective treatment to cope with the acute and chronic consequences of the disease. Although it is an obvious fact that the placenta is essential for fetal development, it is known that epigenetic factors have a role in placental processes such as spiral artery remodeling and trophoblast invasion.

Epigenetic mechanisms leading to changes in placental gene expression in PE mediate processes that contribute to the development of placental malfunction, impaired fetal growth, and IUGR, a critical mission in the onset of PE. Lightening the epigenetic processes that conduce to routine placental growth and the triggering incidents in the etiopathogenesis of PE may contribute to the clear etiology of the disease and may lead to the discovery of new treatments.

This review aims to shed light on the epigenetic relationship with PE in light of these perspectives.

Chapter 26 - Pain and its chronicity in the following process are the main subjects of numerous studies nowadays with the adverse impacts of pain on quality of life, loss of workforce it causes, and still not completely explained pathophysiological mechanisms. The difficulties in treating symptoms that accompany pain and individual differences in response to applied treatment methods have accelerated genetic and epigenetic research. Epigenetics, which we have heard frequently in recent years, is the formation of different genetic variations under the influence of various factors and is now accepted as a significant mechanism in the unknown etiology of numerous diseases. Different epigenetic modifications have been described in the formation, typing, and treatment of pain, and new information is obtained with ongoing studies. The difficulties experienced in treatment due to changes at the molecular level caused by the chronic pain process and the activation of sensitization mechanisms have brought about epigenetic mechanisms both in etiopathogenesis studies and in the development of novel treatment approaches.

Chapter 27 - Connective tissue diseases (CTDs) are defined as chronic inflammatory diseases that can affect all organs and systems, primarily the joints. The underlying genetic background is very important for the development of these diseases, and environmental factors also contribute to this process. The clinical spectrum can vary considerably from patient to patient in individuals with CTDs, and even responses varying from person to person are observed in treatment responses. The emergence of such different phenotypic characteristics in this group of patients with relatively similar genotypic characteristics has caused the need to investigate them in different models that may contribute to the underlying pathogenetic process.

It has been recently revealed that changes in DNA cannot be explained only by genetics, and the role of epigenetic mechanisms is also quite large. In epigenetics, the DNA sequence does not change. However, since the promoter region of the gene changes, differences occur in gene transcription, in other words, in the end product of the gene. There is no clear factor that induces this change, and epigenetic modifications such as histone modification, DNA methylation, and microRNA (miRNA) that probably occur under the influence of environmental factors have led to the emergence of a new field to explain different phenotypic characteristics in patients.

In this chapter, the characteristics of epigenetic mechanisms in general and the reflections of these modifications on common CTDs, both at the cellular level and clinically, will be discussed.

Chapter 28 - Rheumatoid arthritis (RA) is chronic, autoimmune, erosive inflammatory rheumatism that impacts especially the female population between the ages of 20-50. Its prevalence varies between 0.5-1% worldwide. The etiology of rheumatoid arthritis is multifactorial. The risk factors include genetic, epigenetic, allergic, hormonal, neuroendocrine, reproduction-related factors, comorbid conditions, smoking, air pollution, socioeconomic status, lifestyle, diet, inhalation of dusts such as silica-asbestos-glass powder-textile dyes, microbiota, and infectious agents. After the diagnosis is established with physical examination, laboratory, and imaging methods, an appropriate treatment regimen must be quickly arranged to prevent disability. Pharmacological and non-pharmacological treatments are used to treat RA. There are patient education, psychosocial support, orthoses, exercise program, physical therapy agents, nutritional support and diet, prevention of osteoporosis and other comorbidities among non-pharmacological treatments. Pharmacologically, conventional DMARDs (disease-modifying anti-rheumatic drugs) are initially used (methotrexate, leflunomide, sulfasalazine, and hydroxychloroquine). In cases unresponsive to conventional treatments, TNF-a inhibitors (adalimumab, golimumab, infliximab, certolizumab pegol, and etanercept) or non-TNF biologics (rituximab, tocilizumab, anakinra, abatacept, baricitinib, tofacitinib) are utilized. Epigenetics refers to changes in gene expression without any change in DNA sequence. Changes occur in the chromosome, various phenotypes emerge, and the resulting changes can be passed on to the next generations by mitosis or meiosis. Environmental stimuli such as drugs, smoke, and cigarettes can induce epigenetic modifications. Hence, the link between the genome and the environment is ensured by epigenetic mechanisms. Epigenetic mechanisms include DNA methylation, post-translational histone modifications (histone methylation, histone acetylation, histone phosphorylation, histone ubiquitination, histone citrullination, and histone ribosylation), and the expression of non-coding RNAs (ncRNAs) such as microRNA (miRNA). DNA hypomethylation, histone acetylation, histone methylation, micro-RNAs, and long non-coding RNAs are the most accused in the relationship between RA and epigenetics. Nowadays, it is thought that these epigenetic mechanisms detected in RA will be employed as a prognostic factor and will have a role in diagnosis and treatment follow-up and in determining the susceptibility to RA.

Chapter 29 - Inflammatory bowel diseases (IBDs) represent a group of diseases, which have a chronic course, cause a decrease in a person's quality of life, and whose etiopathogenesis is still not fully explained. The risk factors include the environment, smoking, diet, genetic factors, a person's immunological status, and the intestinal microbiota. Epigenetic mechanisms have recently begun to take their place in the occurrence mechanism of diseases. The mechanisms described under three main headings, DNA methylation, histone modification, and miRNA, have taken a significant place in the diagnosis and follow-up of many diseases and the treatment protocol. In light of all this information, the association between epigenetics and inflammatory bowel diseases and its place in the future will gain even more importance with new studies.

Chapter 30 - In spite of the decreasing incidence rates of gastric cancer in many industrialized countries, it is still an important cause of death from cancer around the world. Gastric cancer takes the fourth place among causes of death due to cancer worldwide. Gastric cancer incidence in Turkey was detected at 14.2/100,000 among males and 3.4/100,000 among females. Risk factors for gastric cancer involve numerous unmodifiable variables, e.g., sex, age, and race/ethnicity. The remaining risk factors, including smoking, infection with Helicobacter pylori (Hp) bacteria, and diets with high nitrate and nitrite contents, are among the controllable causes. Hp represents a Gram-negative microaerophilic bacterium infecting almost half of the population in the world and is considered the main etiologic agent of gastric cancer. Dietary habits and different environmental factors, including Hp infection, and irregularities in genetic and epigenetic mechanisms are involved in forming gastric cancer. While genetic changes lead to loss of function or protein expression in metabolic pathways in different ways, epigenetic alterations cause differentiation in the expressions of tumor suppressor genes and oncogenes.

In gastric cancer surgery, the only curative method in localized gastric cancers is the complete resection of the regional lymph nodes and tumors. Functional surgical methods can be preferred in suitable patients. Pancreas and spleen-preserving D2 dissection is preferred as a standard approach in serosa-positive and/or lymph node-positive cases.

Chapter 1

The Concept of Epigenetics

Tunay Karan*
Department of Genetics, Yozgat Bozok University, Yozgat, Turkey

Abstract

Epigenetics is termed as non-sequence deoxyribonucleic acid (DNA) alterations in the gene expression profile that is heritable. With these, cellular identity is preserved, and gene function is transferred from one cell to another. Epigenetic changes occur with the effect of DNA methylation, chromatin structure changes, and non-coding ribonucleic acids, histone modifications. Even though cells in different tissues have the same DNA, differences may occur between the steps that take place during protein synthesis from DNA, and this can be explained by epigenetic regulation. In addition to the genetic basis, it is known that epigenetic differences are also effective in the development of many diseases, especially cancer. Changes in gene expression should be investigated with epigenomics rather than gene analysis in a particular region. In the investigation of diseases of unknown etiology, such as obesity, insulin resistance, neurodegenerative, cardiovascular, and immune system diseases, it has been determined that many internal and external environmental factors directly affect gene expression. Understanding the differences that cause diseases with epigenetic mechanisms makes it possible to develop molecular diagnostic tests and targeted treatment strategies. In this chapter, basic information about epigenetics will be given and the situations where disruptions in epigenetic mechanisms may lead to related gene expression, and the importance of epigenetics in these situations will be emphasized.

Keywords: epigenetics, epigenome, epigenetic regulations, gene expression changes

Introduction

The word epigenetics carries the prefix epi- in ancient Greek, meaning "above", "beyond"; genesis, on the other hand, means "birth", "origin", "creation" or "formation". Epigenetics terminology was coined by Conrad Waddington firstly in 1942 from the words epigenesis genetics, and it was investigated how genotype creates phenotype (Dolinoy et al., 2007). Although it was suggested to indicate the developmental processes in establishing the link between epigenetic genotype and phenotype, in the following years Holliday and Pugh

* Corresponding Author's E-mail: tunay.karan@bozok.edu.tr.

In: Epigenetics: Beyond the Genetics and Medicine
Editors: Sevgi Durna Daştan and Nazan Yurtcu
ISBN: 979-8-88697-228-3

proposed the molecular mechanism of covalent DNA modification, including cytosine-guanine dinucleotide (CpG) methylation (Holliday and Pugh, 1975). Later, with the discovery of genomic imprinting and X inactivation in mammals, it was understood that epigenetics is regulated by formations.

In the 90s, epigenetics was studied by considering heredity at the molecular level with the development of molecular techniques. Chromatin structure modifications and DNA methylation are among the explained hereditary epigenetic alterations that are non-sequence based and lead to variations in the gene expression profile. Thus, epigenetics refers to the regulation of gene expression by various mechanisms in the form of "super-genetic" (Egger et al., 2004).

Epigenetics and Its Importance

Epigenetic changes, unlike mutations and polymorphisms, are changes in expression that can be transferred by mitosis or meiosis without causing any changes in the DNA. In other words, it examines hereditary and non-genetic phenotypic variations (Turek-Plewa and Jagodzinski, 2005; Gallipoli et al., 2015). It can explain how cells and organisms with the same DNA have different phenotypic changes. These changes, which directly affect the cell and the organism, determine where and when the genes will be active without making any differences in the DNA. For example, human and animal tissues and organs consist of many cells, and although the DNA sequence of each cell is the same, the place, time, and duration of the stages that take place during protein synthesis from DNA may differ. For example, the tissues of organs such as the heart, liver, and brain, which differ in shape and function, have the same DNA sequence, but the reason for cellular differentiation is epigenetic, some genes work and some are silenced (Martin and Zhang, 2007; Portela and Esteller, 2010).

The inheritance mechanism of epigenetic changes cannot be fully explained. In individuals with the same DNA sequence, such as identical twins, phenotypic differences occur with an epigenetic variation. The molecular basis of the study of differences in non-genotypic gene expression changes is mixed, and this situation can be compared to an orchestra conductor who ensures that the right instruments are played at the right time and thus a good concert emerges. While important biochemical, molecular, and physiological events take place in the cell, various modifications have a vital role in the interpretation of the relevant gene. When the progression process with a proper mechanism is disrupted, various diseases such as neurological, cancer, and autoimmune-based diseases may occur (Bond and Finnegan, 2007; Meissner et al., 2008).

Although epigenetic changes are quite stable, they are also reversible and can regulate epigenetic gene expression according to changing conditions. In other words, gene expression can be controlled with applications such as drugs, therapy, etc. in which environmental conditions change. This situation has made epigenetics the focus of attention in determining new treatment strategies against diseases. Although epigenetic mechanisms have been revealed by various methods, DNA methylation and histone modification are the best characterized and studied. These two events are interrelated, and DNA methylation markers are noteworthy in the diagnosis and classification of most diseases (Shinjo and Kondo, 2015; Zhang et al., 2018).

Epigenetic Regulations

Epigenetic regulation can be divided into mechanisms that directly or indirectly control gene expression.

Mechanisms that Directly Control Gene Expression

Direct control is modifications at the chromatin and DNA level, and the DNA molecule packaged as chromatin in eukaryotes limits the expression of genes. In transcription, proteins called transcription factors have a role in the expression of genes by binding to checkpoints on DNA. Binding occurs when the chromatin structure is loosened and opened, but in cases where the structure is tight and dense, the expression of the relevant gene cannot be ensured because transcription factors cannot reach the genes to be read. As the structural monomers of the chromatin structure, nucleosomes combine both the DNA, which is 146 bp in length, and the core complex that is formed by histone proteins, which are H2A, H2B, H3, and H4 (Meaney and Szyf, 2005). Histone octamers are linked by histones to linker DNA covering the region between nucleosomes. Methylation, ubiquitination, phosphorylation, deamination, acetylation, and sumoylation are modifications of the tails of histone proteins in the N-terminal end region and are involved in posttranslational gene regulation. These modifications also have important roles in the chromatin structure, gene expression, regulation of genome stability, and formation of heterochromatin and euchromatin forms. In other words, promoter-access by the transcription factors and regulation of interactions between DNA and octamer are provided by histone modifications. Quantitative identification of different histone modifications may contribute to the development of therapies targeting histone-regulating enzymes by providing important insights into epigenetic regulation in pathophysiological conditions (Egger et al., 2004; Chen et al., 2010).

DNA methylation is among the most prevalent one of epigenetic arrangements, which can also be defined as the covalent modification of the cytosine base, which is accurately copied in DNA replication and transmits epigenetic information during cell division. 5-methylcytosine (5-mC) is formed through methyl group (CH3) attachment to the cytosine bases of DNA, and this area is called cytosine guanine phosphate (CpG) islets and is an important epigenetic marker in both prokaryotes and eukaryotes. In bacteria, cytosine methylation allows genomic DNA to cleave from bacteriophage DNA that infects bacteria and to cleave phage DNA by host restriction enzymes, whereas in eukaryotes it can inhibit the binding of regulatory proteins and suppress transcription of coding sequences of genes (Parry and Clarke, 2011). The most typical example of chromosomes whose gene expression is silenced by CpG methylation is the inactivation of an X chromosome in female mammals with a placenta in the early embryonic period however, methylation is not always done for gene silencing. Most of the enzymes involved in DNA methylation are composed of DNA Methyl Transferase (DMNT) enzymes, and S-Adenosine Methionine (SAM) is used as the methyl source. These methylated domains are located in the promoter region of the whole genome, affecting protein-DNA relationships and contributing to genome stability (Subramaniam et al., 2014). Genomic imprinting is another example of epigenetic suppression of an expressible gene without any change in the base sequence in the DNA molecule. In the genetic imprinting mechanism, different gene expression occurs according to the origin and only one of the maternal or paternal genes is genetically imprinted. Defects that may occur in genes under genomic imprinting may predispose to lung, breast, colon, and bladder cancers (Nestler, 2014).

Mechanisms that Indirectly Control Gene Expression

Developing sequencing techniques have revealed that almost %2 of the human proteome contains structural genes, which lead to approximately 20 thousand genes. In the remaining part of the genome, genetic sequences revealed to have no protein-coding sequences and whose end product is the RNA molecule were found (Ricciuti et al., 2014). Non-translated RNAs are involved in many physiological events such as chromosome modeling, gene silencing, and cellular defense as bidirectional promoter transcripts and repetitive sequences. Such RNAs are divided according to their nucleotide lenght as either short or long (Li et al., 2014).

Short non-coding RNAs (Snc-RNA) are 19-28 nucleotides long and double-stranded and have an important function in gene silencing. Micro RNAs (miRNAs), siRNAs, and piwi RNAs (piRNA) are short non-coding RNAs obtained from larger RNA precursor molecules and have a role in epigenetic mechanisms. MiRNAs, which bind to the 3' region of the messenger RNA that are not translated, are the single-stranded ncRNAs that have been the most studied as transcriptional regulators recently. miRNAs inhibit the expression of many genes by suppressing translation at the post-transcriptional stage or regulate them by directly inducing mRNA degradation with the RNA interfering silencing complex (RISC). To date, miRNAs that change gene expression by binding to more than 5000 specific sites have been identified. These regulate the translational efficiency or stability of the targeted mRNA in gene silencing. siRNAs are similar in length to miRNAs, but unlike miRNAs, they are obtained from double-stranded RNAs, while piRNAs are RNAs with a length of 22-33 nucleotides and are obtained from single-stranded precursor molecules. piRNAs provide transposon repression, and they do this by restriction enzymes cleaving in the cytoplasm, then loaded onto piwi proteins and returned to the nucleus. As a result of the overexpression of piRNAs in most different cancers, the resulting mRNAs are fragmented and inhibited, but at low levels, oncogene transcription increases (Mattick and Makunin, 2006; Huang et al., 2013).

Among the non-coding RNAs, those that are greater than 200 nucleotides in length are termed as long non-coding RNAs (lncRNA), which alter the gene expression. lncRNAs are involved in the regulation of oncogene and tumor suppressor genes and signaling pathways. In studies, lncRNA expression was observed at abnormal levels in most cancer types. Hox Transcript Antisense RNA (HOTAIR) at the gene locus called homeobox-C in mammals is an example of lncRNA and is used as a reference in the diagnosis of breast cancer (Gupta et al., 2010).

Epigenome and Epigenetics

All formations that cover epigenetic arrangements and mechanisms are called the epigenome. The epigenome is the determining factor of the specific gene expression profiles of various cells despite the fact that they all carry the same DNA sequence, which is achieved by the formation of a genome-to-environment interface. The epigenome is very important in understanding and solving diseases by dynamically responding to environmental factors and epigenetic regulation that occurs through various mechanisms (Murrell et al., 2005).

Epigenomics is an exciting new discipline that studies epigenetic modifications that occur in the whole genome and combines epigenetics and epigenomic sciences (Callinan and Feinberg, 2006). Epigenomic research is advancing in understanding genetic regulation, its effect on cellular growth and differentiation, and creating new treatment opportunities for aging and diseases. Today, the basis for the necessary experiments with microarray technology has been prepared, and epigenomic data continues to make new contributions to genomic sciences. Thus, there will be possible outcomes in understanding the mechanism of epigenetic diseases, especially cancer, synthesizing the desired molecule or protein from existing cells, and even transforming any somatic cell in our body into another tissue or organ without the need for stem cells (Egger et al., 2004; Gupta et al., 2010).

Epigenetic Diseases and Cancer

Changes in gene expression resulting from deviations in any of the epigenetic mechanisms can cause various diseases. Understanding the etiology of epigenetic diseases that cause excessive increase or suppression of gene expression may provide an opportunity to make necessary interventions against diseases (Rodenhiser and Mann, 2006).

Specifically regulated gene expression profiles of different cells possibly can be attributed to epigenetic regulations, causing metabolic changes and diseases that are present throughout life. Some diseases of epigenetic origin are growth retardation, Silver-Russell syndrome, Beckwith-Wiedemann syndrome, Prader-Willi syndromes, and Angelman syndrome. Systemic lupus erythematosus, an autoimmune disease, is the phenotypic result of a series of mutations in the line of DNA methylation. Gene hypomethylation on the inactivated X-chromosome directly results in upheaval in the expected gene expression profiles, which also leads to the development of a syndrome called ICF that combines clinical disruptions in the immune system, cell cycle, and facial morphology (Richardson et al., 1990; Hansen et al., 1999; Procter et al., 2006). Fragile X syndrome caused by abnormal DNA methylation on the X chromosome is another epigenetic disease (Crawford et al., 2001). It has been determined that both Alzheimer's Disease and Parkinson's Disease, and possibly other neurodegenerative diseases with age correlation, have a connection to the DNA methylation mechanism. The expression of a protein called reelin has been studied to be suppressed as a result of the brain hypermethylation in schizophrenia patients with mood disorders. In addition, genes that undergo hypermethylation have been revealed in different anatomical structures of the brain, such as the hippocampus and prefrontal cortex. Under extreme stress conditions, the cognitive functions of the brain may be adversely affected, and pathological conditions may occur. Abnormal DNA methylation can result in postnatal death or decreased neurogenesis. In another study, it was stated that both acute renal injury and chronic renal failure have decisive connections to epigenetic regulations.

Every event, from the mother's womb to the deathbed, is believed to influence behaviors, personality, and the development of mental disorders (Grayson et al., 2005; Tsankova et al., 2007). Studies that have been conducted or will be conducted together in the field of neuroscience and genetics are very important in the regulation of human behavior and psychiatric diseases. Treatments targeting epigenetic regulation show promise for the treatment of psychiatric disorders, depression, schizophrenia, and substance abuse. Studies have shown that people with the short allele of the serotonin transporter gene are susceptible to depression and stress. Changing gene expression is effective in curing and perhaps preventing psychiatric diseases (Jaenisch and Bird, 2003; Abel and Zukin, 2008).

Some autoimmune and autoinflammatory diseases, whose pathogenesis and disease mechanism are not understood, have been investigated in recent years using epigenetic studies. Rheumatoid arthritis, defined by extracellular matrix destruction, is an autoimmune disease, and although the exact cause of the disease has not been revealed, it has been understood that different methylation states change the gene function of cells (Majithia and Geraci, 2007). Similarly, high methylation rates and low MEFV expression were detected in the MEFV Exon-2 in patients with FMF (Familial Mediterranean Fever), which is an autoinflammatory disease (Kirectepe et al., 2011).

Cancer can be described as a multifactorial disease, which stems from the overmoulding of both genetic and epigenetic disorders. The cancer's connection to the DNA methylation patterns was revealed for the first time in 1983, and hypomethylation was detected in cancer genomes compared to normal cells. Hypomethylation of DNA causes cancer formation by activating oncogenes, and loss of methylation is known to affect the severity of the disease and the possibility of metastasis (Feinberg and Tycko, 2004; Robertson, 2005). Cancer cells also show hypermethylation of cancer-related genes, thereby silencing many genes. For example, genes involved in cell cycle regulators (such as RB1, p14 ARF), genes involved in signal transduction (such as APC, RASSF1, LKB1/STK11), genes involved in apoptosis (such as p53, DAPK, and caspase 8) and DNA repair Hypermethylation of genes (such as BRC1, MLH1, MGMT) contributes to carcinogenesis (Miyamoto and Ushijima, 2005). Studies on cancer cells have generally revealed that gene-specific hypermethylation occurs together with hypomethylation. While hypermethylation is the cause of unwanted silencing in the gene, oncogenes become active in hypomethylation. It has also been reported that irregular histone acetylation/deacetylation affects cancer (Wolffe, 2001).

Cancer and Epigenetics Therapy

Epigenetics makes an innovative contribution not only to the diagnosis of cancer but also to its treatment. Efforts to determine the epigenetic and genetic changes of different types of cancers in the early period are very important in terms of the prevalence and prognosis of the disease. In cancer, epigenetic changes usually occur before genetic changes. Recently, with the realization of how important the epigenetics is in the early diagnosis of cancer, drug research, and development studies have accelerated to correct epigenetic errors (Bishop and Ferguson, 2015).

The most common epigenetic change studied in cancer is the methylation of cytosine guanine (CpG) dinucleotides and occurs before genetic changes. Thus, drug candidates that can improve the methylation and histone modification profile have been developed. For example, the treatment process can be improved by the reactivation of DNA repair mechanisms and tumor suppressor genes. Among the drug candidates developed, DNMT inhibitors and HDAC inhibitors are the most promising compounds. DNMT inhibitors, by using DNMT enzyme inhibitors involved in methylation, re-enable various silenced tumor suppressor genes to express themselves. 5-Aza-2'-deoxycytidine (decitabine) and 5-Fluoro-2'-deoxycytidine (gemcitabine), which are nucleoside analogs of DNMT inhibitors, participate in the structure of the newly synthesized DNA strand by forming a complex and provide hypomethylation of the DNA strand that will extend as they lose their catalysis ability. However, if the integrated decitabine with the genome is not destroyed by the cells, a disadvantageous situation may occur as it will cause mutations in new cells. After the negative effects of nucleoside analogs were discovered, DNMT inhibitors that are not nucleoside analogs were developed. Compounds called (-)-epigallocatechin-3- gallate and RG108, which are abundant in green tea, bind to the active center of DNMT and inhibit the activity of the enzyme, causing a decrease in methylation. HDAC inhibitors, prevent the deacetylation of histones by making the reverse reaction of the histone acetylase (HAT) enzyme and ensuring the continuity of transcription. These inhibitors act simultaneously on multiple pathways such as cell cycle and apoptosis (Miyamoto, and Ushijima, 2005; Suphic et al., 2013; Bishop and Ferguson, 2015). They also provide re-expression of repressed regulatory genes in cancer cells. It has been reported that compounds such as Apcidin, Butyrates, Pyroxamide, Vorinostat, and Valproic acid, which are the most commonly used substances, significantly reduce tumor growth and metastasis by increasing the acetylation of some non-histone proteins, transcription factors, tumor suppressor proteins.

Epigenetic proteins have also been extensively studied in drug discovery, due to the existence of opinions on epigenetic-based diseases. The efficacy of bromodomain proteins, which bind to secondary chromatin modifications or transcriptional mechanism elements of epigenetic marks and assist their recognition, has been demonstrated. Bromodomains appear as readers of acetyl groups on histone tails and regulate gene transcription by binding acetylated lysines to histone tails. There are a total of 61 bromodomains divided into 8 subfamilies according to their sequence and structure in 46 different human proteins. BRD2, BRD3, BRD4, and BRDT, which belong to the bromodomain and extra-terminal protein family, are highly associated with various cancer types. BRD2, BRD3, and BRD4 can be expressed in most places, except BRDT, which is expressed only in testicles and is important for spermatogenesis. BRD2 and BRD3, which are particularly functional in cell growth, specifically recognize the histone acetylation code and assist in the transcription of RNA Pol-II. Considering the functions of BET in transcription and malignancy, inhibitors have been developed. First, two small molecules, JQ1 and IBET762, were synthesized to disrupt the interaction between BET and the BRD of acetyllysine, respectively. After early clinical studies, many studies have been published showing the efficacy of JQ1 in various solid tumors such as hepatocellular carcinoma, pancreatic cancer, lung cancer, colon cancer, and prostate cancer. Following the success achieved with the use of these compounds in myeloma cases, where c-Myc expression and BET dissociation were observed, different compounds were taken into development.

Another bromodomain inhibitor, PLX51107, has been identified in preclinical models as a potent and selective BET inhibitor with its pharmacological properties. The compound PLX51107 impairs chromatin remodeling and gene expression by binding to the acetylated lysine recognition motifs of BRD4 on histones (Parry and Clarke, 2005).

The Relationship between Environment, Nutrition, Aging, and Epigenetics

Environment and lifestyle affect gene expression by interfering with genetic and epigenetic regulation. The effects on DNA methylation of people exposed to cigarette smoke, air pollution, and heavy metals such as lead and mercury or chemical agents have been reported in many studies (Ruiz-Hernandez et al., 2015). Identical twins are genetically the same, but the differences that can be seen in individuals are an example of the environmental factor in epigenetic changes. Unnatural changes in gene expression in the living body create different genetic variations and transfer to newly formed cells is ensured by cell division.

The individual's risk of having a disease has a clear-cut relation to its nutritional balance, which also influences the epigenetic mechanisms. In malnourished or diabetic patients, the epigenetic profile may change and be passed on from parent to offspring. Many studies explaining the relationship of nutrition with the epigenome and metabolic diseases have been conducted by considering the prenatal and postnatal periods. The effect of folate supplementation during pregnancy on methylation in the IGF-2 gene has been reported. It has been determined that not only the mother but also the father influences the epigenetic profile of the progeny, particularly when a protein-poor diet is subjected to the adult father (Hoyo et al., 2011). Disruption of the balance between gene silencing and activation may trigger the emergence of diseases. Some changes in tissues, including adipose tissue, liver, skeletal muscles, and pancreas, result in metabolic diseases (Cheng et al., 2018). Metabolic disorders such as cardiovascular diseases, obesity, and type-2 diabetes are epigenetic diseases that can occur with the effect of the environment and nutrition (Nilsson et al., 2014; Van Dijk et al., 2015). Foods containing compounds such as folate, polyphenols such as epigallocatechin-3-gallate, resveratrol, lignans in flaxseed, vitamin E, selenium, and isothiocyanate in cruciferous vegetables have been reported to prevent the occurrence of epigenetic changes that lead to cancer (Supic et al., 2013; Bishop and Ferguson, 2015). Individuals need to regulate their eating habits along with physical activity tp preventing diseases due to epigenetic changes and create a healthy society (Muduliar et al., 2016).

Aging is an irreversible physiological event based on many exogenous and endogenous factors. The leading causes of aging include telomere shortening, degeneration of cell and organ structures, accumulation of somatic mutations, oxidative DNA damage, and changes in gene expression. Recently, it has been emphasized that gene-environmental disease complexes, which can be caused by malnutrition and a sedentary lifestyle, are also related to aging through epigenetics. The fact that female honeybee larvae are short-lived and worker bee larvae are long-lived can be given as an example of the relationship between nutrition, aging, and epigenetic changes (Kucharski et al., 2008). DNA methylation, noncoding RNAs, and histone modifications are the major epigenetic mechanisms that affect genetic expression in aging. Many studies have shown that DNA methylation levels change with aging. In studies conducted for the first time in salmon and later in mice, hamsters, cattle, and humans, results pointed out an aging-related decrease in DNA methylation ratios in repeating sequences of the genome. Age-related decrease in DNA methylation in the mammalian genome was shown by different studies, while the level of methylation in CpG islets in blood, heart, and liver cells increases with age (Bacalini et al., 2014). In addition, in which regions of the genome the methylation level changes in young and old cells can be determined by microarray or various other methods. Thus, understanding the determination of aging through epigenetic mechanisms will be extremely important in the development of protective measures against aging in the future.

Conclusion

Changes in gene expressions can be observed starting from the embryo and throughout the lifespan. Epigenetics is in a crucial position for non-sequence alterations in gene regulation. All entities involved in epigenetic mechanisms include the epigenome, and genes are expressed in specific cells and at times as needed. As one of the epigenetic mechanisms, genomic suppression causes gene activation and gene-silencing, which leads to parental expression of certain gender-specific genes.

Errors or irregularities caused by an excessive increase or suppression of the expression of certain genes constitute epigenetic diseases. DNA methylation is seemingly essential in gene regulation, and methylation of different regions in the genome has been promising in the treatment of some diseases whose mechanisms are not fully understood. It will provide exciting developments in the early diagnosis of cancer, which is one of the most important diseases of our age, or in the development of drugs for treatment.

It has been determined that the environment and nutrition also have effects on the emergence of diseases due to epigenetic changes. Especially, bad eating habits and unhealthy environmental conditions trigger changes in gene expression. Diabetes mellitus, cardiovascular diseases, and obesity are metabolic diseases that occur due to the irregularities that may be developed in mechanisms involved in DNA methylation and/or histone modifications. For a healthy society and generation, regulating the nutritional habits of humans together with physical activity will reduce the incidence of diseases in children to be born and prevent the occurrence of epigenetic changes that lead to cancer.

For many years, the functions of many hereditary diseases and cancer types in the fields of medicine, biology, and genetics have not been fully understood. Today, there are many cases where genetics is insufficient but can be explained beyond the boundaries of genetics. Now, many phenomena can be explained by mechanisms under the name of epigenetic regulation. The discovery of epigenetic events has accelerated to a great extent with the advancing technologies, and especially with the discovery of their effects on humans, their relationship with diseases has been understood. In line with all this information, it can be said that with the science of epigenetics, a new and respected profession such as 'epigenetic engineering' will be born soon and Nobel Prizes will be awarded to studies in this field in the future.

References

Abel, T., & Zukin, R. S. (2008). Epigenetic targets of HDAC inhibition in neurodegenerative and psychiatric disorders. *Current Opinion in Pharmacology*, *8*(1), 57-64.

Bacalini, M. G. Friso, S., Olivieri, F., Pirazzini, C., Giuliani, C., Capri, M., & Garagnani, P. (2014). Present and future of anti-ageing epigenetic diets. *Mechanisms of Ageing and Development*, *136*, 101-115.

Bishop, K. S., & Ferguson, L. R. (2015). The interaction between epigenetics, nutrition and the development of cancer. *Nutrients*, *7*(2), 922-947.

Bond, D. M., & Finnegan, E. J. (2007). Passing the message on: inheritance of epigenetic traits. *Trends in Plant Science*, *12*(5), 211-216.

Callinan, P. A., & Feinberg, A. P. (2006). The emerging science of epigenomics. *Human Molecular Genetics*, *15*(suppl_1), R95-R101.

Chen, Z., Wang, L., Wang, Q., & Li, W. (2010). Histone modifications and chromatin organization in prostate cancer. *Epigenomics*, *2*(4), 551-560.

Cheng, Z., Zheng, L., & Almeida, F. A. (2018). Epigenetic reprogramming in metabolic disorders: nutritional factors and beyond. *The Journal of Nutritional Biochemistry*, *54*, 1-10.

Crawford, D. C., Acuña, J. M., & Sherman, S. L. (2001). FMR1 and the fragile X syndrome: human genome epidemiology review. *Genetics in Medicine*, *3*(5), 359-371.

Dolinoy, D. C., Weidman, J. R., & Jirtle, R. L. (2007). Epigenetic gene regulation: linking early developmental environment to adult disease. *Reproductive Toxicology*, *23*(3), 297-307.

Egger, G., Liang, G., Aparicio, A., & Jones, P. A. (2004). Epigenetics in human disease and prospects for epigenetic therapy. *Nature*, *429*(6990), 457-463.

Feinberg, A. P., & Tycko, B. (2004). The history of cancer epigenetics. *Nature Reviews Cancer*, *4*(2), 143-153.

Gallipoli, P., Giotopoulos, G., & Huntly, B. J. (2015). Epigenetic regulators as promising therapeutic targets in acute myeloid leukemia. *Therapeutic Advances in Hematology*, *6*(3), 103-119.

Grayson, D. R., Jia, X., Chen, Y., Sharma, R. P., Mitchell, C. P., Guidotti, A., & Costa, E. (2005). Reelin promoter hypermethylation in schizophrenia. *Proceedings of the National Academy of Sciences*, *102*(26), 9341-9346.

Gupta, R. A., Shah, N., Wang, K. C., Kim, J., Horlings, H. M., Wong, D. J., & Chang, H. Y. (2010). Long non-coding RNA HOTAIR reprograms chromatin state to promote cancer metastasis. *Nature*, *464*(7291), 1071-1076.

Hansen, R. S., Wijmenga, C., Luo, P., Stanek, A. M., Canfield, T. K., Weemaes, C. M., & Gartler, S. M. (1999). The DNMT3B DNA methyltransferase gene is mutated in the ICF immunodeficiency syndrome. *Proceedings of the National Academy of Sciences*, *96*(25), 14412-14417.

Holliday, R., & Pugh, J. E. (1975). DNA Modification Mechanisms and Gene Activity During Development: Developmental clocks may depend on the enzymic modification of specific bases in repeated DNA sequences. *Science*, *187*(4173), 226-232.

Hoyo, C., Murtha, A. P., Schildkraut, J. M., Jirtle, R. L., Demark-Wahnefried, W., Forman, M. R., & Murphy, S. K. (2011). Methylation variation at IGF2 differentially methylated regions and maternal folic acid use before and during pregnancy. *Epigenetics*, *6*(7), 928-936.

Huang, T., Alvarez, A., Hu, B., & Cheng, S. Y. (2013). Noncoding RNAs in cancer and cancer stem cells. *Chinese Journal of Cancer*, *32*(11), 582.

Jaenisch, R., & Bird, A. (2003). Epigenetic regulation of gene expression: how the genome integrates intrinsic and environmental signals. *Nature Genetics*, *33*(3), 245-254.

Kirectepe, A. K., Kasapcopur, O., Arisoy, N., Celikyapi Erdem, G., Hatemi, G., Ozdogan, H., & Tahir Turanli, E. (2011). Analysis of MEFV exon methylation and expression patterns in familial Mediterranean fever. *BMC Medical Genetics*, *12*(1), 1-6.

Kucharski, R., Maleszka, J., Foret, S., & Maleszka, R. (2008). Nutritional control of reproductive status in honeybees via DNA methylation. *Science*, *319*(5871), 1827-1830.

Li, P. F., Chen, S. C., Xia, T., Jiang, X. M., Shao, Y. F., Xiao, B. X., & Guo, J. M. (2014). Non-coding RNAs and gastric cancer. *World Journal of Gastroenterology: WJG*, *20*(18), 5411.

Majithia, V., & Geraci, S. A. (2007). Rheumatoid arthritis: diagnosis and management. *The American Journal of Medicine*, *120*(11), 936-939.

Martin, C., & Zhang, Y. (2007). Mechanisms of epigenetic inheritance. *Current Opinion in Cell Biology*, *19*(3), 266-272.

Mattick, J. S., & Makunin, I. V. (2006). Non-coding RNA. *Human Molecular Genetics*, *15*(suppl_1), R17-R29.

Meaney, M. J., & Szyf, M. (2005). Maternal care as a model for experience-dependent chromatin plasticity? *Trends in Neurosciences*, *28*(9), 456-463.

Meissner, A., Mikkelsen, T. S., Gu, H., Wernig, M., Hanna, J., Sivachenko, A., & Lander, E. S. (2008). Genome-scale DNA methylation maps of pluripotent and differentiated cells. *Nature*, *454*(7205), 766-770.

Miyamoto, K., & Ushijima, T. (2005). Diagnostic and therapeutic applications of epigenetics. *Japanese Journal of Clinical Oncology*, *35*(6), 293-301

Mudaliar, U., Zabetian, A., Goodman, M., Echouffo-Tcheugui, J. B., Albright, A. L., Gregg, E. W., & Ali, M. K. (2016). Cardiometabolic risk factor changes observed in diabetes prevention programs in US settings: a systematic review and meta-analysis. *PLoS medicine*, *13*(7), e1002095.

Murrell, A., Rakyan, V. K., & Beck, S. (2005). From genome to epigenome. *Human Molecular Genetics*, *14*(suppl_1), R3-R10.

Nestler, E. J. (2014). Epigenetic mechanisms of drug addiction. *Neuropharmacology*, *76*, 259-268.

Nilsson, E., Jansson, P. A., Perfilyev, A., Volkov, P., Pedersen, M., Svensson, M. K., & Ling, C. (2014). Altered DNA methylation and differential expression of genes influencing metabolism and inflammation in adipose tissue from subjects with type 2 diabetes. *Diabetes*, *63*(9), 2962-2976.

Parry, L., & Clarke, A. R. (2011). The roles of the methyl-CpG binding proteins in cancer. *Genes & Cancer*, *2*(6), 618-630.

Pérez-Salvia, M., & Esteller, M. (2017). Bromodomain inhibitors and cancer therapy: From structures to applications. *Epigenetics*, *12*(5), 323-339.

Portela, A., & Esteller, M. (2010). Epigenetic modifications and human disease. *Nature Biotechnology*, *28*(10), 1057-1068.

Procter, M., Chou, L. S., Tang, W., Jama, M., & Mao, R. (2006). Molecular diagnosis of Prader–Willi and Angelman syndromes by methylation-specific melting analysis and methylation-specific multiplex ligation-dependent probe amplification. *Clinical Chemistry*, *52*(7), 1276-1283.

Ricciuti, B., Mecca, C., Crinò, L., Baglivo, S., Cenci, M., & Metro, G. (2014). Non-coding RNAs in lung cancer. *Oncoscience*, *1*(11), 674.

Richardson, B., Scheinbart, L., Strahler, J., Gross, L., Hanash, S., & Johnson, M. (1990). Evidence for impaired T cell DNA methylation in systemic lupus erythematosus and rheumatoid arthritis. *Arthritis & Rheumatism: Official Journal of the American College of Rheumatology*, *33*(11), 1665-1673.

Robertson, K. D. (2005). DNA methylation and human disease. *Nature Reviews Genetics*, *6*(8), 597-610.

Rodenhiser, D., & Mann, M. (2006). Epigenetics and human disease: translating basic biology into clinical applications. *Cmaj*, *174*(3), 341-348.

Ruiz-Hernandez, A., Kuo, C. C., Rentero-Garrido, P., Tang, W. Y., Redon, J., Ordovas, J. M., & Tellez-Plaza, M. (2015). Environmental chemicals and DNA methylation in adults: a systematic review of the epidemiologic evidence. *Clinical Epigenetics*, *7*(1), 1-24.

Shinjo, K., & Kondo, Y. (2015). Targeting cancer epigenetics: Linking basic biology to clinical medicine. *Advanced Drug Delivery Reviews*, *95*, 56-64.

Subramaniam, D., Thombre, R., Dhar, A., & Anant, S. (2014). DNA methyltransferases: a novel target for prevention and therapy. *Frontiers in Oncology*, *4*, 80.

Supic, G., Jagodic, M., & Magic, Z. (2013). Epigenetics: a new link between nutrition and cancer. *Nutrition and Cancer*, *65*(6), 781-792.

Tsankova, N., Renthal, W., Kumar, A., & Nestler, E. J. (2007). Epigenetic regulation in psychiatric disorders. *Nature Reviews Neuroscience*, *8*(5), 355-367.

Turek-Plewa, J., & Jagodzinski, P. P. (2005). The role of mammalian DNA methyltransferases in the regulation of gene expression. *Cellular and Molecular Biology Letters*, *10*(4), 631.

Van Dijk, S. J., Molloy, P. L., Varinli, H., Morrison, J. L., & Muhlhausler, B. S. (2015). S Members of Epi: Epigenetics and human obesity. *Int J Obes (Lond)*, *39*(1), 85-97.

Wolffe, A. P. (2001). Chromatin remodeling: why it is important in cancer. *Oncogene*, *20*(24), 2988-2990.

Zhang, H., Lang, Z., & Zhu, J. K. (2018). Dynamics and function of DNA methylation in plants. *Nature Reviews Molecular Cell Biology*, *19*(8), 489-506.

Chapter 2

The Relationship between Epigenetics and Diseases/Disorders

Nilsun Kuas*, **MD**
Department of Pediatric Surgery - Pediatric Urology,
Ankara University, Ankara, Turkey

Abstract

Epigenetic changes occur in the phenotype due to differences in the expression of genes while remaining the same in the existing DNA sequence. Disruptions in the promoter methylation pattern, histone modifications, and non-coding RNA irregularities can be given as examples of epigenetic changes. The positive or negative effects of lifestyle changes lead to epigenetic mechanisms and these mechanisms often work together to cause changes that affect all organ systems. These changes can result in autoimmune diseases or syndromes. Therefore, further research on epigenetic mechanisms can significantly contribute to the diagnosis, follow-up, and the treatment of many organ systems diseases.

Keywords: epigenetics, Down syndrome, Genomic Stigma, Charge syndrome, DiGeorge syndrome

Introduction

Epigenetic changes result in a difference in the expression of genes, that is, a change in the phenotype, without changing the existing DNA sequence, that is, without a change in the genotype. Disruptions in the promoter methylation pattern, histone modifications, and non-coding RNA irregularities can be given as examples of epigenetic changes (Loscalzo & Handy, 2014). Since nucleosomes are subject to constant remodeling and histones are known to be modified, all discovered DNA and histone markers are understood to be reversible. However, the stability of these markers and rate of change are variable in different genomic domains (Allis & Jenuwein, 2016).

Epigenetics has a critical role in the management of disease, from diagnosis to treatment and prognosis. Given the fundamental nature of gene expression, it is not surprising that epigenetic abnormalities lead to consequences that affect all systems of the body, from intestinal disorders to cardiovascular disorders and dermatological diseases (Goardon et al.,

* Corresponding Author's E-mail: dr.nilsun@hotmail.com.

In: Epigenetics: Beyond the Genetics and Medicine
Editors: Sevgi Durna Daştan and Nazan Yurtcu
ISBN: 979-8-88697-228-3

2011). For example, mutations in various enzymes have been associated with neurodegenerative processes in Alzheimer's conditions, such as learning disability and memory formation (Desplats et al., 2011; Millis, 2011). Some brain disorders, such as autism, schizophrenia, and Rett's syndrome, also appear to have significant epigenetic components (Ellis et al., 2009). The mechanisms that lead to epigenetic changes work together. Epigenetic control of gene expression, among these mechanisms, is both the most significant part and an essential component of medical diseases.

Lifestyle changes, such as the quality of a person's diet or exercise, are known to positively or negatively affect their health. Although much has been learned about epigenetic changes in medicine, it is not fully known how the changes in the first years of life will affect adulthood or how they will affect lifespan. Studies of monozygotic twins show that phenotypic changes increase with the aging of organism. This increase is due to environmental factors that can partially change the epigenetic mechanism (Goardon et al., 2011). A study used machine learning to measure chronological and biological age indicators from high-throughput DNA methylation data. Changes in CpG methylation in the genomic region were highly correlated with age between tissues (Horvath, 2013). In addition, studies have found that epigenetic age accelerates with high body mass index (we age) and decreases with increased education, physical activity, low body mass index, and consumption of fish, vegetables, and fruits (Quach et al., 2017). By elucidating the epigenetic mechanisms, many diseases can be stopped before they start or at least do not progress. In addition, it can make it easier to diagnose diseases more practically and to predict their results more accurately (Goardon et al., 2011).

DNA is initially wrapped around histone proteins (Can, 2016). Later, these histone-DNA complexes form chromosomes (Karaçay, 2009). Histone modifications include acetylation, methylation, ubiquitination, phosphorylation, sumoylation, citrullination, ADP-ribosylation, and proline isomerization (Nestler, 2014). These modifications regulate the transcription process (Cañas et al., 2016; Hewagama & Richardson, 2009). Depending on the nature of the change, they are associated with both gene silencing and activation (Can, 2016). Acetylation and deacetylation of lysine residues are the most common histone modifications (Hughes & Sawalha, 2011). The attachment of acetyl to lysine residues is mediated by histone acetyltransferase (HAT). This event stimulates gene expression (Kouzarides, 2007). The enzyme that deacetylates lysine residues in histones is histone deacetyltransferases (HDAT). This event results in the suppression of gene expression. Methylases and demethylases also mediate the addition and removal of methyl groups to histones (Wang et al., 2017).

S-adenosylmethionine (SAM), acetyl-coenzyme A (acetyl-CoA), and nicotinamide adenine dinucleotide (NAD+) are important metabolites that can cooperate with epigenetic modifying enzymes such as DNMT, HDAC, and HAT to modify chromatin (Sawalha et al., 2019). SAM is produced from adenosine triphosphate (ATP) and methionine by methionine adenosyltransferase (MAT) (Oaks & Perl, 2014; Wang et al., 2018). It is the methyl donor in DNA and histone methylation. In addition, folate, vitamins B6 and B12 induce SAM production, and DNA and histone methyltransferases depend on SAM as a methyl donor (Cavalli & Heard, 2019). Decreased SAM levels may negatively affect histone demethylase activity (Etchegaray & Mostoslavsky, 2016). SAM and methyltransferases can synergistically inhibit transmethylation in lymphocytes, thereby attenuating T-cell manifestations in lupus (Yang et al., 2013). Alpha-ketoglutarate is required for DNA and histone demethylation, while succinate and fumarate inhibit demethylases (Cavalli & Heard, 2019). Methionine metabolism level; It can regulate SAM and adenosyl homocysteine. Therefore, it is helpful to assess histone methylation levels (Wang et al., 2018).

Acetyl-CoA is an essential metabolite for the cellular energy cycle and fatty acid metabolism. It is produced from glucose and fatty acids in the TCA cycle (Guay et al., 2011). The HAT uses Acetyl-CoA as an acetyl source for lysine acetylation (Sawalha et al., 2019). Therefore, the high glucose in the medium increases the level of intracellular Acetyl-CoA and histone acetylation. Thus, gene expression is subsequently promoted (J. Fan et al., 2015). Thus, a high level of Acetyl-CoA is associated with a high amount of histone acetylation (Shi & Tu, 2015). In this case, Acetyl-CoA functions as a biosensor of the cellular metabolic state. The outcome of dietary habits through epigenetic changes, such as histone acetylation affects specific genes (Etchegaray & Mostoslavsky, 2016).

NAD+ is an essential cofactor that mediates deacetylation reactions catalyzed by the sirtuin HDAC family and the substrate glycolytic pathway (Veech, 1969). NADH is the reducing agent of NAD+ (Etchegaray & Mostoslavsky, 2016). Sirtuin levels depend on the NADH/NAD+ balance (Li & Kazgan, 2011). NAD+-dependent sirtuins provide a vital link between metabolism and epigenetic modifications. For example, circadian fluctuation of NAD+ activates surges of SIRT1-mediated deacetylation in promoter regions of genes (Nakahata et al., 2008). When the relationship between sirtuin, a nutrient, and the level of NAD+ was investigated, it was found that there was a relationship between insufficient SIRT1 activity due to NAD+ depletion in mice fed a high-fat diet. Histone acetylation can be affected by a high-fat diet and calorie restriction through NAD+ levels (Sawalha et al., 2019).

Inheritance of epigenetic marks requires DNA replication and survival in mitosis. Histone modifications are unaffected by mitosis and DNA replication. The reason is that nucleosomes do not have a replication system based on the DNA template. Barker et al., reported that exposure to environmental factors such as drugs, stress, chemicals, or infections during sensitive periods of pregnancy might predispose to diseases in childhood or adulthood (Cavalli and Heard., 2019). Subsequent studies suggested that this predisposition may be mediated by epigenetic mechanisms (Malhotra et al., 2014). Long-term changes in the epigenome that affect cancer susceptibility and biological age have been reported in many studies (Palumbo et al., 2018). Metabolic diseases such as diabetes, obesity, and neurological conditions such as Parkinson's and Alzheimer's have also been investigated many times (Cavalli & Heard, 2019). The intrauterine period and the first years of life have been defined as two critical periods in which the genome is susceptible to epigenetic changes (McGowan et al., 2009).

Overall, epigenetic mechanisms allow modifiable responses in extreme environmental conditions while buffering ecological diversity. Most organisms buffer environmental variations in physiology and heredity. Therefore, phenotypes are the result of genome composition, epigenetic components, and environmental stimuli (Cavalli & Heard, 2019). The increasing trend in non-communicable chronic diseases has become a significant health problem in developed and developing countries. According to the Developmental Origins of Health and Disease hypothesis, exposure to adverse factors in early childhood can program the individual to adapt to illness immediately or increase the risk of pathological conditions, including metabolic disorders later in life (Kohn et al., 2003). Although not fully elucidated, epigenetic modifications likely mediate the mechanism of action of changes in early life conditions, such as saturated fat-rich foods or refined sugar, in the modern world. The mammalian epigenome is subject to significant epigenetic changes during early development.

Among the most studied epigenetic mechanisms is DNA methylation. For many years, it has enabled us to understand the power of epigenetics in many events such as mitotic inheritance and X chromosome inactivation. DNA methylation studies have taught us that even if the change seems simple, it can have a massive impact on health (Bergman & Cedar, 2013). Changes in DNA methylation and modifications of DNA methylation patterns at the cytosine and guanine residues of the existing DNA sequence are some of the main mechanisms of epigenetic modulations (Khan et al., 2018). Exposure to toxic substances is related to changes in DNA methylation patterns in both humans and other animal models (Wright et al., 2010). It occurs by adding a methyl group to the 5th carbon of cytosine-guanine (CpG) dinucleotides to make 5-methylcytosine residues (Meda et al., 2011). This reaction is mediated by methyltransferase enzymes (Sawalha et al., 2019). DNA methyltransferases synthesize 5-methylcytosine and transfer a methyl group donor from S-adenosylmethionine (SAM) to cytosine (Wang et al., 2017). DNA methyltransferases are responsible for maintaining epigenetic covalent modifications during DNA replication and repair. Some subtypes participate in de nova methylation during embryonic development (Z. X. Chen et al., 2005). Thus, methylation of cytosine bases reduces the binding affinity of transcription factors (Sawalha et al., 2019). It contains methylated CpG sequences and methylated DNA binding domain to alter chromatin structure to form a co-repressor complex, promoting gene transcription (S. Fan & Zhang, 2009; Hughes & Sawalha, 2011). DNA methylation can be passively induced during replication by inhibiting methyltransferases (Sawalha et al., 2019). It can also be caused by various molecules such as DNA glycosylases, demethylases, or glucocorticoids (Fitzpatrick and Wilson, 2003).

The rate of mutations that can occur entirely by chance in DNA is only 0.01%. For this reason, the problems caused by toxic substances such as Vinclozolin transmitted from generation to generation cannot be explained by random mutations in the structure of DNA (Can, 2016; Karaçay, 2009). Genome-wide DNA demethylation occurs during germ cell maturation, followed by remethylation before fertilization. The second wave of genome-wide demethylation characterizes early embryogenesis, and methylation patterns are re-established after implantation. The epigenetic window of developmental plasticity in humans begins before pregnancy and includes childhood. In these developmental periods, epigenetic changes triggered by environmental factors in susceptible individuals can continue throughout life and result in various pathological conditions in adult life. Studies in twin humans have shown that although the instability of the epigenome appears to decrease with age, the epigenetic regulatory mechanisms remain less labile throughout life than during development. Such fine-tuning of epigenetic modification can allow an organism to adapt to changing environmental conditions. However, a such modification may also increase the risk of pathology in the next generation (Blancafort et al., 2013). Skinner et al., stated that surprising results emerged when considered together with epigenetic mechanisms. For example, they suggested that endocrine inhibitors, which constitute an important group from the group of environmental compounds, alter the hormone signal by inhibiting or mimicking the functions of hormones. They stated that endocrine damage could have severe consequences due to the critical role of hormones in development (Skinner, 2009).

Nestler argues that the combination of genetic factors originating from some specific genes that have not yet been identified and non-genetic factors such as random events during development and environmental exposure may cause sensitivity to substance addiction in some individuals, and this situation can be examined under the name of neural flexibility in individuals with this sensitivity. Stable changes in gene expression, through the epigenetic regulation of specific genes, in adolescence or adulthood, are said to overlap with exposure to an addictive substance in individuals with a high addiction susceptibility. Nestler claims that studies on epigenetic regulation in addiction models will teach basic principles about epigenetics in the growth stage and adult nervous system and will open a vital door for studying transcription mechanisms in the brain (Nestler, 2014).

X Chromosome Inactivation

The most studied epigenetic phenomena in mammals are X chromosome inactivation and genomic imprinting. Whether a particular chromosome is of maternal or paternal origin, its phenotypic expression is altered. In female mammals, the dosage of sex chromosome is determined by epigenetic inactivation and stabilization through a transcriptionally silenced X chromosome. An X chromosome is randomly selected and inactivated during early embryogenesis by heterochromatinization. The transcription gene-specific for X chromosome inactivation is Xist, and the antisense gene Tisx also controls its inactivation. X chromosome inactivation is conserved by DNA methylation and histone acetylation. Xist is hypermethylated on the active X, while it is not methylated on the inactive X. Inactive x is hypermethylated in the CpG islets and the gene promoter regions. Another disease due to abnormal methylation of the X chromosome is Fragile X syndrome (Can, 2016).

Genomic Stigma

Genomic imprinting is a form of gene editing that applies cascading gene expression (Can, 2016). Most are discrete clusters, about 1 Mb long, containing maternally and paternally expressed genes (Kalish et al., 2014). Since insulin-like growth factor 2 (Igf2) and the insulin-like growth factor 2 receptor (Igf2r) have been identified, numerous imprinted genes have been placed in mice and humans (Can, 2016). The regulation of clustered genes is controlled by short DNA sequences called imprinting control regions (ICRs). These ICRs are mostly regions where DNA is methylated on a parental allele (DMRs). Most of these sites are methylated in the oocyte before ovulation. In contrast, several ICRs are methylated in the prenatal male germline (Kalish et al., 2014).

In addition to increased susceptibility to cancer, imprinted gene mutation or disordered expression has been associated with many disorders, including the pediatric genetic disease Prader-Willi syndrome, the neurogenetic disease Angelman syndrome, and the overgrowth disease Beckwith Wiedemann syndrome (bladder, lung, ovary, and others) and Neuronatin (pediatric leukemia). Genetic stigma has been associated with atopic diseases, behavioral and psychological disorders, and genetic stigma. The loss of imprinted Igf2 is thought to increases the frequency of intestinal tumors (Can, 2016).

For instance, failure to express the paternal allele of genes within the SNRPN engraved domain affects Prader-Willi Syndrome (PWS), and failure to express the maternal allele results in Angelman Syndrome (AS). Similarly, genetic and epigenetic changes in the H19/IGF2 or KCNQ1 domains result in Beckwith-Wiedemann Syndrome (BWS) or Russell-Siver (RSS), depending on which parental allele is affected. The key to allelic imprinting in clusters is the consistent parent-specific marking of the ICR. Differential DNA methylation is the modification best described to confer parental identity (Kalish et al., 2014).

Autoimmune Diseases

Autoimmune diseases are defined by immune cells' abnormal production of autoantibodies against healthy cells. The roles of B lymphocytes and CD4+ T lymphocytes have been described. With increasing evidence, CD8+ T cells (Cytotoxic T lymphocytes) have been shown to have an essential role in the pathogenesis of diseases. Many inflammatory cytokines, transcription factors, and chemokines can affect the activation of CD8+ T cells. In addition to its protective function in viral infections and tumors, CD8+ cells have been shown to have an essential role in the progression of autoimmune diseases such as experimental autoimmune encephalomyelitis, multiple sclerosis, systemic lupus erythematosus, type 1 diabetes, rheumatoid arthritis, and vitiligo (Sawalha et al., 2019). For example, Graves' disease is characterized by goiter and hyperthyroidism, which occur when circulating autoantibodies stimulate receptors in the thyroid gland. Limbach et al., studied genome-wide DNA methylation in CD8+ T cells in Graves' patients and identified 3322 distinct methylated DNA regions. These regions also contain parts involved in suppressing the activation of CD8+ T cells.

Multiple sclerosis is an autoimmune disease of the central nervous system characterized by loss and inflammation of the axonal. CD8+ T cells are found 3-10 times more than CD4+ T cells in acute and chronic lesions of patients with multiple sclerosis (Friese and Fugger, 2009). In addition, increasing evidence indicates that CD8+ T cells have DNA methylation profiles that are 95% different from control groups in patients with multiple sclerosis (Maltby V. E., 2015). Systemic sclerosis is an autoimmune disease of the connective tissue. It is characterized by immune system dysregulation due to the development of fibrosis in the skin, organs, and tissues and endothelial cell dysfunction resulting from excessive extracellular matrix deposition. In addition, global hypomethylation of interferons, which have a critical role in skin fibrosis, has been demonstrated.

Down Syndrome

Down Syndrome (Trisomy 21) is one of the most common congenital chromosomal disorders, with a frequency of 1/700 in live births. It affects many organs and systems, as well as intellectual disability. It is considered a gene expression disorder. Not only genes like HSA21, but also genes on other chromosomes are defective. Defects in more than one gene can disrupt the interaction between chromosomes. Deregulated genes are regulated in regulatory domains of gene expression. These areas are associated with LAD. However, LADs are not affected in patients with Trisomy 21. The H3K4me3 epigenetic mark in gene regulatory domains is involved in the fibroblasts from these patients. This effect suggests that the disease is partially a chromatin disorder. Overexpression of genes on chromosome 21 may be the source of chromatin modifications. For instance, the HMG1 gene (high mobility group nucleosome binding site), which encodes an element that alters histones and affects the structure of chromatin, is dysregulated in these patients (Moore-Morris et al., 2018).

CHARGE Syndrome

CHARGE syndrome (ocular colobomas, heart diseases, choanal atresia, severe growth and developmental retardation, ear anomalies, genital anomalies) is seen in 1/10000 live births. CHD7, a chromatin remodeling factor (CRF) and a chromatin-helix DNA-binding family of ATP-dependent chromatin remodeling enzymes, is mutated in these patients. Nonsense and frameshift mutations can lead to protein loss (Basson & van Ravenswaaij-Arts, 2015). The CRF subsets participate in maintaining proteins and clearing nucleosomes from their gene regulatory regions to allow the binding of transcription factors. Activation or inhibition of proteins depends on the genomic environment (Klement et al., 2014; Schulz et al., 2014). CHD7 is mainly recruited from distant enhancers and is associated with H3K4me epigenetic markers, indicating the role of CRF in gene activation (Schnetz et al., 2010; Zentner et al., 2010).

DiGeorge Syndrome

DiGeorge Syndrome is a congenital disease that includes craniofacial and cardiac disorders secondary to 22q11 deletion. Tbx1 at the locus is the primary gene candidate for the syndrome (Moore-Morris et al., 2018). To begin with, the histone chaperone protein HIRA, including WDrepeats, has been implicated in the 22q11 syndrome (Lorain et al., 1996). HIRA regulates gene transcription by affecting the structure of chromatin. It is an essential chaperone for nucleosome regulation (Ray-Gallet et al., 2002). Tbx1 has been found to regulate the activity of histone methyltransferase LSD1 and exerts its effect on gene expression through this enzyme (L. Chen et al., 2012). TBX1 also interacts with chromatin-modifying monomethyltransferase genes and regulates many target genes, such as Wnt5 in the heart region. Tbx1 was found to positively regulate monomethylation of histone3lisin4 (H3K4me1) (Fulcoli et al., 2016). These data suggest that DiGeorge syndrome has many epigenetic components and is a more complex disease than expected.

Conclusion

Many changes in the phenotype can be created by changing the active and passive regions of DNA without a change in the genotype. However, they appear with many differences in daily life thanks to these changes. Although progress has been made on the relationship between epigenetic changes and diseases, still some points need to be clarified. With further studies, significant contributions can be made to the diagnosis, follow=up, and the treatment of many organ systems diseases.

References

Allis, C. D., & Jenuwein, T. (2016). The molecular hallmarks of epigenetic control. In *Nature Reviews Genetics* (Vol. 17, Issue 8, pp. 487-500). https://doi.org/10.1038/nrg.2016.59.

Basson, M. A., & van Ravenswaaij-Arts, C. (2015). Functional Insights into Chromatin Remodelling from Studies on CHARGE Syndrome. *Trends in Genetics*, 31(10), 600-11. https://doi.org/10.1016/j.tig.2015.05.009.

Bergman, Y., & Cedar, H. (2013). DNA methylation dynamics in health and disease. *Nature Structural & Molecular Biology*, 20, 274-281. https://doi.org/10.1038/nsmb.2518.

Blancafort, P., Jin, J., & Frye, S. (2013). Writing and rewriting the epigenetic code of cancer cells: From engineered proteins to small molecules. In *Molecular Pharmacology* (Vol. 83, Issue 3). https://doi.org/10.1124/mol.112.080697.

Can, M. İ. & Aslan, A. (2016). Epigenetic Mechanisms and Some Recent Studies. *Karaelmas Fen ve Mühendislik Dergisi*, 6(2), 445-452.

Cañas, C. A., Cañas, F., Bonilla-Abadía, F., Ospina, F. E., & Tobón, G. J. (2016). Epigenetics changes associated to environmental triggers in autoimmunity. *Autoimmunity*, 49(1), 1-11. https://doi.org/10.3109/08916934.2015.1086996.

Cavalli, G., & Heard, E. (2019). Advances in epigenetics link genetics to the environment and disease. *Nature*, 571(7766), 489-499. https://doi.org/10.1038/s41586-019-1411-0.

Chen, L., Fulcoli, F. G., Ferrentino, R., Martucciello, S., & Illingworth, E. A. (2012). Transcriptional Control in Cardiac Progenitors: Tbx1 Interacts with the BAF Chromatin Remodeling Complex and Regulates Wnt5a. *PLoS Genet*, 8(3), 1-11. https://doi.org/10.1371/journal.pgen.1002571.

Chen, Z. X., Mann, J. R., Hsieh, C. L., Riggs, A. D., & Chédin, F. (2005). Physical and functional interactions between the human DNMT3L protein and members of the de novo methyltransferase family. *Journal of Cellular Biochemistry*, 95(5), 902-917. https://doi.org/10.1002/jcb.20447.

Desplats, P., Spencer, B., Coffee, E., Patel, P., Michael, S., Patrick, C., Adame, A., Rockenstein, E., & Masliah, E. (2011). α-Synuclein Sequesters Dnmt1 from the Nucleus: A Novel Mechanism for Epigenetic Alterations in Lewy Body Diseases. *Journal of Biological Chemistry*, 286(11), 9031-9037. https://doi.org/10.1074/JBC.C110.212589.

Ellis, L., Atadja, P. W., & Johnstone, R. W. (2009). Epigenetics in cancer: Targeting chromatin modifications. In *Molecular Cancer Therapeutics* (Vol. 8, Issue 6). https://doi.org/10.1158/1535-7163.MCT-08-0860.

Etchegaray, J. P., & Mostoslavsky, R. (2016). Interplay between Metabolism and Epigenetics: A Nuclear Adaptation to Environmental Changes. *Molecular Cell*, 62(5), 695-711. https://doi.org/10.1016/j.molcel.2016.05.029.

Fan, J., Krautkramer, K. A., Feldman, J. L., & Denu, J. M. (2015). Metabolic Regulation of Histone Post-Translational Modifications. *ACS Chem. Biol*, 10, 95-108. https://doi.org/10.1021/cb500846u.

Fan, S., & Zhang, X. (2009). CpG island methylation pattern in different human tissues and its correlation with gene expression. *Biochemical and Biophysical Research Communications*, 383(4), 421-425. https://doi.org/10.1016/J.BBRC.2009.04.023.

Fitzpatrick, D. R., & Wilson, C. B. (2003). Methylation and demethylation in the regulation of genes, cells, and responses in the immune system. *Clinical Immunology*, 109(1), 37-45. https://doi.org/10.1016/S1521-6616(03)00205-5.

Friese, M. A., & Fugger, L. (2009). Pathogenic CD8 + T cells in multiple sclerosis. *Annals of Neurology*, 66(2), 132-141. https://doi.org/10.1002/ana.21744.

Fulcoli, F. G., Franzese, M., Liu, X., Zhang, Z., Angelini, C., & Baldini, A. (2016). Rebalancing gene haploinsufficiency *in vivo* by targeting chromatin. *Nature Communications*, 7. https://doi.org/10.1038/ncomms11688.

Goardon, N., Marchi, E., Atzberger, A., Quek, L., Schuh, A., Soneji, S., Woll, P., Mead, A., Alford, K. A., Rout, R., Chaudhury, S., Gilkes, A., Knapper, S., Beldjord, K., Begum, S., Rose, S., Geddes, N., Griffiths, M., Standen, G., Sternberg, A., Cavenagh, J., Hunter, H., Bowen, D., Killick, S., Robinson, L., Price, A., Macintyre, E., Virgo, P., Burnett, A., Craddock, C., Enver, T., Jacobsen, E. W., Porcher, C., Vyas P., (2011). Coexistence of LMPP-like and GMP-like Leukemia Stem Cells in Acute Myeloid Leukemia. *Cancer Cell*, 19(1), 138-152. https://doi.org/10.1016/J.CCR.2010.12.012.

Guay, C., Roggli, E., Nesca, V., Jacovetti, C., & Regazzi, R. (2011). Diabetes mellitus, a microRNA-related disease? *Translational Research*, 157(4), 253-264. https://doi.org/10.1016/j.trsl.2011.01.009.

Hewagama, A., & Richardson, B. (2009). The genetics and epigenetics of autoimmune diseases. *Journal of Autoimmunity*, 33(1), 3-11. https://doi.org/10.1016/J.JAUT.2009.03.007.

Horvath, S. (2013). DNA methylation age of human tissues and cell types. *Genome Biology*, 14(10), 1-19. https://doi.org/10.1186/gb-2013-14-10-r115.

Hughes, T., & Sawalha, A. H. (2011). The role of epigenetic variation in the pathogenesis of systemic lupus erythematosus. *Arthritis Research and Therapy*, 13(5), 1-11. https://doi.org/10.1186/ar3 484.

Kalish, J. M., Jiang, C., & Bartolomei, M. S. (2014). Epigenetics and imprinting in human disease. *International Journal of Developmental Biology*, 58(2-4), 291-298. https://doi.org/10.1387/ijdb.140077 mb.

Karaçay, B. (2009). Kalıtımın Yeni Boyutu: Epigenetik [*The New Dimension of Heredity: Epigenetics*]. *Bilim ve Teknik*, 505, 32-37.

Khan, F., Momtaz, S., & Abdollahi, M. (2018). The relationship between mercury exposure and epigenetic alterations regarding human health, risk assessment and diagnostic strategies. *Journal of Trace Elements in Medicine and Biology*, 52, 37-47. https://doi.org/10.1016/j.jtemb.2018.11.006.

Klement, K., Luijsterburg, M. S., Pinder, J. B., Cena, C. S., del Nero, V., Wintersinger, C. M., Dellaire, G., van Attikum, H., & Goodarzi, A. A. (2014). Opposing ISWI- and CHD-class chromatin remodeling activities orchestrate heterochromatic DNA repair. *Journal of Cell Biology*, 207(6), 717-733. https://doi.org/10.1083/jcb.201405077.

Kohn, D. B., Sadelain, M., & Glorioso, J. C. (2003). Occurrence of leukaemia following gene therapy of X-linked SCID. *Nature Reviews Cancer*, 3(7), 477-488. https://doi.org/10.1038/nrc1122.

Kouzarides, T. (2007). Chromatin Modifications and Their Function. *Cell*, 128(4), 693-705. https://doi.org/10.1016/j.cell.2007.02.005.

Li, X., & Kazgan, N. (2011). Mammalian sirtuins and energy metabolism. *International Journal of Biological Sciences*, 7(5), 575-587. https://doi.org/10.7150/ijbs.7.575.

Lorain, S., Demczuk, S., Lamour, V., Toth, S., Aurias, A., Roe, B. A., & Lipinski, M. (1996). Structural organization of the WD repeat protein-encoding gene HIRA in the DiGeorge syndrome critical region of human chromosome 22. *Genome Research*, 6(1), 43-50. https://doi.org/10.1101/gr.6.1.43.

Loscalzo, J., & Handy, D. E. (2014). Epigenetic modifications: Basic mechanisms and role in cardiovascular disease (2013 Grover Conference series). *Pulmonary Circulation*, 4(2), 169-174. https://doi.org/10.1086/675979.

Malhotra, N., Malhotra, J., Bora, N. M., Bora, R., & Malhotra, K. (2014). Fetal origin of adult disease. *Donald School Journal of Ultrasound in Obstetrics and Gynecology*, 8(2), 164-177. https://doi.org/10.5005/jp-journals-10009-1352.

Maltby, V. E., Moira C. Graves, Rodney A. Lea, Miles C. Benton, Katherine A. Sanders, Lotti Tajouri, Rodney J. Scott and Jeannette Lechner-Scott.. (2015). Genome-wide DNA methylation profiling of CD8+T cells shows a distinct epigenetic signature to CD4+T cells in multiple sclerosis patients. *Clin Epigenetics*, 7(118), 1-6.

McGowan, P. O., Sasaki, A., D'Alessio, A. C., Dymov, S., Labonté, B., Szyf, M., Turecki, G., & Meaney, M. J. (2009). Epigenetic regulation of the glucocorticoid receptor in human brain associates with childhood abuse. *Nature Neuroscience*, 12(3), 342-348. https://doi.org/10.1038/nn.2270.

Meda, F., Folci, M., Baccarelli, A., & Selmi, C. (2011). The epigenetics of autoimmunity. *Cellular & Molecular Immunology*, 8, 226-236. https://doi.org/10.1038/cmi.2010.78.

Millis, R. M. (2011). Epigenetics and Hypertension. *Current Hypertension Reports*, 13, 21-28. https://doi.org/10.1007/s11906-010-0173-8.

Moore-Morris, T., van Vliet, P. P., Andelfinger, G., & Puceat, M. (2018). Role of epigenetics in cardiac development and congenital diseases. *Physiological Reviews* 98(4), 2453-2475. https://doi.org/10.1152/physrev.00048.2017.

Nakahata, Y., Kaluzova, M., Grimaldi, B., Sahar, S., Hirayama, J., Chen, D., Guarente, L. P., & Sassone-Corsi, P. (2008). The NAD+-Dependent Deacetylase SIRT1 Modulates CLOCK-Mediated Chromatin Remodeling and Circadian Control. *Cell*, 134(2), 329-340. https://doi.org/10.1016/j.cell.2008.07.002.

Nestler, E. J. (2014). Epigenetic mechanisms of drug addiction. In *Neuropharmacology* (Vol. 76, Issue PART B, pp. 259-268.). https://doi.org/10.1016/j.neuropharm.2013.04.004.

Oaks, Z., & Perl, A. (2014). Metabolic control of the epigenome in systemic Lupus erythematosus. *Autoimmunity*, 47(4), 256-264. https://doi.org/10.3109/08916934.2013.834495.

Palumbo, S., Mariotti, V., Iofrida, C., & Pellegrini, S. (2018). Genes and aggressive behavior: Epigenetic mechanisms underlying individual susceptibility to aversive environments. *Frontiers in Behavioral Neuroscience*, 12, 1-9. https://doi.org/10.3389/fnbeh.2018.00117.

Quach, A., Levine, M. E., Tanaka, T., Lu, A. T., Chen, B. H., Ferrucci, L., Ritz, B., Bandinelli, S., Neuhouser, M. L., Beasley, J. M., Snetselaar, L., Wallace, R. B., Tsao, P. S., Absher, D., Assimes, T. L., Stewart, J. D., Li, Y., Hou, L., Baccarelli, A. A., Eric A Whitsel and Horvath, S. (2017). Epigenetic clock analysis of diet, exercise, education, and lifestyle factors. *Aging*, 9(2), 419-446. https://doi.org/10.18632/aging.101168.

Ray-Gallet, D., Quivy, J. P., Scamps, C., Martini, E. M. D., Lipinski, M., & Almouzni, G. (2002). HIRA is critical for a nucleosome assembly pathway independent of DNA synthesis. *Molecular Cell*, 9(5), 1091-1100. https://doi.org/10.1016/S1097-2765(02)00526-9.

Sawalha, A., Perl, A., Noss, E. H., Ding, Y., Xiao, R., Deng, Q., Luo, Y., Chang, C., & Wu, H. (2019). The Emerging Epigenetic Role of CD8+T Cells in Autoimmune Diseases. *A Systematic Review. Front. Immunol*, 10(856), 1-15. https://doi.org/10.3389/fimmu.2019.00856.

Schnetz, M. P., Handoko, L., Akhtar-Zaidi, B., Bartels, C. F., & Pereira, C. F. (2010). CHD7 Targets Active Gene Enhancer Elements to Modulate ES Cell-Specific Gene Expression. *PLoS Genet*, 6(7), 1-15. https://doi.org/10.1371/journal.pgen.1001023.

Schulz, Y., Wehner, P., Lennart Opitz, Salinas-Riester, G., Bongers, E. M. H. F., Conny, van Ravenswaaij-Arts, M. A., Wincent, J., Schoumans, J., Kohlhase, J., Borchers, A., Pauli, S., Schulz, Y., Pauli, S, Wehner, P., Borchers, A, Bongers, E. M. H. F., & Kohlhase, J. (2014). CHD7, the gene mutated in CHARGE syndrome, regulates genes involved in neural crest cell guidance. *Hum Genet*, 133, 997-1009. https://doi.org/10.1007/s00439-014-1444-2.

Shi, L., & Tu, B. P. (2015). Acetyl-CoA and the regulation of metabolism: mechanisms and consequences. *Current Opinion in Cell Biology*, 33, 125-131. https://doi.org/10.1016/J.CEB.2015.02.003.

Skinner, M. K., Manikkam, M., and Guerrero-Bosagna, C., (2009). Epigenetic transgerenational actions of environmental factors in disease etiology. *NIH Public Access*, 21(4), 214-222.

Veech, R. L., Eggleston, L. V., Krebs H. A. (1969). The redox state of free nicotinamide–adenine dinucleotide phosphate in the cytoplasm of rat liver. *Biochem J*, 115(4), 609-619.

Wang, Z., Long, H., Chang, Christopher, Zhao, M., & Lu, Q. (2018). Crosstalk between metabolism and epigenetic modifications in autoimmune diseases: a comprehensive overview. *Cellular and Molecular Life Sciences*, 75, 3353-3369. https://doi.org/10.1007/s00018-018-2864-2.

Wang, Z., Lu, Q., & Wang, Z. (2017). Epigenetic Alterations in Cellular Immunity: New Insights into Autoimmune Diseases. *Cellular Physiology and Biochemistry*, 41(2), 645-660. https://doi.org/10.1159/000457944.

Wright, R. O., Schwartz, J., Wright, R. J., Bollati, V., Tarantini, L., Park, S. K., Hu, H., Sparrow, D., Vokonas, P., & Baccarelli, A. (2010). Biomarkers of lead exposure and DNA methylation within retrotransposons. *Environmental Health Perspectives*, 118(6), 790-795. https://doi.org/10.1289/ehp.0901429.

Yang, M.-L., Gee, A. J. P., Gee, R. J., Zurita-Lopez, C. I., Khare, S., Clarke, S. G., & Mamula, M. J. (2013). Lupus autoimmunity altered by cellular methylation metabolism) Lupus autoimmunity altered by cellular methylation metabolism Lupus autoimmunity altered by cellular methylation metabolism. *Autoimmunity*, 46(1), 21-31. https://doi.org/10.3109/08916934.2012.732133.

Zentner, G. E., Hurd, E. A., Schnetz, M. P., Handoko, L., Wang, C., Wang, Z., Wei, C., Tesar, P. J., Hatzoglou, M., Martin, D. M., & Scacheri, P. C. (2010). CHD7 functions in the nucleolus as a positive regulator of ribosomal RNA biogenesis. *Human Molecular Genetics*, 19(18), 3491-3501. https://doi.org/10.1093/hmg/ddq265.

Chapter 3

The Role of DNA Methylation and Histone Modifications in Oncogenesis

Gözde Öztan*, **PhD**
Department of Medicine, Istanbul University, Istanbul, Turkey

Abstract

Epigenetic modifications include DNA methylation and covalent modifications of histones. In spite of the fact that they are reversible, these alterations have an unavoidable effect on gene expression and are very stable. Cytosines are more frequently methylated than guanine nucleotides or CpG sites in DNA. In addition to regulating tissue-specific gene expression, DNA methylation also affects genomic imprinting and the inactivation of X chromosomes. It is possible that DNA methylation in different genomic regions may influence gene activity differently depending on the genetic sequence.

Methylation changes in the promoter or first exon can mimic the effects of mutations in various tumor suppressor genes (TSGs) or protooncogenes. Cancer may also develop from abnormal DNA methylation, such as hyper- or hypomethylation of cancer-related genes' promoters or first exons. The transcriptional silencing of a variety of TSGs is caused by hypermethylation of their promoters. Activating the transcription of protooncogenes, retrotransposons, and genes that encode proteins that have a role in genome instability and malignant cell metastasis is accomplished by hypomethylating regulatory DNA sequences.

In carcinogenesis, DNA methylation has a critical role in gene expression. In this chapter, hypo- and hyper-DNA methylation on cancer as well as recurrence risk of human cancers are discussed along with the mechanisms and cell-regulating effects of both hypo- and hyper-methylation.

Keywords: epigenetic, oncogenesis, DNA methylation, histone modifications

Introduction

Epigenetic Mechanisms

The chromatin structure explains the way genetic information is organized within cells in the form of DNA. An octamer of four core histone proteins (H3, H4, H2A and H2B) is wrapped around 146 base pairs of DNA to form an octamer of nucleosomes, which are repeating units

* Corresponding Author's E-mail: gozdeoztan@yahoo.com.

In: Epigenetics: Beyond the Genetics and Medicine
Editors: Sevgi Durna Daştan and Nazan Yurtcu
ISBN: 979-8-88697-228-3

of chromatin. Epigenetic mechanisms control chromatin structure, including DNA methylation, covalent modifications of histones, as well as noncovalent mechanisms including histone variants, and nucleosome remodeling. Modifications affect mainly accessibility and compactness within the genome by modifying the dynamics of the local structure of the chromatin within the genome (Sharma et al., 2010).

The process through which epigenetic changes of the genome are transmitted during cell divisions is called epigenetic inheritance. It is accomplished either within an individual, through mitosis, defined as persistence, or between generations, through meiosis, defined as inheritance. While epigenetic modifications can alter gene expression, the DNA sequence is unchanged. Modifies the way genes are transcribed and expressed by mechanisms such as methylation of CpG sites, noncoding RNAs, or chromatin remodeling. Various stimuli result in epigenetic modifications, ranging from the immediate external environment of a cell to the cell's immediate surroundings (Spencer, 2016).

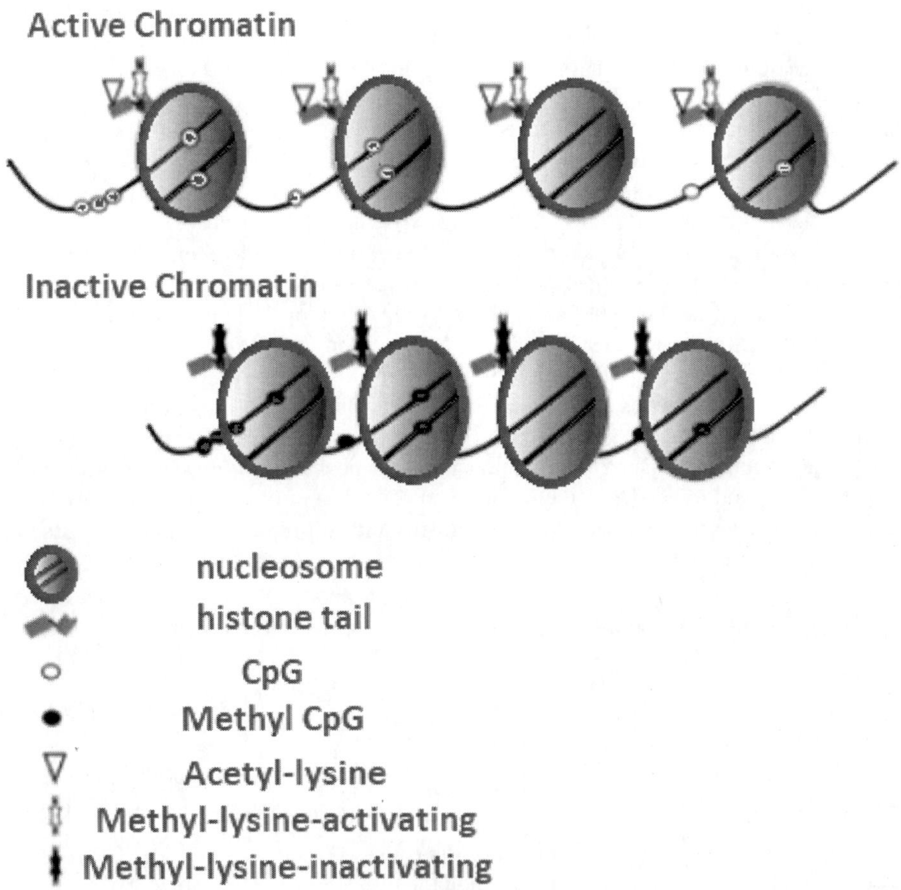

Figure 1. Chromatin structure and epigenetic tags. Nucleosomes are formed by packaging DNA around histone cores. Post-translational modifications of histone tails, such as lysine acetylation and specific lysine methylation, are necessary for the maintenance of open nuclear structures that are accessible to nuclear factors. Gene promoters can be overlapped by CpG islands, which are unequally distributed among the CpG dinucleotides on chromosomal DNA (Handy et al., 2011).

A chromatin is an association of chromosomal DNA and proteins found in the nucleus. Chromatin consists of DNA packaged around histone proteins, called nucleosomes. DNA containing 147 base pairs is attached to a nucleosome by two H3-H4 dimers, passing through two H2A-H2B dimers. Histone N-terminal tails are released from nucleosomes and are associated with the nuclear lumen. The histone H1 binds to the DNA residing between nucleosomes. The chromatin structure is defined by the spacing of nucleosomes, also known as heterochromatin or euchromatin. Both DNA and histone tail modifications regulate the structure of the chromatin and gene access to the transcriptional machinery (Figure 1) (Handy et al., 2011).

DNA methylation biomarkers can be used for detection, diagnosis, and risk assessment. According to data obtained, cancer cells do not exhibit the typical complex chromatin structure and DNA methylation organization, resulting in aberrant gene expression profiles. Furthermore, evidence suggests that hypermethylation of GC-rich DNA regions contributes significantly to tumor growth largely because it is responsible for the inactivation and silencing of tumor suppressor genes. The abnormal methylation of cytosine residues within these CpG islands has been found to be a basis for both mutations and cytogenetic abnormalities within cancer cells. Even though thc findings strongly associate hypermethylation in the CpG islands with cancer development, they also reveal a strong association between hypomethylation in the global genome and carcinogenesis (Ziech, et al., 2010).

Epigenetic DNA Modifications

Eukaryotic cells use chromatin, a highly controlled, dynamic, and complex structure in the nucleus, to control gene expression. The chromatin structure undergoes some structural and chemical changes and affects gene expressions. When the chromatin structure, which is a very tightly packed form of DNA, is opened during DNA replication, the structural and chemical modifications existing in the template chain, in other words, "epigenetic marks" are transferred to the newly synthesized chains and thus are protected from cell to cell during each replication (Jiang, et al., 2004).

The epigenetic system consists of several types of chemical modifications in DNA or histones. A wide variety of biological events can cause these genes to produce cellular outcomes, but they are stable without changing the genomic sequence. DNA methylation on CpG islands is a common epigenetic modification in mammals, as it functions as a repressive chromatin modification, which functions long-term to silence genes. A CpG island methylation abnormality can contribute to disease (Furuya et al., 2019).

DNA methylation is the process of covalently attaching a methyl group (CH3) to either the cytosine or the adenine of DNA molecules (Liao & Xu, 2019). The DNA methyltransferases (DNMTs) catalyze this chemical process. The enzymes responsible for S-adenosyl-L-methionine (SAM) transfer methyl groups to the 5th carbon of cytosine. There are five DNA methyl transferase enzymes in mammals; DNMT1, DNMT3A, DNMT3B, DNMT3L, and DNMT2 (Denis et al., 2011). The DNMT1, DNMT3A, and DNMT3B DNA methyltransferases catalyze this modification (Liao & Xu, 2019). DNMT1 is responsible for transferring established methylation patterns in the DNA chain to new strands. De novo methyltransferases DNMT3A and DNMT3B are responsible for setting up the first methylation patterns during development (Denis et al., 2011).

The methylation of DNA is critical for the epigenetic regulation of gene expression. When high levels of methylation are present at or near transcription start sites, this often leads to transcriptional silencing. As evidenced by the insensitivity of methylated chromatin to nuclease digestion and the significantly reduced acetylation of histone proteins, DNA methylation leads to a closed chromatin structure (Liao & Xu, 2019). Nitrogenous bases in DNA are chemically manipulated to regulate gene expression. A base of DNA known as methylated cytosine (5-mC) has been established long before DNA has been recognized as a genetic material. Although recent discoveries of additional DNA modifications have raised interest in epigenomics, attention has tended to focus on the conventional modified DNA base 5-methylcytosine (5-mC). In order to understand the regulation of epigenetic gene, epigenetic marks must be removed (Kumar et al., 2018).

Histone Modifications

Histones can be post-translationally modified, and these modifications are typically located on the tails of the histones. It is through these modifications that the chromatin structure can be regulated and frequently used to recruit various non-histone proteins on chromatin. Histones are modified by acetylation, methylation, phosphorylation, and ubiquitylation during post-translational processing. Histones or a combination of histones of transcriptionally active and silent chromatin differ in their post-translational modifications. The H3 and H4 tails of active genes are typically acetylated, H3 lysine 4 is trimethylated, H3 lysine 79 is trimethylated, H2B is ubiquitylated, and H3 lysine 36 is trimethylated. Among the genes repressed by trimethylation, ubiquitylation of H2A on lysine 119, trimethylation of H3 on lysine 9, is associated with trimethylation of lysine 27 (Figure 2) (Zhang et al., 2015).

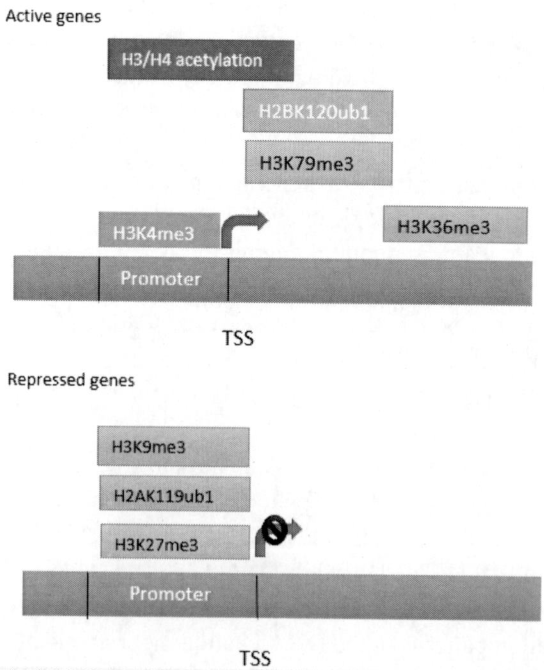

Figure 2. Genes that are active or repressed based on the distribution of histone modifications.

Besides modifying histones, histone modifications can also serve as epigenetic passengers that can be passed down through daughter cells to maintain lineage-specific transcription profiles. Histone modifications can directly affect the structure of chromatin. It is possible to decrease the positive charge of histones with acetylation, which can weaken the interaction between them and negatively charged DNA and contribute to nucleosome fluidity. According to this hypothesis, post-translational modifications operate as signal platforms for locating local effector modules, and it is these readers or effectors that determine the functional outcome of the modifications (Yun et al., 2011).

A large amount of chromatin function depends on the post-translational modifications of histones, which include adding, removing, and recognizing them. Histone proteins are modified by post-translational modifications such as ubiquitin and ubiquitin-likes (UBLs) that act as signal molecules by facilitating protein–protein interactions. By identifying novel ubiquitin and UBL sites and identifying writers, erasers, and readers, researchers are discovering that ubiquitin signaling influences a wide range of chromatin functions. As a result of UBL attachment, functional consequences can be recognized through the UBL-interacting domains, resulting in a specific charge on the surface of the UBL. Nucleosome structures have existed containing ubiquitin molecules and ubiquitin reader proteins, possibly limiting the flexibility of ubiquitin attachment (Vaughan et al., 2020).

Methylation of DNA and Histones in Cancer

A heritable way to control gene expression is achieved by covalent modification of DNA and histone proteins, which are the core parts of chromatin (Jin et al., 2011). Changing the nucleosome (histones) through covalent modification affects the structure and function of the chromatin, which in turn affects gene expression. Chromatin is classified into six categories based on histone modifications: promoter, enhancer, insulator, transcribed, repressed, and inactive chromatin (Kamińska et al., 2019). Covalent modifications to histone tails, such as acetylation, methylation, phosphorylation, ubiquitination, and sumoylation, contribute to gene transcription, DNA replication, and DNA repair. The alteration of DNA methylation and specific histone modifications appears to induce reverse effects during the development of mammals and cancer (Jin et al., 2011). Acetylation and methylation of histone are often associated with a more relaxed chromatin conformation, and they serve as the most important indicators of active chromatin. Chromatin condensation is linked to histone deacetylation and phosphorylation, which is a marker of inactive chromatin (Kamińska et al., 2019).

Normal cells and tumor cells exhibit different DNA methylation patterns. Cancerous cells have an inverted CpG methylation profile compared to normal cells. The methylation of DNA has been reported to have a role in many tumor genes, and two epigenetic mechanisms have been demonstrated. These methylation changes are caused by global hypomethylation and hypermethylation of generally unmethylated CpG islands at an early stage in the progression of neoplasia. DNA hypomethylation contributes to oncogene transcription and chromosome instability. Hypermethylation of promoters causes the silence of certain genes, including tumor suppressor genes. As a consequence of silencing the genes that control the cell cycle, cells will grow and reproduce uncontrollably, causing a tumor to form (Wu & Ni, 2015).

The human genome consists of long interspersed nucleotide elements-1 (LINE-1) and repetitive elements contributed by the ALU. LINE-1, ALU, and SAT2 may have an important role in liver carcinogenesis through hypomethylation. As early as stages of hepatocellular carcinoma (HCC), the loss of methylation in SAT2 precedes the loss in LINE-1 and ALU. Chromosomal instability and a poorer prognosis are associated with genome-wide loss of methylation in HCC. HCC patients with hypomethylated LINE-1 elements in circulating DNA have a poor prognosis when they have been diagnosed in advanced stages. (Anwar & Lehmann, 2014). Acute Myeloid Leukemia (AML) is prone to DNA methylation abnormalities, which are among the most common alterations found in AML. AML is characterized by specific DNA methylation patterns that can be used to distinguish subtypes of AML. The leukemic transformation is partially influenced by interactions between mutations in transcription factors and epigenetic networks. EZH2 and DNMT3A mutations have been reported to be found in diseases leading to secondary leukemia and acute myeloid leukemia (Schoofs & Müller-Tidow, 2011).

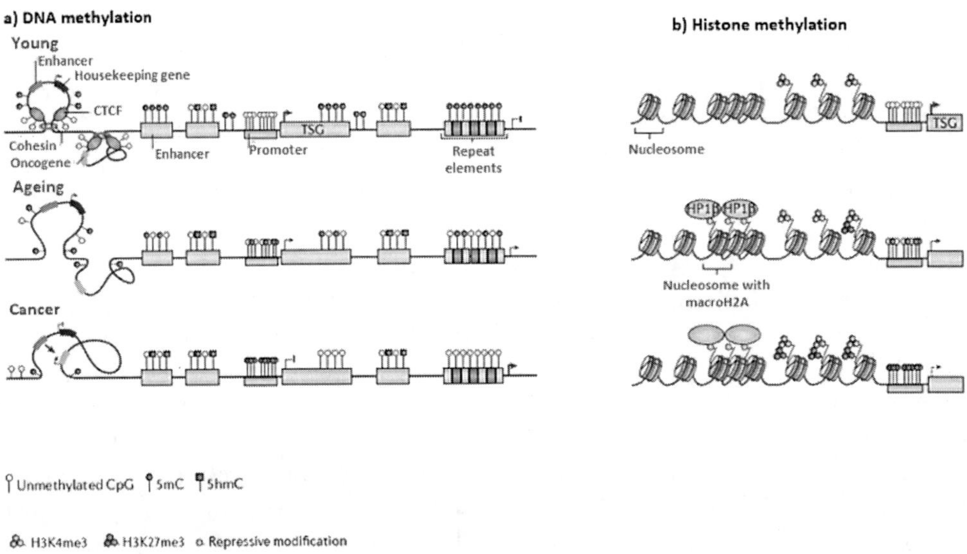

Figure 3. The methylation of DNA and histones in cancer cells. a) DNA methylation. Young, normal cells have low levels of 5-methylcytidine (5mC) methylation in promoter regions, but it is highly methylated in the genic (coding and noncoding) and intergenic (upstream and downstream) regions. In the presence of boundary factors such as CCCTC-binding factor (CTCF) and cohesin, large-scale chromatin loops can be deregulated by altered enhancer methylation. During aging and cancer, DNA methylation occurs at selected genomic loci where tumor suppressor genes (TSGs) and polycomb-repressed genes are expressed, leading to gene silencing. The demethylation of retrotransposons and satellite repeats as well as their transcription have been observed in human cancer and aged cells (Michalak et al., 2019). b) Histone methylation. Replicatively senescent cells possess a changed chromatin structure, as well as a higher level of heterochromatin factors such as the H2A histone variant macroH2A and heterochromatin-binding protein 1β. In cancer cells, some of these characteristics can lead to gene silencing. In normal cells, DNA methylation levels around promoters in intended bivalent loci are lowest; aging alters this and leads to DNA hypermethylation, which is linked to several cancers and decreases the expression of TSGs (Michalak et al., 2019).

S-adenosylmethionine (SAM) is a methyl donor which is used by enzymes called methyltransferases ('writers') during methylation. There are also methyl demethylases and methyl 'readers.' There is a connection between methylation pathways and many diseases, which emphasizes their importance. Mammalian genomes show a high level of DNA methylation, with 70% of CpG dinucleotides methylated. CpG-rich regions are typically unmethylated in the promoters of active genes in this model. DNA methylation silences many tumour suppressor genes in cancer. Mammalian genomes contain primarily repetitive elements, and many of them contain methyl groups. Cancer cells hypomethylate these repetitive elements during early embryogenesis and tumor development. In this way, endogenous retroviral elements can be activated and transposed, leading to genomic instability (Figure 3a) (Michalak et al., 2019).

Histone methylation is primarily controlled by recruiting or inhibiting histone-binding proteins. Activating proteins, such as transcription factors, are recruited into gene promoters by H3K4me3, while transcription repressors such as the nucleosome remodeling and deacetylase complex are inhibited by H3K4me3. In mammalian heterochromatin, members of HP1 family, particularly HP1β, are specifically bound to H3K9me2 and H3K9me3, which have a key role in generating higher-order heterochromatin architectures (Figure 3b) (Michalak et al., 2019).

DNA hypomethylation occurs on a genome-wide level rather than based on a gene-by-gene basis in many malignancies. The amount of global hypomethylation increases as the stage of prostate cancer progresses, according to a number of studies. In benign and early stage PCa, the gene for plasminogen activator (PLAU) promoter is heavily methylated. Nevertheless, the gene is demethylated in highly invasive malignant tumors. Hypomethylation of DNA contributes to oncogenesis and cancer progression by causing genomic instability and mutations (Liao & Xu, 2019).

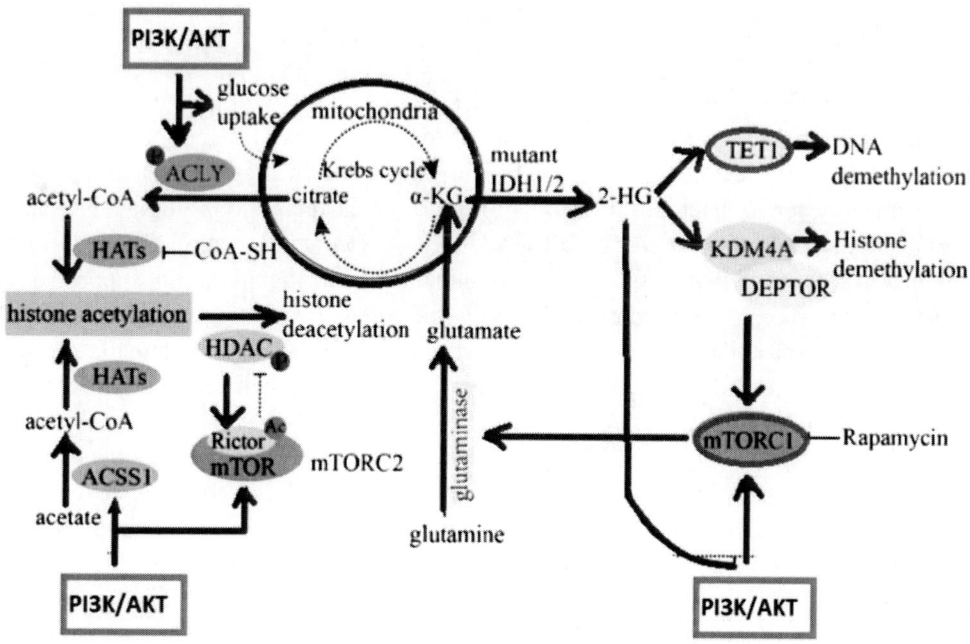

Figure 4. The PI3K/AKT pathway regulates histone acylation and DNA/histone methylation associated with TET. Cancer cells can also synthesize acetyl-CoA from acetate by utilizing acetyl-CoA synthases (ACSS1/ACSS2). Acetyl-CoA pool is replenished by the two enzymes to meet HAT activity demands.

The tumor microenvironment (TME) contributes significantly to cancer progression. In a TME, tumor cells, the stroma that surrounds them, and the extracellular matrix are all present.

The interaction between the TME components contributes to tumorigenesis. Tumor-associated stromal cells have been studied by various research studies on DNA methylation. It has been shown that DNA methylation influences the activation of stromal cells, and methylated genes contribute to the procancerous activity of stromal cells. Interactions between tumor cells and tumor cell-derived molecules trigger the activation of cancer-associated fibroblasts (CAFs) within the TME. A large proportion of tumor stroma is composed of CAFs. These CAFs interact with tumor cells to regulate intercellular signaling and mechanically remodel the cancerous tissue by secreting various factors (Zhang, et al., 2017).

Acetylation and deacetylation of histones explain how the N-terminal tails of nucleosomes are modified by acetylation and deacetylation at lysine residues. As a result of deacetylation, chromatin can become tightly packed and referred to as heterochromatin. Histone acetyltransferase (HAT) or histone deacetylase (HDAC) is the enzyme responsible for acetylating or deacylating histones. There has been a correlation between global histone acetylation levels and patient prognosis in several studies along a wide range of cancer types. In prostate cancer, glucose is preferred over glutamine and fatty acids as a source of acetyl-CoA. It has been shown that under hypoxia stress, cancer cells can activate ACSS1 through AKT signaling, exhibiting hyperactivity of acetyl-CoA synthetases (ACSS1/ACSS2) that use acetate to make acetyl-CoA. The mechanism by which PI3K/AKT regulates histone acetylation has been appropriately modeled (Yang et al., 2019) (Figure 4).

Conclusion

The field of epigenetics deals with how chemical compounds can affect gene expression, for example, by modifying DNA methylation, histone modifications, and noncoding RNA. Genomic imprinting and inactivation of chromosome X are mediated by DNA methylation, which in turn leads to heterochromatin and transcriptional repression. Studies have reported that mutations in the genes that control DNA methylation and demethylation lead to faulty methylation patterns in lymphomas. A mutation that causes malignant tumor suppressor genes to be silenced can cause genomic instability, while a mutation that causes gene-wide DNA hypomethylation can silence tumor suppressor genes. A measure of the patient's response to chemotherapy or a demethylating agent may be able to predict their response to personalized therapies (Chebly et al., 2021).

Each of the four histone tails, H2A, H2B, H3, and H4, is exposed outside the nucleosome and undergoes various post-translational modifications. Modifications that occur most commonly are methylation, acetylation, glycosylation, ubiquitination, sumoylation, and phosphorylation. Most of the histone modifications studied in lymphomas involve histone methylation and histone acetylation. A number of genes that regulate histone modifications have been identified to have abnormal methylation or acetylation patterns. The majority of studies have examined genes responsible for global histone modifications (Chebly et al., 2021).

Malignant cells show significantly altered DNA methylation patterns compared to normal cells. It is usually hypomethylation that results from repeated DNA sequences, typically long interspersed nuclear elements, and hypermethylation that results from CpG islands. Hypermethylation of the CpG islands can be prevented by a variety of mechanisms. There are several mechanisms that prevent access to DNA methyltransferase, including transcription activity, active demethylation, replication timing, and local chromatin structure. In over 90%

of prostate cancers, GSTP1 is hypermethylated. However, in acute myeloid leukemias, it is largely unmethylated. Leukemias and other hematologic diseases are frequently associated with hypermethylation. The ER gene, p21Cip1/Waf1, the Calcitonin gene, p15INK4B, SDC4, MDR genes have been found to be hypermethylated in various hematological cancers. Among the types of methylation defects associated with malignancy, hypomethylation is the second most common type. Hypomethylation is frequently observed in cervical cancer, metastatic hepatocellular cancer, prostate tumors, and hematological malignancies (Das & Singal, 2004).

The role of histone modifications in the coordination of gene expression is critical. The abnormal post-translational modifications of histone tails that occur with leukemogenesis are also associated with genetic mutations that cause DNA sequence changes. Histone methyltransferases (HMTs) can covalently modify lysine residues in histone tails. The Set1 (COMPASS) family of proteins catalyzes the methylation of H3K4, of which the KMT2A protein has a direct role in aggressive forms of acute leukemia. Hematological malignancies have been shown to be affected by H3K27 methylation, as in T-cell acute lymphoid leukemia, where mutations in the H3K27 demethylase UTX or other components of PRC2, SUZ12 and EED contribute to the methylation changes (Birch & Shilatifard, 2020).

In this chapter, various mechanisms by which the effects of DNA methylation and histone modifications on oncogenesis are presented. DNA methylation and histone modifications both exhibit variable patterns of distribution in cancer cells. The DNA methylation patterns of cancer cells differ greatly from those of normal cells upon comparison. Methylation-induced cancer development can be explained by three different mechanisms: genome-wide hypomethylation, tumor suppressor gene inactivation due to hypermethylation in CpG islands, and mutations in CpG dinucleotides. Since DNA methylation has an important place in carcinogenesis, methods to detect this condition are widely used today to support the clinical diagnosis and to choose the appropriate treatment method in the presence of methylation. At the same time, they can be useful in the follow-up of cases after treatment and in the periodic screening of people at high risk for cancer. Various histone modifications at the level of individual cells have been found to predict the outcome of cancer. Atypical histone modification patterns are observed in cancers. It is consistent with the observations that histone-modifying enzymes impair activity in various cancers which is the cellular levels of histone modifications deviate.

It should be considered that other regulations such as histone modifications and chromatin structure may be effective in addition to DNA methylation in elucidating epigenetic inheritance mechanisms. Understanding all of these mechanisms will contribute to the elucidation of the pathogenesis of multifactorial diseases and the epigenetic factors that predispose to the disease, and to the development of possible new treatment molecules.

References

Anwar, S. L., Lehmann, U. (2014). DNA methylation, microRNAs, and their crosstalk as potential biomarkers in hepatocellular carcinoma. *World Journal of Gastroenterology*, 20:7894-7913.

Birch, N. W., & Shilatifard, A. (2020). The role of histone modifications in leukemogenesis. *Journal of Biosciences*, 45:6. https://doi.org/ 10.1007/s12038-019-9969-0.

Chebly, A., Chouery, E., Ropio, J., Kourie, H. R., Beylot-Barry, M., Merlio, J. P., Tomb, R., Chevret, E. (2021). Diagnosis and treatment of lymphomas in the era of epigenetics. *Blood Reviews*, 48:100782. https://doi.org/10.1016/j.blre.2020.100782.

Das, P. M., & Singal, R. (2004). DNA Methylation and Cancer. *Journal of Clinical Oncology*, 22:4632-42. https://doi.org/10.1200/JCO.2004.07.151.

Denis H., Ndlovu M. N., Fuks, F. (2011). Regulation of mammalian DNA methyltransferases: a route to new mechanisms. *EMBO reports*, 12: 647-56.

Furuya, K., Ikura, M., Ikura, T. (2019). Epigenetic interplays between DNA demethylation and histone methylation for protecting oncogenesis. *The Journal of Biochemistry,* 165:297–299. https://doi.org/ 10.1093/jb/mvy124.

Handy, D. E., Castro, R., Loscalzo, J. (2011). Epigenetic Modifications: Basic Mechanisms and Role in Cardiovascular Disease. *Circulation,* 123:2145–2156. https://doi.org/10.1161/CIRCULATIONAHA.110.956839

Jiang, Y., Bressler, J., Beaudet, L. A. (2004). Epigenetics and human disease. *Annual Review of Genetics*. 5:479-510.

Jin, B., Li, Y., Robertson, K. D. (2011). DNA Methylation: Superior or Subordinate in the Epigenetic Hierarchy? *Genes & Cancer,* 2:607-617. https://doi.org/ 10.1177/1947601910393957.

Kamińska, K., Nalejska, E., Kubiak, M., Wojtysiak, J., Żołna, L., Kowalewski, J., Lewandowska, M. A. (2019). Prognostic and Predictive Epigenetic Biomarkers in Oncology. *Molecular Diagnosis & Therapy*, 23:83–95. https://doi.org/ 10.1007/s40291-018-0371-7.

Kumar, S., Chinnusamy, V., Mohapatra, T. (2018). Epigenetics of Modified DNA Bases: 5 Methylcytosine and Beyond. *Frontiers in Genetics*, 9:640. https://doi.org/10.3389/fgene.2018.00640.

Liao, Y., & Xu, K. (2019). Epigenetic regulation of prostate cancer: the theories and the clinical implications. *Asian Journal of Andrology,* 21:279-290. https://doi.org/10.4103/aja.aja_53_18.

Michalak, E. M., Burr, M. L., Bannister, A. J., Dawson, M. A. (2019). The roles of DNA, RNA and histone methylation in ageing and cancer. *Nature Reviews Molecular Cell Biology,* 20, 573–589. https://doi.org/ 10.1038/s41580-019-0143-1.

Schoofs, T., Müller-Tidow, C. (2011). DNA methylation as a pathogenic event and as a therapeutic target in AML. *Cancer Treatment Reviews*, 37:13-18.

Sharma, S., Kelly, T. K., Jones, P. T. (2010). Epigenetics in cancer. *Carcinogenesis*, 31:27–36. https://doi.org/ 10.1093/carcin/bgp220.

Spencer, H. G. (2016). Epigenetic Inheritance. *Encyclopedia of Evolutionary Biology,* 2:1-5. https://doi.org/ 10.1016/B978-0-12-800049-6.00050-0.

Vaughan, R. M., Kupai, A., Rothbart, S. B. (2021). Chromatin Regulation through Ubiquitin and Ubiquitin-like Histone Modifications. *Trends in Biochemical Sciences*. 46:258-269. https://doi.org/10.1016/j.tibs.2020.11.005.

Wu, Q & Ni, X. (2015). ROS-Mediated DNA Methylation Pattern Alterations in Carcinogenesis. *Current Drug Targets*. 16, 13-19.

Yang, Q., Jiang, W., Hou, P. (2019). Emerging role of PI3K/AKT in tumor-related epigenetic regulation. *Seminars in Cancer Biology*. 59:112-124. https://doi.org/10.1016/j.semcancer.2019.04.001.

Yun, M., Wu, J., Workman, J. L., Li, B. (2011). Readers of histone modifications. *Cell Research*. 21:564-578. https://doi.org/ 10.1038/cr.2011.42.

Zhang, M. W., Fujiwara, K., Che, X., Zheng, S., Zheng, L. (2017). DNA methylation in the tumor microenvironment. *Journal of Zhejiang University Science B*. 18:365-372. https://doi.org/10.1631/jzus.B1600579.

Zhang, T., Cooper, S., Brockdorff, N. (2015). The interplay of histone modifications - writers that read. *EMBO Reports*. 16: 1467–1481. https://doi.org/10.15252/embr.201540945.

Ziech, D., Franco, R., Pappa, A., Malamou-Mitsi, V., Georgakila, S., Georgakilas, A. G., Panayiotidis, M. I. (2010). The role of epigenetics in environmental and occupational carcinogenesis. *Chemico-Biological Interactions*. 188:340-9. https://doi.org/10.1016/j.cbi.2010.06.012.

Chapter 4

Epigenetic Effects of MicroRNAs in Oncogenesis

Muhammed Recai Akdoğan[1,*], MD and Necip Nas[2], MD

[1]Department of Internal Medicine, Ataturk University, Erzurum, Turkey
[2]Department of Internal Medicine, Private Siirt Hayat Hospital, Siirt, Turkey

Abstract

Epigenetics refers to changes that do not affect the DNA sequence but can affect gene expression. Healthy cells transform into malignant cells through some complex mechanisms. The simultaneous evaluation of tumor suppressor genes and oncogenesis with epigenetics makes it easier for us to understand this complex process. Among epigenetic mechanisms, there are two mechanisms that directly control gene expression, which are DNA methylation and histone modification. DNA methylation is involved in cellular control, while histone modifications have functions in transcriptional activity and modifications at the chromatin structure level. It has been determined that epigenetic mechanisms such as DNA methylation and histone modifications also regulate the expression of miRNAs. miRNAs are non-coding RNA molecules composed of twenty-two nucleotide sequences that are short and involved in the development of both physiological and important diseases such as malignancies. Tumor-associated abnormalities in miRNA or epigenetic mechanisms are commonly found in human cancers. Abnormal proliferation, apoptosis, and genetics are involved in the development of malignant cells. miRNAs are considered to be actively involved in the regulation of these processes. Available data reveal that miRNAs, which can be used as biomarkers, are biomarkers that can be used in early diagnosis, tumor subtyping, early treatment, prognosis prediction, and treatment resistance. Thus, it is considered that they can increase the disease-free lifetime and quality of life of cancer patients. In this paper, it was attempted to describe the relationship between dysregulated miRNA and epigenetic mechanisms in cancer.

Keywords: cancer, epigenetic, miRNA

Introduction

Cancer is the disease that causes the most deaths after heart diseases around the world. According to the data for 2018, 18 million cancer cases, including 36 types of cancer, were

* Corresponding Author's E-mail: mrakdogan2163@gmail.com.

In: Epigenetics: Beyond the Genetics and Medicine
Editors: Sevgi Durna Daştan and Nazan Yurtcu
ISBN: 979-8-88697-228-3

diagnosed in 185 countries around the world, and 9.5 million deaths were recorded. Studies on cancer are highly important when these data are taken into account. It will be inspiring to find out how cancer occurs and develops in the evolutionary process and how cancer mechanisms work in the treatment of cancer. Along with functional changes in oncogenes or tumor suppressor genes in the occurrence of cancer, the existence of epigenetic mechanisms causes cancer to become a complex disease. Epigenetics refers to changes that do not affect the DNA sequence but can affect gene expression (Bird, 2007). Epigenetic mechanisms are classified into two as those that directly control gene expression (DNA methylation and histone modification) and those that indirectly control gene expression (RNA interference). It is uncertain which of the above-mentioned mechanisms will affect which type of cancer cells, and each mechanism is considered to have a significant role in the development of cancer.

In the case of oncogenesis, gene expression may be affected by changes in the nucleotide and DNA levels. It is considered that especially RNA interference, DNA methylation, and the modification of histone proteins lead to the transformation of cells into malignant cells.

DNA Methylation

The genes that allow DNA methylation are normally involved in the expression of tissue-specific genes and inactivation of the x-chromosome in healthy individuals (Csankovszki et al., 2001). DNA methylation is possible through the DNA methyltransferase enzyme, which is found at the cytosine base in the CpG dinucleotide. Abnormal DNA methylation is the most common epigenetic mechanism in patients with cancer. Abnormal DNA methylation also causes tumor suppressor genes to be silenced (Bird, 2002). Three enzymes that allow DNA methylation are available. Among them, the DNA methyltransferase 1 enzyme ensures the continuation of methylation. The DNA methyltransferase 1 enzyme performs the methylation function by adding methyl groups to CpG regions.

Histone Modifications

In histone modification, one of the mechanisms that directly control gene expression among epigenetic mechanisms, the main mechanism is modifications at the chromosome level. Two important enzymes are involved in histone modifications, which are acetyltransferase and methyltransferase. It is considered that they are responsible for acetylation and methylation, respectively (Klose et al., 2006).

RNA Interference (RNAi)

They are non-coding RNA molecules that indirectly express genes among epigenetic mechanisms. miRNA (microRNA) has transcriptional and post-translational silencing functions in the RNA interference group (Jiang et al., 2004). In the present studies, the expression of protein-coding genes is regulated by DNA methylation and histone modifications, which are capable of direct gene expression among epigenetic mechanisms, and it is also considered that miRNA can regulate gene expression. miRNAs cannot directly encode proteins; however, they are subjected to similar processes with epigenetic mechanisms that can directly encode proteins (Malumbres, 2013).

MicroRNA

miRNAs are non-coding RNA molecules composed of twenty-two nucleotide sequences that are short and involved in the development of both physiological and important diseases such as malignancies. miRNAs lead to translational repression by binding to mRNA in the target gene. Furthermore, they can also post-transcriptionally regulate gene expression (Siomi et al., 2010). RNA polymerase II and III occur as a result of the transcriptional function of miRNAs. Drosha is an RNAse enzyme complex located in the nucleus. This enzyme complex is transformed into pre-miRNA by DGCR8/Pasha. Pre-miRNA enters the cytoplasm with the exportin-5 protein, and the maturation process starts. Two miRNA strands become independent of each other during this process. One of these independent strands connects with the Argonaut 2 (AGO2) protein located in the RISC (RNA-induced silencing complex) complex. This connection acts as a guide to suppress target mRNAs (Niwa et al., 2007).

MicroRNAs and Cancer

Normal cells can be transformed into malignant cells when they proliferate undesirably and lose their cell death function. Abnormal proliferation, apoptosis, and genetics are involved in the development of malignant cells. It is considered that miRNAs are actively involved in the regulation of these processes. The 3'UTR region is located on protein-coding genes. Nearly more than half of the genes in this region have conserved miRNA binding sites. It can be controlled by target miRNAs due to this conserved site. Based on the available information, despite the lack of comprehensive data on known miRNAs, information can be obtained on the examination of miRNA gene expression, regulatory functions of miRNAs, and their roles. Studies have demonstrated that miRNA expression differs between healthy individuals and malignant cells, which supports the ideas that miRNA may affect the occurrence and spread of cancer cells. Despite the limited knowledge about miRNA, it has been concluded that miRNA expression is associated with the diagnosis, spread, and prognosis of cancer, and drug resistance. Calin et al., first determined in 2002 that miR-15a and miR-16-1 were deleted in the majority of their region and downregulated at a significant rate in patients with chronic lymphocytic leukemia. miRNAs were separated into two groups as tumor suppressor and oncogenic miRNAs after this determination. There was an increase in miRNA studies on cancer-associated gene regions in later periods. Oncogenic miRNAs are generally upregulated; however, tumor suppressor miRNAs are generally down-regulated. Thus, the overexpression of tumor suppressor miRNAs and the inhibition of oncogenic miRNAs are important for the development of targeted treatments, in which miRNAs are critical in cancer treatment. Different rates of miRNA expression were found when cells from healthy individuals and malignant cells were compared. These modified and differentially expressed miRNAs are also encountered in the most common types of breast, colon, lung, head and neck, and brain cancers.

Available data reveal that miRNAs, which can be used as biomarkers, are biomarkers that can be used in early diagnosis, tumor subtyping, early treatment, prognosis prediction, and treatment resistance. Thus, it is considered that they can increase the disease-free lifetime and quality of life of patients with cancer.

miRNAs and Epigenetics

Epigenetic miRNAs that are defined as miRNAs aimed at regulating polycomb repressive complexes with the DNA methyltransferase enzyme, which is involved in methylation, and histone deacetylase, which is involved in histone modification, have their own specific functions. The expression of these epi-miRNAs may lead to significant consequences in the epigenetic regulation of many cellular pathways and processes. miRNAs epigenetically control gene expression indirectly. However, the accumulation of promoter-specific protein complexes that control the expression of genomic DNA suggests that miRNAs may also have functions that directly regulate gene expression. Therefore, epigenetic pathways and miRNA are formed in a complex regulatory cycle. In case of any disturbance in this cycle, it leads to the occurrence of some important diseases such as malignancies (Malumbres, 2013). According to the obtained data, it has been reported that many miRNAs are regulated by epigenetic mechanisms, and they are specifically methylated to the most common cancers in these mechanisms (Kunej et al., 2011). miRNAs can be deregulated due to the abnormal expression of histone deacetylase, which is involved in histone modification, and polycomb repressive complexes. Polycomb-group proteins are transcriptional repressors that control lineage selection during differentiation and development. Two polycomb repressive complexes (PRCs), including PRC1 and PRC2, are available. PRC1 is formed by Ring Cbx, Bmi-1, Me118, and Mph units, and PRC2 consists of Suz12, Eed, and Ezh2 subunits (Richly et al., 2011).

miRNAs Regulated by Epigenetic Mechanisms and Their Expression and the Associated Cancers

miR-9

Through extracellular studies, it has been revealed that the exposure of miR-9 synthesized from CpG islands to xenoestrogen may affect abnormal epigenetic formations (Hsu et al., 2009), which suggests that it is possible to use epigenetic silencing of the mir-9 gene region in the early diagnosis of breast cancer. Mir-9 affects the development of many cancer cells via nuclear factor-kappa B (Guo et al., 2009). The hypermethylation of the miR-9 locus was found in various malignant tissues, including head and neck, lung, colon, melanoma, acute leukemia, and breast cancer (Bandres et al., 2009). The release of miR-9 is increased in patients diagnosed with non-small cell cancer. Erlotinib used in treatment reduces the expression of miR-9 (Chen et al., 2015).

miR-34 (A and B/C)

The targeted mechanism of action of miR-34 in malignant cells epigenetically occurs via p53. It is effective in the regulation of p53. MiR-34 has 3 subtypes, such as a/b/c. The first is monocistronic, and the other two are polycistronic (Lodygin et al., 2008). miR-34 has been reported to be dysregulated in various human cancers and is considered a tumor suppressor microRNA due to its synergistic effect with the well-known tumor suppressor p53. Mature miR-34 targets various genes that are associated with the spread of cancer, such as E2F3, MYC, and MET. The epigenetic mechanism of action of miR-34 a/b/c is to stop the cell cycle, and it exerts this effect by silencing the target genes it will affect. Another mechanism of action is to inhibit cell proliferation and abnormal cell spread, by inducing apoptosis (Sato et al., 2011). The loss of miR-34 expression has been associated with resistance to apoptosis caused by p53-activating agents used in chemotherapy (Hermeking, 2010).

miR-124

MiR-124, with a key role in neurological diseases and neurogenesis, is regarded to be a miRNA with the highest number in the human brain (Cao et al., 2007). The miR-124 gene locus has 3 types. Mir-124 is mostly found in brain cells and is epigenetically silent in brain tumors. Moreover, it has also been found epigenetically in colon (75%), lung (48%), breast (32-50%), lymph cancer (42%), and leukemia (36%) cancer types (Sun et al., 2012). miR-124, miR-137, and miR-340 were found to be associated with the poor prognosis of colorectal cancer (Zhu et al., 2013).

miR-137

The ectopic expression of miR-137 leads to downregulation by targeting Cdc42, CDK6. Mir-137 epigenetically arrests the cell cycle at the G1 point. It induces apoptosis, which is a cell death mechanism. Mir-137 exerts this effect through overexpression (Lujambio et al., 2008).

miR-148

It has been observed to be associated with malignant metastases (Imoto et al., 2000). MiR-148 targets the induced transcription factor 2. miR-148 is overexpressed in ovarian cancer. It is considered that the silencing of miR-148 epigenetically increases the induced transcription factor 2 (Calin et al., 2000).

Let-7a-3

The Let-7 gene locus is a miRNA with many subtypes. In this group, while Let-7a-3 functions as miRNA with oncogenic function, other subtypes of the group function as tumor suppressor miRNA (Calin et al., 2000). Unlike other subtypes, the Let-7a-3 gene locus with an oncogenic function is hypomethylated in lung and colon cancers (Brueckner et al., 2007). The data indicating that let-7 miRNA is effective in the pathogenesis of lung cancer are increasingly more observed. In their study, Takamizawa et al., found that the level of Let-7 significantly decreased in patients with cancer, regardless of the stage of cancer and whether the tumor became metastatic. It was found that Let-7 reduced cell proliferation, especially in cell lines with adenocarcinoma (Takamizawa et al., 2004).

Epi-miRNA

Epi-miRNA is defined as miRNAs aimed at regulating polycomb repressive complexes with the DNA methyltransferase enzyme, which is involved in methylation, and histone deacetylase, which is involved in histone modification. The first identified epi-miRNA was miR-29. MiR-29 targets DNA methyltransferase 3A-3B in lung cancer cells. Some effector epi-miRNAs that regulate the epigenetic mechanism are presented in the Table 1.

Table 1. Effector epi-miRNAs that regulate the epigenetic mechanism

miRNA	Target	Cancer or tissue
miR-29a/b/c	DNMT3a, DNMT3b, DNMT1, YY1	Lung, AML
miR-101	Ezh2	Prostate, bladder
miR-128	Bmi1	Glioma, pancreatic and colorectal cancer
miR-148a/b	DNMT3b, DNMT1	Cervical
miR-152	DNMT1	Endometrial, liver
miR-185	DNMT1	Glioma
miR-200a,b	Suz12, Sirt1, HDAC4	Liver tumors
miR-203	Bmi1	Pancreatic and colorectal cancer cells
miR-214	Ezh2	Skeletal muscle and embryonic stem cells
miR-449a	HDAC1	Prostatic

Conclusion

In conclusion, epigenetics is extremely important for understanding oncogenesis and developing new treatment plans. It has an important position in determining new strategies for prevention, diagnosis, and treatment. Healthy cells transform into malignant cells through some complex mechanisms. The simultaneous evaluation of tumor suppressor genes and oncogenesis with epigenetics makes it easier for us to understand this complex process. Epigenetic modifications that directly control gene expression (DNA methylation and histone modification) and indirectly control gene expression (miRNA) and treatment approaches are the most important treatment targets. The knowledge of epigenetic changes before the transformation of healthy cells into malignant cells in advance can provide early diagnosis, development of new treatment modalities, and even early cancer prevention.

References

Bandres, E., Agirre, X., Bitarte, N., Ramirez, N., Zarate, R., Roman-Gomez, J., Prosper, F., & Garcia-Foncillas, J. (2009). Epigenetic regulation of microRNA expression in colorectal cancer. *Int. J. Cancer, 125*(11), 2737–2743. https://doi.org/10.1002/ijc.24638.

Bird, A. (2002). DNA methylation patterns and epigenetic memory. *Genes & Development, 16*(1), 6–21. https://doi.org/10.1101/gad.947102.

Bird, A. (2007). Perceptions of epigenetics. *Nature, 447*(7143), 396–398. https://doi.org/10.1038/nature05913.

Brueckner, B., Stresemann, C., Kuner, R., Mund, C., Musch, T., Meister, M., Sultmann, H., & Lyko F. (2007). The human let-7a-3 locus contains an epigenetically regulated. *Cancer Res.*, 15, *67*(4), 1419-1423. https://doi.org/10.1158/0008-5472.CAN-06-4074.

Calin, G. A., Dumitru, C. D., Shimizu, M., Bichi, R., Zupo, S., Noch, E., Aldler, H., Rattan, S., Keating, M., Rai, K., Rassenti, L., Kipps, T., Negrini, M., Bullrich, F., & Croce, C. (2002). Frequent deletions and down-regulation of micro- RNA genes miR15 and miR16 at 13q14 in chronic lymphocytic leukemia. *Proc Natl. Acad. Sci. U.S.A., 99*(24), 15524-15529. https://doi.org/10.1073/pnas.242606799.

Calin, G. A., Ferracin, M., Cimmino, A., Leva, G., Shimizu, M., Wojcik, S., Iorio, M., Visone, R., Ilfer-Sever, N., Fabbri, M., Iuliano, R., Palumbo, T., Pichiorri, F., Roldo, C., Garzon, R., Sevignani, C., Rassenti, L., Alder, H., Volinia, S.,... & Croce, C. (2005). A microRNA signature associated with prognosis and progression in chronic lymphocytic leukemia. *N. Engl. J. Med., 353*(17), 1793-1801. https://doi.org/10.1056/NEJMoa050995.

Calin, G. A., Sevignani, C., Dumitru, C. D., Hyslop, T., Noch, E., Yendamuri, S., Shimizu, M., Rattan, S., Bullrich, F., Negrini, M., & Croce, C. (2000). Human microRNA genes are frequently located at fragile sites and genomic regions involved in cancers. *Proc. Natl. Acad. Sci. U.S.A., 101*(9), 2999–3004. https://doi.org/10.1073/pnas.0307323101.

Cao, X., Pfaff, S. L., & Gage, F. H. (2007). A functional study of miR-124 in the developing neural tube. *Genes & Development, 21*(5), 531–536. https://doi.org/10.1101/gad.1519207.

Chang, T. C., Yu, D., Lee, Y. S., Wentzel, E., Arking, D., West, K., Dang, C., Thomas-Tikhonenko, A., & Mendell, J. (2008). Widespread microRNA repression by Myc contributes to tumorigenesis. *Nat Genet, 40*(1), 43-50. https://doi.org/10.1038/ng.2007.30.

Chen, X., Zhu, L., Ma, Z., Sun, G., Luo, X., Li, M., Zhai, S., Li, P., & Wang, X. (2015). Oncogenic miR-9 is a target of erlotinib in NSCLCs. *Scientific Reports, 5,* 17031. https://doi.org/10.1038/srep17031.

Csankovszki, G., Nagy, A., & Jaenisch, R., (2001). Synergism of Xist RNA, DNA methylation, and histone hypoacetylation in maintaining X chromosome inactivation. *J. Cell Biol., 153*(4), 773–784. https://doi.org/10.1083/jcb.153.4.773.

Guo, L. M., Pu, Y., Han, Z., Liu, T., Li, Y.X., Liu, M., Li, X., & Tang, H. (2009). MicroRNA-9 inhibits ovarian cancer cell growth through regulation of NF-kappaB1. *FEBS J., 276*(19), 5537–5546. https://doi.org/10.1111/j.1742-4658.2009.07237.x.

Hermeking, H. J. C. D. (2010). The miR-34 family in cancer and apoptosis. *Cell Death & Differentiation, 17*(2), 193-199. https://doi.org/10.1038/cdd.2009.56.

Hsu, P. Y., Deatherage, D. E., Rodriguez, B. A., Liyanarachchi, S., Weng, Y. I., Zuo, T., Liu, J., Cheng, A. S., & Huang, T. H. (2009). Xenoestrogen-induced epigenetic repression of microRNA-9-3 in breast epithelial cells. *Cancer Res., 69*, 5936– 5945.

Imoto, I., Pimkhaokham, A., Watanabe, T., Saito-Ohara, F., Soeda, E., & Inazawa, J. (2000). Amplification and overexpression of TGIF2, a novel homeobox gene of the TALE superclass, in ovarian cancer cell lines. *Biochem Biophys Res. Commun., 276*(1), 264–270. https://doi.org/10.1006/bbrc.2000.3449.

Jiang, Y., Bressler, J., & Beaudet, L. A. (2004). Epigenetics and human disease. *Annu. Rev. Genomics Hum. Genet., 5*, 479-510. https://doi.org/10.1146/annurev.genom.5.061903.180014.

Klose, R.J., & Bird, A.P. (2006). Genomic DNA methylation: the mark and its mediators. *Trends Biochem. Sci., 31*(2), 89– 97. https://doi.org/10.1016/j.tibs.2005.12.008.

Kunej, T., Godnic, I., Ferdin, J., Horvat, S., Dovc, P., & Calin, G.A. (2011). Epigenetic regulation of microRNAs in cancer: an integrated review of literature. *Mutat. Res., 717* (1–2), 77–84. https://doi.org/10.1016/j.mrfmmm.2011.03.008.

Lodygin, D., Tarasov, V., Epanchintsev, A., Berking, C., Knyazeva, T., Korner, H., Knyazev, P., Diebold, J., & Hermeking, H. (2008). Inactivation of miR-34a by aberrant CpG methylation in multiple types of cancer. *Cell Cycle, 7*(16), 2591–2600. https://doi.org/10.4161/cc.7.16.6533.

Lu, J., Getz, G., Miska, E. A., Alvarez-Saavedra, E., Lamb, J., Peck, D., Sweet-Cordero, A., Ebert, B.L., Mak, R.H., Ferrando, A.A., Downing, J.R., Jacks, T., Horvitz, H.R., & Golub, T.R. (2005). MicroRNA expression profiles classify human cancers. *Nature, 435*(7043), 834-838. https://doi.org/10.1038/nature 03702.

Lujambio, A., Calin, G. A., Villanueva, A., Ropero, S., Sanchez-Cespedes, M., Blanco, D., Montuenga, L. M., Rossi, S., Nicoloso, M. S., Faller, W. J., Gallagher, W. M., Eccles, S. A., Croce, C. M., & Esteller, M. (2008). A microRNA DNA methylation signature for human cancer metastasis. *Proc. Natl. Acad. Sci. U.S.A., 105*(36), 13556–13561. https://doi.org/10.1073/pnas.0803055105.

Malumbres, M. (2013). miRNAs and cancer: An epigenetics view. *Molecular Aspects of Medicine, 34*(4), 863–874. https://doi.org/10.1016/j.mam.2012.06.005.

Nicoloso, M.S., Spizzo, R., Shimizu, M., Rossi, S., & Calin G. A. (2009). MicroRNAs—the micro steering wheel of tumour metastases. *Nat. Rev. Cancer, 9*(4), 293-302. https://doi.org/10.1038/nrc2619.

Niwa, R., & Slack, F. J. (2007). The evolution of animal microRNA function. Current Opinion in *Genetics & Development, 17*(2), 145-150. https://doi.org/10.1016/j.gde.2007.02.004.

Richly, H., Aloia, L., & Di Croce, L. (2011). Roles of the Polycomb group proteins in stem cells and cancer. *Cell Death Dis., 2*(9), e204. https://doi.org/10.1038/cddis.2011.84.

Sato, F., Tsuchiya, S., Meltzer, S.J., & Shimizu, K. (2011). MicroRNAs and epigenetics. *FEBS J., 278*(10), 1598- 1609. https://doi.org/10.1111/j.1742-4658.2011.08089.x.

Siomi, H., & Siomi, M.C. (2010). Posttranscriptional regulation of microRNA biogenesis in animals. *Mol. Cell, 38*(3), 323- 332. https://doi.org/10.1016/j.molcel.2010.03.013.

Sun, Y. A. N., Zhao, X., Zhou, Y., & Hu, Y. U. (2012). miR-124, miR-137 and miR-340 regulate colorectal cancer growth via inhibition of the Warburg effect. *Oncology reports, 28*(4), 1346-1352. https://doi.org/10.3892/or.2012.1958.

Takamizawa, J., Konishi, H., Yanagisawa, K., Tomida, S., Osada, H., Endoh, H., Harano, T., Yatabe, Y., Nagino, M., Nimura, Y., Mitsudomi, T., & Takahashi, T. (2004). Reduced expression of the let-7 microRNAs in human lung cancers in association with shortened postoperative survival. *Cancer Res., 64*(11), 3753-3756. https://doi.org/10.1158/0008-5472.CAN-04-0637.

Zhu, X., Li, Y., Shen, H., Li, H., Long, L., Hui, L., & Xu, W. (2013). miR-137 inhibits the proliferation of lung cancer cells by targeting Cdc42 and Cdk6. *FEBS Letters, 587*(1), 73-81. https://doi.org/10.1016/j.febslet.2012.11.004.

Chapter 5

The Concepts of Epigenomics and Cell Epigenomes

Taner Daştan[1], PhD and İnanç Baral[2,]*, PhD

[1]Department of Biochemistry, Faculty of Science,
Sivas Cumhuriyet University, Sivas, Turkey
[2]Department of Zootechnics and Animal Nutrition,
Faculty of Veterinary Medicine,
Sivas Cumhuriyet University, Sivas, Turkey

Abstract

Genetics cannot solely explain genetic variations in humans and disease developments. We see varying differences in phenotypes and disease susceptibility in organisms that have the same genetic make-up, e.g., monozygotic twins and cloned animals. The information carried by the genomic sequence is the blueprint, but the final product requires environmental determinants. Here comes the concept of epigenetics, as it is the framework where biochemical interactions between the genome and the environment blend. We can describe epigenetics as mechanisms that are beyond genetics, as such mechanisms alter the result of the genomic blueprint without altering the information itself, i.e., the sequence. Both epigenetics and epigenomics are trending research fields to better evaluate the genotype and the phenotype. The methylation of genetic material is a well-studied and well-known epigenetic marker. The epigenome, as a term, describes the inheritable changes in both the DNA and histone molecular structures, where the methylation and acetylation mechanisms are studied extensively. As the building blocks of the chromatin structure, nucleosomes depend on epigenetic changes, which lead to becoming either tight or loose, based on the particular mechanisms. Chromatin structure changes directly affect the gene expression, e.g., particular gene expression becomes silenced if the gene position has DNA hypermethylation and histone hypoacetylation that leads to the condensed form of the chromatin. Inversely, if the said changes were removed, genes in that position would express themselves again. Therefore, epigenetics provides a vigorous and remarkably malleable means for gene expression regulations. Epigenomics includes both the epigenetic mechanisms on the DNA and histones and complicated interactions between the genotype and the phenotype. There are well-known epigenomic changes in DNA, RNA, and protein levels. DNA base changes in somatic cells and chromosome positioning are among the aspects determining the epigenomic scene. Alternative splicing mechanism, RNA processing (editing, capping, Poly-A tailing, etc.), RNA methylation, and regulations conferred by the non-coding RNAs (ncRNAs) are RNA level epigenomic changes. Epigenomic changes at the protein level include various mechanisms of the post-translational modification. Epigenomics research includes total hypomethylation profile of the genome, identification of hypermethylated genes, microRNA-driven gene silencing

* Corresponding Author's E-mail: ibaral@cumhuriyet.edu.tr.

In: Epigenetics: Beyond the Genetics and Medicine
Editors: Sevgi Durna Daştan and Nazan Yurtcu
ISBN: 979-8-88697-228-3

with DNA methylation, epigenome projects, and DNA-based clinical therapies for different biomedical conditions. This chapter will detail fundamental concepts and basic approaches to both epigenomics and epigenomes.

Keywords: DNA modifications, epigenetics, epigenome, epigenomics, epigenotype, RNA regulations

Abbreviations

HPLC:	High-performance Liquid Chromatography
HPCE:	High-performance Capillary Electrophoresis
LUMA:	Luminometric Methylation Assay
MAPKs:	Mitogen-activated protein kinases
PI3K:	Phosphatidylinositide- 3-kinase
AKT:	Protein kinase B isozymes
PLK1:	Polo-like kinase 1
PARP:	Poly (ADP-ribose) polymerase
HATs:	P300/CBP CREB binding protein coactivators.

Introduction

A terminology overview would be beneficial for a better understanding of the concept of epigenomics by providing the conceptual similarities and differences. Epigenetics as a whole encompasses all the mechanisms that result in inheritable changes without sequence alterations. These mechanisms are responsible for the creation of different cell lines at the stage of developmental differentiation, of which X-chromosome inactivation (Barr body) and genomic imprinting in mammalian organisms are particularly pronounced in disease developments. The epigenetic code denotes the scheme of genomic methylation and histone modifications related with the expression regulation. The epigenetic code combines with the genetic code to provide an effective modulation of gene expression patterns. Epigenetic inheritance describes the heritable patterns of the somatic cell lines and epigenetic information transmitted through the germ-line cells. Epigenetic marks indicate region-specific DNA and histone modifications that are inheritable and able to regulate the expression of localized genes (Meissner and Walter, 2015). Epigenetic reprogramming describes the returning of epigenetic marks into a neutral state, which would then lead to transitioning into another cell line or developmental stage, e.g., reverting into the ground state of primordial germ-line cells. Such reprogramming course is also seen in the nuclear transfer of somatic cells. Global epigenetic status represents the epigenome, which is different in each developing cell line during the embryonic development phase. Epigenome maps are virtual representations of the chromosomes that reveal DNA methylation and other modifications seen in the chromatin structure. The Epigenotype describes the entire epigenetic marks found in a specific cell line or during a specific developmental phase. Epimutations indicate deviations from normally expected epigenetic marks in a given region that would alter gene expression (Meissner and Walter, 2015).

Epigenetics research currently focuses on the following methodologies for revealing changes in gene expression profiles or chromatin restructuring; DNA methylation patterns, histone modifications, nuclear positioning, ncRNA-driven regulations, and microRNA regulations (Chen and Rajewsky, 2007; Fraser and Bickmore, 2007; Martin-Subero and Siebert, 2009; Esteller, 2009; Qui, 2006). On the other hand, if the research efforts are for revealing epigenetic marks in a specific sequence, then epigenomics would indicate the separation of possible modifications from the rest of the genome (Callinan and Feinberg, 2006; Fazzari and Greally, 2004; Pennisi, 2005; Martin-Subero and Siebert, 2009). Various research point to the susceptibility of the epigenome to environmental determinants that would make it more prone to change than the robust genome, such as nutritional factors (e.g., royal jelly, folic acid, etc.), chemical pollutants, external stimulation of neurons, and psychiatric conditions such as stress (Martin-Subero and Siebert, 2009; Esteller, 2009). Initial studies on cancer revealed that DNA methylation changes gradually throughout the lifespan; however, recent studies suggest different results by showing the alterability of the DNA methylation during the first week following the birthing in mice and sustained DNA methylation patterns in brain tissue associated with aberrant behaviors (Sato et al., 2003; Callinan and Feinberg, 2006). Research revealed that epigenetic changes formed by fetal malnutrition in rats lead to disease developments in the adult stage (Fazzari and Greally, 2004; Qui, 2006; Weaver et al., 2004). Epigenomic changes are present in humans, as revealed by comparative epigenomics conducted in monozygotic twins (Pennisi, 2005; Esteller, 2007; Martin-Subero and Siebert, 2009; Suzuki et al., 2013). The reversible nature of epigenetic mechanisms makes them a verifiable alternative to genomic imprinting, where the maternal epigenetic marks in a given imprinted gene are shown to return to paternal epigenetic marks in the progeny (Weaver et al., 2009; Fraga and Esteller, 2002; Laird, 2003; VanSteensel and Henikoff, 2003; Lillycrop et al., 2005; 2008; Fraga et al., 2005). This reversible nature of epigenetic changes is also apparent in genes in neural tissue that can be induced by medications for mental conditions, which reverts epigenetic marks into neutral states (Kubato et al., 2014, Payne, 2014; Tsankova et al. 2006; Jessberger et al., 2007; Dong et al., 2008; 2010; Wang et al., 2011). Possible restoration of methylation patterns in autism-related genomic positions by folic acid administration in autistic children is postulated (James et al., 2004; Moretti et al., 2005). Recent advances increasingly point to the possibility of genomic site-specific epigenetic drugs, which is seen in contemporary compounds such as pyrrole-imidazole polyamide (Kubato et al., 2014, Payne, 2014; Ohtsuki et al., 2009; Matsuda et al., 2011). The rise of the epigenetics stoutly contests the agreed-upon idea that the acquired nature cannot be inherited by the progeny, which is further supported by the epigenetic changes formed due to the psychiatric conditions passed into the progeny as far as the third generation via spermatogenesis (Hackett et al., 2013; Franklin et al., 2010; Sato et al., 2003). While still a postulation for humans, it is possible to restore deviations in epigenetic marks by external interventions by drugs, nutritional supplements, and environmental conditioning (Kubato et al., 2014, Payne, 2014).

It is now established that nutritional factors and environmental determinants have effects on epigenetic changes, which are most pronounced in smoking, where alterations induced by smoking are reported to have potential for malignancies that can be alleviated by dietary and lifestyle improvements. Advances in molecular methodologies enable the discovery of anticancer traits of the wide array of natural compounds (Spencer et al., 2004; Orlikova and Diederich, 2012; Stepanic et al., 2014), which mostly revealed that such traits function through chromatin remodeling to protect the integrity of the cellular epigenome (Reuter et al., 2011).

Among these compounds, polyphenols induce chromatin remodeling by affecting the gene expression of chromatin remodeling enzymes (Suzuki and Miyata, 2011). Polyphenols are potently modifying cellular processes related to survival and death by targeting numerous kinases, which are listed as MAPKs, PI3K, AKT, Aurora B, PLK1, PARP, and some epigenome modifying enzymes like HATs. Along with their diverse effects in various bio-signaling pathways, it can be suggested that polyphenols are significant representatives of what are called polypharmacological substances (Stepanic et al., 2014).

Novel findings and significant signs of progress in epigenetics research are directly related to advances in molecular methodologies, and recent years provided the characterization efforts for the epigenome by different methodologies (Fazzari and Greally, 2004; Callinan and Feinberg, 2006; Esteller, 2007; Fraga and Esteller, 2002; Laird, 2003; Martin-Subero and Siebert, 2009; Esteller, 2009). With the utilization of microarrays in epigenetics, an increasing number of studies are directed towards epigenome characterization both in normal and aberrant conditions (Martin-Subero and Siebert, 2009). In the current study, the DNA methylation data from The Cancer Genome Atlas (TCGA) Project (Zhang and Zhang, 2022), especially the 450K array data from different cancer types (Sandoval et al., 2011), were analyzed and highly informative CpG sites located in more than 150 centrosomal genes were presented. This study is one of those that helps scientists understand the epigenetic- epigenomics mechanism underlying cancers for utilizing these epigenetic modifications as novel cancer biomarkers (Zhang and Zhang, 2022).

Epigenome Characterization

Genome regulation is being better understood by the researchers with the successful utilization of epigenomic methodology in whole genomes, which invariably leads to the discovery of disease-related patterns by revealing normal patterns (Esteller, 2009; Martin-Subero and Siebert, 2009). Recently, DNA methylation patterns revealed in different healthy tissues have been investigated by sequence analysis, conservation, and effects on gene expression for correlation. Human Epigenome Project revealed two-way modes of distribution for DNA methylation in more than 2500 genes that were sequenced by bisulfite sequencing in amplicons from example human tissues (Martin-Subero and Siebert, 2009). Overall, they surfaced that 5'UTR regions with a high amount of CpG islands are unmethylated, whereas 5'UTR regions with a lower amount of CpG islands are mostly methylated, which is supported by other research (Weber et al., 2007; Smiraglia et al., 2001; Martin-Subero and Siebert, 2009). Microarray analysis on peripheral human blood revealed that approximately 4% of CpG islands located on promoters are methylated (Shen et al., 2007; Martin-Subero and Siebert, 2009). Of the limited set of genes investigated, DNA methylation patterns did not provide significant differences between gender and age groups. A striking study, which utilized chromatin immunoprecipitation on chips (ChIP-on-Chip), comparatively investigated DNA methylation patterns in promoter regions that have low, intermediate, and high density of CpG islands by correlating with the gene expression, which revealed high DNA methylation in promoter regions with a lower density of CpG islands and unmethylation in promoter regions that have a high amount of CpG islands (Weber et al., 2007; Martin-Subero and Siebert, 2009). In terms of RNA Polymerase recruitment by the promoters, researchers revealed that a high density of CpG islands in promoters (66% of the studied promoter regions) enhanced the recruitment activity, whereas a low density of CpG islands in promoters (11% of the studied promoter regions) have redundant recruitment activity. By this account, the relationship related to methylation and expression compared between promoters with a higher and an intermediate density of CpG islands revealed a negative correlation. Of particular note is the finding of no correlation between methylation and expression in promoters having lower CpG island densities. Summarily, it is evident that methylation is in close association with the expression suppression in promoters having no significant amount of CpG island presence (Blelloch et al., 2007). Investigation of stem and differentiated cells by using CpG-specific bead array analysis revealed significant data in methylation models between embryonic stem cells and differentiated cells in 23 genes, which provided 25 discernible sets of CpG islands (Bibikova et al., 2006; Martin-Subero and Siebert, 2009).

The ChIP-on-Chip methodology also enables the genome-wide detection and characterization of histone protein modifications (Bernstein et al., 2004; Huebert et al., 2006). Various research utilizing the ChIP-on-Chip method revealed fine aspects of the so-called histone code by discovering the patterns and combinations of histone modifications associated with a given transcriptional phase or a structural stage of chromatins (Jenuwein and Allis, 2001). Certain research efforts also revealed the structural characterization of chromatin in cell lines (Bernstein et al., 2006; Bracken et al., 2006; Lee et al., 2006; Martin-Subero and Siebert, 2009). The highly conserved nature of epigenetic marks of histone proteins, even in modest amounts in orthologous genomic regions, spanning a diverse array of species strongly suggests their universality in transcriptional regulation (Bernstein et al., 2005). From this on, comparative epigenomics would be a feasible approach to reveal regulatory factors that are not included in the conserved genomic regions. The ability of the ChIP-on-Chip method to expose histone modification differences in genomic regions, especially the transcriptional start sites (TSSs), has driven the attention of researchers to the embryonic stem cells, since these cells can be changed into any of the differentiated tissues of the organism, thus forming the cell line identity (Buszczak and Spradling, 2006). As of late, Polycomb Group (PcG) proteins are in attention due to their maintenance roles in stem cell pluripotency by their ability to suppress genes responsible for cell-line differentiation (Martin-Subero and Siebert, 2009).

Derangements of the epigenetic mechanisms, mostly more than one aberration, are best attributed to cancerous cells, which are also markers for their characterization and include DNA methylation, histone modifications, and nucleosome restructuring (Esteller, 2007; Jones and Baylin, 2007; Laird, 2005). Until now, DNA methylation, especially on tumor suppressor genes, is among the most extensively studied mechanism in cancer types (Esteller, 2007), which revealed 50+ genes silenced in cancerous differentiation and differences in methylation patterns discernible in distinct cancer types. Advances in epigenomics gradually increase the precision of accessibility of cancer cell epigenomes, which are progressing to the next generation of biomarkers for cancerous cell lines. Additionally, researchers are now able to better evaluate carcinogenesis by comparing DNA methylation patterns at the genome, development, and transcriptional levels. Having the most diverse set of cell types, the hemopoietic system cancers include many distinct leukemias and lymphomas classified by morphology, immunohistochemistry, and genetics. Recently, researchers have focused on heterogeneous diseases like those seen in the hemopoietic system cancers to utilize microarray methodology to profile methylation patterns and to reveal possible epigenetic marks having diagnostic precision (Martin-Subero and Siebert, 2009).

The Profiling Whole Genome Methylation Models

Two general approaches are available for genome-wide profiling of methylation, (1) whole-genome scanning of global DNA methylation patterns; and (2) genome-wide sequence-specific methylation profiling by microarray analysis. The former can be done by conducting different instrumentation such as HPLC, HPCE, or LUMA, but they are all limited to DNA methylation (Laird, 2003; Martin-Subero and Siebert, 2009)]. The latter is a more powerful yet biased approach for profiling with the promise of discovering new marks but is biased due to its dependence on using methylation-specific enzymes to bind to CpG islands, which may not always include recognition sequences for enzyme binding. Consequently, it is limited in scope as to which CpG islands present in the possibly investigated genome. Recently, a quadruple-enzyme approach to effectively investigate 41% of total CpG islands in a given genome was published, which also recommends including unmethylated DNA fragments to better discern methylation differences between samples. Antibody elucidation of methylcytosine is a less biased alternative for identifying methylated DNA sequences but it is limited in its ability to be sequence-specific. Certain modification efforts are available for this approach to alleviate limitations, which include sodium bisulfite treatment to induce transition of unmethylated cytosines to uracils and leave methylcytosine intact. Consequently, there are already existing analysis approaches for SNPs where differential binding of oligonucleotides into methylated (C) and unmethylated (U/T) alleles can be utilized (Bibikova et al., 2006). Again, there are numerous microarray approaches for methylation profiling differing in their resolution, capacity, and sequence specificity. In addition to the aforementioned approaches, there are also epigenomic-based oligonucleotide assays that include promoter and CpG island assays, which are yielding high-density results. Recently, a combination of both genetic and epigenetic profiles is shown to be revealed through the use of SNP-ChIP coupled with methylation-specific endonucleases (Yuan et al., 2006). Lastly, high resolution of whole-genome coverage is made possible with the advent of oligonucleotide tiling arrays, which span several millions of oligonucleotides. As it can be seen, despite the development of newer microarray approaches, there is no consensus and universal integrity in the validation of obtained data from conducting any of the methods that are all different in their technical aspects, capabilities, precisions, and analysis complexity, which naturally suggest the need of developing a universal, flexible, and undisputable validation framework encompassing all approaches for epigenomic research (Martin-Subero and Siebert, 2009).

Analysis of the Genome-wide Histone Modification Patterns

ChIP is currently the standard methodology for revealing histone modifications in a given genomic region, which utilized specific antibodies for different modifications. This method summarily includes DNA cross-linking by formaldehyde treatment, chromatin trimming, and incubation with modification-specific antibodies. Once the modified histone-antibody complex is formed, chromatins are isolated with a suitable method, e.g., Protein A or Protein G coated agarose beads, and cross-links are removed to separate the DNA, and finally, DNA is extracted. Extracted DNA can be utilized in microarray analysis for a specific histone modification by sequence enrichment (Bernstein et al., 2004; Hubert et al., 2006). The main drawbacks of the ChIP are the requirement for high-specificity antibodies, high sample integrity, and excessive sample amounts. Recent developments enabled the ChIP to be used in smaller amounts of sample cells for histone modification profiling (Martin-Subero and Siebert, 2009).

A New Frontier in Epigenomics: High-Throughput Sequencing

The next-generation sequencing (NGS) technology enables newer frontiers in epigenomics research in addition to their substantial roles in genomics. In summary, the next-generation sequencing technology enables researchers to sequence as much as 2 Gbps sequence in a single run with different techniques deployed by the sequencing platform. Initial applications of NGS in epigenomics revealed 20 distinct profiles of histone methylation marks (Mikkelsen et al., 2007). The NGS is utilized in a recent development called the 5C method (Chromosome Conformation Capture Carbon Copy) to discover DNA to regulatory factor interactions (Simonis et al., 2007). Together with the NGS, a 3D investigation of the nuclear environment revealed intricate communication networks between different parts of the chromatin landscape (Fraser and Bickmore, 2007). A particular problem arises in sodium bisulfite treatment for the definition of methylation, where normally 4 unmethylated base pairs reduce to 3 unmethylated base pairs, which results in uncertainty in sequence origin (Martin-Subero and Siebert, 2009).

Epigenomic Marks

DNA modifications, e.g., methylation and hydroxymethylation, histone protein modifications of tails, e.g., acetylation, phosphorylation, methylation, sumoylation, ubiquitination, and ncRNA-driven regulations constitute the epigenomic marks in a genome. However, reproducibility and conservation traits currently limit these conceptual marks to methylation and histone modifications (Berger et al., 2009; Bell, 2012; Tollefsboll, 2012). Reproducibility and conservation traits are essential in the preservation of cell-line identities and cell epigenomes, especially in somatic cells having the same genomes (Richards, 2006). The methylation is the attachment of a methyl group into a 5' Carbon atom of the cytosine base to produce methylcytosine, which results in the formation of CpG islands since cytosines are followed by guanines in the genome. DNA methylation is the robust epigenetic mark. Gene expression suppression by methylation is required to be removed from specific sequences, sometimes even at a genome-wide level, depending on the developmental stage of the organism. The known stages are the post-fertilization period and the germ-line cell differentiation in both genders. Especially in the post-fertilization period, global demethylation of the entire genome is present in the embryo, which is followed by the reinstallation of global DNA methylation just before the embryonic implantation, making the embryo particularly susceptible to all kinds of environmental agitation (Faulk and Dolinoy, 2011; Bell, 2012; Tollefsbol, 2012).

Epigenome-Wide Association Studies (EWAS)

Advanced microarray methodologies with their comprehensive coverages enable the discerning of the disease-associated epigenetic alterations in humans (Rakyan et al., 2011; Bibikova,

2016). Target-specific and site-specific methods focusing on candidate genes are largely replaced by the EWAS to solicit the epigenetic effect between health and disease states in a highly systematic way. A standardized experimental framework for EWAS has yet to be achieved and the fundamental principles of whole genome association analysis (GWAS) are mostly incompatible with the EWAS (Michels et al., 2013; Bibikova, 2016). EWAS typically focuses on the epigenetic state of a great number of loci of a specific tissue to associate them with a trait. Mostly, the epigenetic state in question is DNA methylation and the trait in question is diseases or environmental conditions. Both the NGS and the microarray methodologies find themselves places in EWAS, each with its drawbacks (Plongthongkum et al., 2014; Bock et al., 2010; Harris et al., 2010; Bibikova, 2016).

Future Perspectives for Epigenomics

Currently, epigenomics is a highly thrilling subject promising many breakthroughs in the field of medical biology, so much so that researchers in the field are calling for international coordination for the human epigenome project (Esteller, 2006; Garber, 2006; Jones and Martienssen, 2005; Rauscher, 2005; Bibikova, 2016; Zhang and Zhang, 2022). Similar to the human genome project, the human epigenome project would be a real scientific challenge, which may be more so compared to the human genome project due to the very nature of epigenetics. Indeed, its dynamic adaptability, highly specified mechanisms, and the inter-variability between tissues and organisms make such an endeavor one of the truly formidable scientific achievements (Martin-Subero and Siebert, 2009; Zhang and Zhang, 2022). It is said that there are initiatives aiming to characterize the epigenome by using the power of the NGS to reveal the methylation profiles of millions of CpGs. Yet, heterogeneity of the epigenetics across the individuals still makes the microarray methodologies a necessity in epigenomics research (Zhang and Zhang, 2022). Otherwise, the requirement of multiple samples to overcome the heterogeneity would make the characterization efforts unaffordable at best. On the other hand, it is possible to reveal tissue-specific consensus of cell epigenomes per sample basis by combining the microarray approaches and the NGS. Still, the precise revelation of a cellular epigenome requires an indisputable method to detect the cell-specific DNA methylation patterns of CpG islands per cell basis. Again, the need for a unified cellular analysis system covering genomics, transcriptomics, proteomics, and epigenomics is increasingly pronounced to differentiate all the possible states of a given cell, which would substantially change the way how any alterations are associated with what kind of physiological state (VanSteensel, 2005). While the majority of the studies focused on cancer, it should be stressed that epigenetics is associated with all aspects of life due to its universality in the integration of external and internal stimuli into the genome proper (Jirtle and Skinner, 2007). Advances in the field will certainly progress to genome-wide levels and reveal genomic regions that are specifically prone to epigenetic modifications by the external stimuli, which will be pivotal in deciphering how the genetic code precisely manifests itself in the phenotype (Martin-Subero and Siebert, 2009; Zhang and Zhang, 2022).

Conclusion

Even though many different epigenetic mechanisms are known and some have been studied extensively, there are still many unanswered questions that need answers. Epigenomics is more sophisticated than epigenetics as it represents the genotype-to-phenotype transitioning in a non-linear way. The first of the challenges to overcome will be deciphering the obscurity of epigenomic programming to reveal associations of both genetic and epigenetic factors to the final phenotype. Epigenomic variation is much greater than genetic variation in cells since its dynamically adaptable and cell-line-specific traits. The nature of the data obtained from epigenomic research is multifaceted, which means that it has meaning at multiple levels, and even how to collect meaningful data is a challenge itself. The complexity of the data makes the integration and analysis of findings more complicated than genomic data. Despite the presence of reviews about epigenomic programming, essential aspects are still unknown (Smith and Huang, 2012).

Various research strongly suggests polyphenols as an effective epigenetic modulator by pointing out their ability to re-establish normal epigenomic landscape in aberrant patterns seen in cancerous cells. As natural substances, polyphenols are known to affect more than one target, in this case, epigenome modulatory enzymes. Of particular note is the curcumin, which is shown to affect antagonistic enzymes. Consequently, a debate about the difference between epigenetic balance and epigenetically balanced cell concepts has arisen. Right now, there is no telling of how such polymodal mechanisms would provide and which consequences. As expected, the effect obtained from polyphenol administration depends on the concentration, administration period, and epigenomic landscape of the administered tissue, especially in cancerous cells. Polyphenols are targets of different metabolic pathways and are processed by a multitude of enzymes, which are variable depending on the concentration and the cell. Therefore, instead of preferring their natural substance forms, their most active biological form should be clarified by chemical characterization (Stepanic et al., 2014). Lastly, further research into chromosomal band structures to reveal chromosome-specific epimutation hotspots and epigenomic marks would contribute to the understanding of disease associations with the epimutations in cell epigenomes.

References

Bell, C. G. (2012). Epigenomic factors in human obesity. In T. O. Tollefsbol (Ed.). *Epigenetics in Human Disease* (pp. 273-296). Elsevier, San Diego, CA, USA.

Berger, S. L. Kouzarides, T. Shiekhattar, R. Shilatifard, A. (2009). An operational definition of epigenetics. *Genes Development*, 23,781-783.

Bernstein, B. E. Humphrey, E. L. Liu, C. L. et al. (2004). The use of chromatin immunoprecipitation assays genomewide analyses histone modifications. *Methods in Enzymology*, 376, 349-360.

Bernstein, B. E. Kamal, M. Lindblad, K. et al. (2005). Genomic maps and comparative analysis of histone modifications in human and Mouse. *Cell,* 120, 169-181.

Bernstein, B. E. Mikkelsen, T. S. Xie, X. et al. (2006). A bivalent chromatin structure marks key developmental genes in embryonic stem cells, *Cell,* 125, 315-326.

Bibikova, M. (2016). DNA methylation microarrays. In M. F. Fraga and A. F. Fernandez (Eds.) *Epigenomics in Health and Disease* (pp. 19- 46) Elsevier, San Diego, CA, USA.

Bibikova, M. Chudin, E. Wu, B. et al. (2006). Human embryonic stem cells have a unique epigenetic signature. *Genome Research*, 16, 1075-1083.

Bibikova, M. Lin, Z. Zhou, L. et al. (2006). High-throughput DNA methylation profiling using universal bead arrays. *Genome Research,* 16, 383-393.

Blelloch, R. Wang, Z. Meissner, A. et al. (2006). Reprogramming efficiency following somatic cell nuclear transfer is influenced by the differentiation and methylation state of the donor nucleus, *Stem Cells,* 24, 2007-2013.

Bock, C. Tomazou, E. M. Brinkman, A. B. Muller, F. Simmer, F. Gu, H. et al. (2010). Quantitative comparison of genome-wide DNA methylation mapping technologies. *Nature Biotechnology* 28(10), 110614.

Bracken, A. P. Dietrich, N. Passini, D. et al. (2006). Genome-wide mapping of Polycomb target genes unravels their roles in cell fate transitions *Genes Development*, 20, 1123-1136.

Buszczak, M. Spradling, A. C. (2006). Searching chromatin for stem cell identity. *Cell*, 125, 233-236.

Callinan, P. A. Feinberg, A. P. (2006). The emerging science of epigenomics, *Human Molecular Genetics*, 15 Suppl 1, R95-R101.

Chen, K. Rajewsky, N. (2007). The evolution of gene regulation by transcription factors and microRNAs, *Nature Review Genetics*, 8, 93-103.

Dong, E. Chen, Y. Gavin, D. P. Grayson, D. R. Guidotti, A. (2010). Valproate induces DNA demethylation in nuclear extracts from adult mouse brain. *Epigenetics*, 5(8),730-735.

Dong, E. Nelson, M. Grayson, D. R. Costa, E. Guidotti, A. (2008). Clozapine and sulpiride but not haloperidol or olanzapine activate brain DNA demethylation. *Proceedings of National Academy of Sciences, USA*, 105(36), 13614-13619.

Esteller, M. (2007). Cancer epigenomics: DNA methylomes and histone-modification maps. *Nature Review Genetics,* 8, 286-298.

Esteller, M. (2007). Epigenetic gene silencing in cancer: the DNA hypermethylome. *Human Molecular Genetics,* 16, 1, R50-59.

Esteller, M. (2006). The necessity of a human epigenome project. *Carcinogenesis*, 27, 1121-1125.

Esteller, M. (2009). *Epigenetics in Biology and Medicine*. CRC Press, Taylor & Francis Group, New York, USA.

Faulk, C. Dolinoy, D. C. (2011). Timing is everything: The when and how of environmentally induced changes in the epigenome of animals. *Epigenetics*, 6.

Fazzari, M. J. Greally, J. M. (2004). Epigenomics: beyond CpG islands. *Nature Review Genetics,* 5, 446-455.

Fraga, M. F. Ballestar, E. Paz, M. F. et al. (2005). Epigenetic differences arise during lifetime monozygotic twins. *Proceedings of National Academy of Sciences, USA*, 102(30), 10604-10609.

Fraga, M. F. Esteller, M. (2002). DNA methylation: a profile of methods and applications. *Biotechniques,* 33, 636-649.

Franklin, T. B. Russig, H. Weiss, I. C. Gräff, J. Linder, N. Michalon, A. Vizi, S. Mansuy, I. M. (2010). Epigenetic transmission of the impact of early stress across generations. *Biological Psychiatry,* 68(5), 408-415.

Fraser, P. Bickmore, W. (2007). Nuclear organization of the genome and the potential for gene regulation. *Nature*, 447, 413-417.

Garber, K. (2006). Momentum building for human epigenome project. *Journal of the National Cancer Institute,* 98, 84-86.

Hackett, J. A. Sengupta, R. Zylicz, J. J. Murakami, K. Lee, C. Down, T. A. Surani, M. A. (2013). Germline DNA demethylation dynamics and imprint erasure through 5-hydroxymethylcytosine. *Science,* 339(6118), 448-452.

Harris, R. A. Wang, T. Coarfa, C. et al. (2010). Comparison of sequencing-based methods to profile DNA methylation and identification of monoallelic epigenetic modifications. *Nature Biotechnology*, 28(10), 1097105.

Huebert, D. J. Kamal, M. O'Donovan, A. et al. (2006). Genome-wide analysis of histone modifications by ChIP-on-chip. *Methods,* 40, 365369.

James, S. J. Cutler, P. Melnyk, S. Jernigan, S. Janak, L. Gaylor, D. W. Neubrander, J. A. (2004). Metabolic biomarkers of increased oxidative stress and impaired methylation capacity in children with autism. *American Journal of the Clinical Nutrition,* 80(6),1611-1617.

Jenuwein, T. Allis, C. D. (2001). Translating the histone code. *Science,* 293, 1074-1080.

Jessberger, S. Nakashima, K. Clemenson, G. D. Mejia, E. Mathews, E. Ure, K. Ogawa, S. Sinton, C. M. Gage, F. H. Hsieh, J. (2007). Epigenetic Modulation of Seizure-Induced Neurogenesis and Cognitive Decline. *Journal of Neuroscience*, 27(22),5967-5975.

Jirtle, R. L. Skinner, M. K. (2007). Environmental epigenomics and disease susceptibility. *Nature Reviews Genetics*, 8, 253-262.

Jones, P. A. Baylin, S. B. (2007). The epigenomics of cancer. *Cell,* 128, 683-692.

Kubota, T. Miyake, K. Hirasawa, T. (2014). Current Understanding of Epigenomics and Epigenetics in Neurodevelopmental Disorders. In C. J. Payne (Ed.). *Epigenetics and Epigenomics*. (pp. 77-96).

Laird, P. W. (2003). The power and the promise of DNA methylation markers, *Nature Reviews Cancer,* 3, 253-266.

Laird, P. W. (2005). Cancer epigenetics. *Human Molecular Genetics*, 14,1, R65-76.

Lee, T. I. Jenner, R. G. Boyer, L. A. et al. (2006). Control of developmental regulators by Polycomb in human embryonic stem cells. *Cell,* 125, 301-313.

Lillycrop, K. A. Phillips, E. S. Jackson, A. A. Hanson, M. A. Burdge, G. C. (2005). Dietary protein restriction of pregnant rats induces and folic acid supplementation prevents epigenetic modification of hepatic gene expression in the offspring. *Journal of Nutrition,*135(6),1382-1386.

Lillycrop, K. A. Phillips, E. S. Torrens, C. Hanson, M. A. Jackson, A. A. Burdge, G. C. (2008). Feeding pregnant rats a protein-restricted diet persistently alters the methylation of specific cytosines in the hepatic PPAR alpha promoter of the offspring. *British Journal of Nutrition,* 100(2), 278-282.

Matsuda, H. Fukuda, N. Ueno, T. Katakawa, M. Wang, X. Watanabe, T. Matsui, S. Aoyama, T. Saito, K. Bando, T. Matsumoto, Y. Nagase, H. Matsumoto, K. Sugiyama, H. (2011). Transcriptional inhibition of progressive renal disease by gene silencing pyrroleimidazole polyamide targeting of the transforming growth factor-β1 promoter. *Kidney International*, 79(1),46-56.

Martin-Subero, J. I. Siebert, R. (2009). Epigenetics and epigenomics. In M. Esteller (Ed.) *Epigenetics in Biology and Medicine*. (pp. 261-285). CRC Press, Taylor & Francis Group, New York, USA.

Meissner, A. Walter, J. (2015). *Epigenetic Mechanisms in Cellular Reprogramming*. Springer, New York, USA. ISBN: 978-3-642-31974-7.

Michels, K. B. Binder, A. M. Dedeurwaerder, S. et al. (2013). Recommendations for the design and analysis of epigenome-wide association studies. *Nature Methods*, 10(10),94955.

Mikkelsen, T. S. Ku, M. Jaffe, D. B. et al. (2007). Genome-wide maps of chromatin state in pluripotent and lineage-committed cells. *Nature,* 448, 553-560.

Miyake, K. Yang, C. Minakuchi, Y. Ohori, K. Soutome, M. Hirasawa, T. Kazuki, Y. Adachi, N. Suzuki, S. Itoh, M. Goto, Y. I. Andoh, T. Kurosawa, H. Oshimura, M. Sasaki, M. Toyoda, A. Kubota, T. (2013). Comparison of genomic and epigenomic expression in monozygotic twins discordant for Rett syndrome. *PLoS One, 8*(6),e66729.

Moretti, P. Sahoo, T. Hyland, K. Bottiglieri, T. Peters, S. Roa, B. Curry, S. Zhu, H. Finnell, R. H. Neul, J. L. Ramaekers, V. T. Blau, N. Bacino, C. A. Miller, G. Scaglia, F. (2005). Cerebral folate deficiency with developmental delay; autism; and response to folinic acid. *Neurology,* 64(6),1088-1090.

Ohtsuki, A. Kimura, M. T. Minoshima, M. Suzuki, T. Ikeda, M. Bando, T. Nagase, H. Shinohara, K. Sugiyama, H. (2009). Synthesis and properties of PI polyamide–SAHA conjugate. *Tetrahedron Letters*; 50, 7288-7292.

Orlikova, B. Diederich, M. (2012). Power from the garden: plant compounds as inhibitors of the hallmarks of cancer. *Current Medicinal Chemistry,* 19(14), 2061-2087.

Payne, C. J. (2014). *Epigenetics and Epigenomics*. AvE4EvA. ISBN-10 9535113631.

Pennisi, E. (2005). Environmental epigenomics meeting. Supplements restore gene function via methylation. *Science,* 310, 1761.

Plongthongkum, N. Diep, D. H. Zhang, K. (2014). Advances in the profiling of DNA modifications: cytosine methylation and beyond. *Nature Reviews*, 15(10), 64761.

Qiu J. (2006). Epigenetics: unfinished symphony. *Nature*, 441(7090), 143-145.

Rakyan, V. K. Down, T. A. Balding, D. J. Beck, S. (2011). Epigenome-wide association studies for common human diseases. *Nature Reviews*, 12(8), 52941.

Rauscher, F. J. (2005). It is time for a human epigenome project. *Cancer Research,* 65, 11229.

Reuter, S. Gupta, S. C. Park, B. Goel, A. Aggarwal, B. B. (2011). Epigenetic changes induced by curcumin and other natural compounds. *Genes Nutrition,* 6(2), 93-108.

Richards, E. J. (2006). Inherited epigenetic variation soft inheritance. *Nature Reviews Genetics*, 7, 395-401.

Sandoval, J. Heyn, H. Moran, S. Serra-Musach, J. Pujana, M. A. Bibikova, M. Esteller, M. (2011). Validation of a DNA methylation microarray for 450,000 CpG sites in the human genome. *Epigenetics,* 6, 692-702.

Sato, S. Yoshimizu, T. Sato, E. Matsui, Y. (2003). Erasure of methylation imprinting of Igf2r during mouse primordial germ-cell development. *Molecular Reproduction and Development*, 65(1), 41-50.

Shen, L. Kondo, Y. Guo, Y. et al. (2007). Genome-wide profiling of DNA methylation reveals a class of normally methylated CpG island promoters. *PLoS Genetics*, 3, 2023-2036.

Simonis, M. Kooren, J. Laat, W. (2007). An evaluation of 3C-based methods to capture DNA interactions. *Nature Methods,* 4, 895-901.

Smiraglia, D. J. Rush, L. J. Frühwald, M. C. et al. (2001). Excessive CpG island hypermethylation in cancer cell lines versus primary human malignancies. *Human Molecular Genetics,* 10, 14131419.

Smith, C. L. Huang, K. (2012). Epigenomics in Neurobehavioral Diseases. In. T. O. Tollefsbol (Ed.) *Epigenetics in Human Disease*. (pp. 127-153). Elsevier, San Diego, CA, USA.

Spencer, J. P. Abd-el-Mohsen, M. M. Rice-Evans, C. (2004). Cellular uptake and metabolism of flavonoids and their metabolites: implications for their bioactivity. *Archives Biochemistry Biophysics*, 423(1), 148-161.

Stepanic, V. Kujundzic, R. N. Troselj, K. G. (2014). Epigenome, Cancer Prevention and Flavonoids and Curcumin. In C. J. Payne (Ed.). *Epigenetics and Epigenomics*. (pp. 173-210). AvE4EvA.

Suzuki, T. Miyata, N. (2011). Lysine demethylases inhibitors. *Journal of Medicinal Chemistry*, 54(24), 8236-8250.

Tollefsbol, T. O. (2012). *Epigenetics in Human Disease.* (pp. 1-7). Elsevier, San Diego, CA, USA.

Tsankova, N. M. Berton, O. Renthal, W. Kumar, A. Neve, R. L. Nestler, E. J. (2006). Sustained hippocampal chromatin regulation in a mouse model of depression and antidepressant action. *Nature Neuroscience,* 9(4), 519-525.

Van Steensel, B. (2005). Mapping of genetic and epigenetic regulatory networks using microarrays. *Nature Genetics,* 37 Suppl, 18-24.

Van Steensel, B. Henikoff, S. (2003). Epigenomic profiling using microarrays. *Biotechniques,* 35, 346-357.

Wang, Q. Xu, X. Li, J. Liu, J. Gu, H. Zhang, R. Chen, J. Kuang, Y. Fei, J. Jiang, C. Wang, P. Pei, D. Ding, S. Xie, X. (2011). Lithium, an anti-psychotic drug, greatly enhances the generation of induced pluripotent stem cells. *Cell Research,* 21(19), 1424-1435.

Weaver, I. C. Cervoni, N. Champagne, F. A. D'Alessio, A. C. Sharma, S. Seckl, J. R. Dymov, S. Szyf, M. Meaney, M. J. (2004). Epigenetic programming by maternal behavior. *Nature Neuroscience*, 7(8), 847-854.

Weaver, J. R. Susiarjo, M. Bartolomei, M. S. (2009). Imprinting and epigenetic changes in the early embryo. *Mammalian Genome*, 20(9-10), 532-543.

Weber, M. Hellmann, I. Stadler, M. B. et al. (2007). Distribution, silencing potential and evolutionary impact of promoter DNA methylation in the human genome. *Nature Genetics*, 39, 457-466.

Yuan, E. Haghighi, F. White, S. et al. (2006). A single nucleotide polymorphism chip-based method for combined genetic and epigenetic profiling: validation in decitabine therapy and tumor/normal comparisons. *Cancer Research,* 66, 3443-3451.

Zhang, Z. and Zhang, W. (2022). Epigenetic signatures of centrosomes are novel targets in cancer diagnosis: insights from an analysis of the cancer genome atlas. *Epigenomes*, 6, 14. https://doi.org/10.3390/epigenomes6020014.

Chapter 6

The Role of Epigenetics in Cancers

İkbal Cansu Barış*
Department of Medical Biology, University of Pamukkale, Denizli, Turkey

Abstract

Epigenetic changes are important mechanisms that have a role in the etiology and/or progression of cancer by causing the activation of oncogenes or the silencing of tumor suppressor genes. Epigenetic mechanisms that alter chromatin structure can be separated into four categories: histone modifications, DNA methylation, nucleosome remodeling, and non-coding RNAs (e.g., miRNAs). These mechanisms work together to organise the functioning of the genome by regulating the accessibility of chromatin and altering the structural dynamics of chromatin. These epigenetic mechanisms are necessary for normal mammalian development and regulation of gene expression. Disorders in epigenetic regulators have been determined in both blood and solid cancers, and the significance of epigenetic changes in cancer cells has been emphasized by several groups in different types of cancer.

Keywords: epigenetic, DNA methylation, histone modifications, nucleosome remodeling, miRNAs, cancer

Introduction

Although great advances have been made in cancer research and the identification of genetic changes underlying tumor development, there are many mechanisms that have not yet been elucidated on the roles of different molecular changes between cancer types in the etiology and/or progression of cancer. Inherited or sporadic mutations, inactivation of tumor suppressor genes or activation of oncogenes, and changes in the epigenome (both DNA and histones) can cause cancer initiation and progression (Ilango et al., 2020). Epigenetic changes are important mechanisms that have a role in the etiology and/or progression of cancer by causing the activation of oncogenes or the silencing of tumor suppressor genes.

The term 'epigenetics' was first used by Conrad Waddington. It is used to describe changes in the conformational structure of DNA other than changes in the DNA sequence. Epigenetic mechanisms are the principal for mammalian development (Sharma et al., 2009). These

* Corresponding Author's E-mail: ibaris@pau.edu.tr.

In: Epigenetics: Beyond the Genetics and Medicine
Editors: Sevgi Durna Daştan and Nazan Yurtcu
ISBN: 979-8-88697-228-3

mechanisms that change chromatin structure can be separated into four categories: histone modifications, DNA methylation, non-coding RNAs, and nucleosome remodeling. They work together to change the structural dynamics of chromatin. Thus, gene expression profiles change. The interaction of these modifications creates an "epigenetic landscape" in different cell types, developmental stages, and in some diseases such as cancer (Jones and Baylin, 2007; Jiang and Pugh, 2009). DNA methylation, nucleosome remodeling, histone modification, and micro RNA's targeting organise many biochemical pathways that are the principle to the regulated tumorigenesis (Dawson and Kouzarides, 2012). In human cancers, these epigenetic modifications affect gene expression. Reversing these modifications has been shown to be very successful in the treatment of many hematological malignancies and a subset of solid tumors (Ilango et al., 2020).

Human Epigenome Project

The Human Epigenome Project (HEP) is the first international epigenome initiative established in 1999 (Beck et al., 1999). The purpose of this project was to establish reference DNA methylation profiles and to record the methylation profiles in healthy human cells and tissues. This project was supported by many cancer researchers around the world (Esteller, 2006; Rauscher, 2005). The HEP initiated high-resolution DNA methylation profiling for three chromosomes in 12 cell types and tissues in humans, proving among other scientific findings that DNA methylation is tissue-specific, mostly changed in evolutionarily conserved regions (Eckhardt et al., 2006; Rakyan et al., 2004). Post-HEP attempts comprised the generation of genome-wide DNA methylation profiles of 16 cell types/tissues and the first whole-genome (methylome) profile (Down et al., 2008; Rakyan et al., 2008). These data represent the human DNA methylation reference data in the Ensembl genome browser (Flicek et al., 2010).

International Human Epigenome Consortium

The International Human Epigenome Consortium (IHEC) is an initiative launched in 2010. It is modeled on The International Cancer Genome Consortium (ICGC) and aims to serve as an umbrella organisation for national and international epigenome projects. The purpose of this project is to constitute 1000 comprehensive human and nonhuman epigenome maps as part of reference cell types/tissues, disease, stem cells, environment, and aging. It has three main purposes: (1) to improve scientific evidences through a joint research program; (2) to band together young colleagues through the Network of Excellence Training program; and (3) to constitute an open dialog by establishing interactive Web sites for both the general public and the scientific community (Lechner et al., 2010).

Epigenetic Mechanisms in Cancer Cells

Malignant cells arise as a result of a multistage process with the increase in genetic and epigenetic lesions in healthy cells. Similarly to genetic lesions, the accumulation of epigenetic lesions also alters the function and structure of the genome, leading to the unrestricted, uncontrolled growth of a cell. Besides, it has also been suggested that epigenetic changes may have a more prominent role in tumor development (Ushijima and Asada, 2010).

Tumorigenesis is a multifactorial and complex transformation process of normal cells into malignant cells. It is identified by resistance to cell death, proliferative signaling, prevention of growth suppression, genomic instability, deregulation of energy metabolism, replicative immortality, inflammatory response, activation of invasion, and induction of angiogenesis finally resulting in metastases (Hanahan and Weinberg, 2011). These cancer-specific changes are stimulated by mutational/non-mutational events in the genome that affects gene expression, leading to tumorigenesis (Hanahan and Weinberg, 2011; Jones and Baylin, 2007). Epigenetic modifications alter the methylation patterns of cytosines in DNA, the nucleosome positioning along DNA, and modification of DNA-binding proteins (Kim et al., 2008).

Disorders in chromatin regulators have been determined in both blood and solid cancers, and the significance of epigenetics in cancer cells has been demonstrated by several groups in different types of cancer (Jones et al., 2019; Toh et al., 2017; Gagliano and Brancolini, 2021).

Role of DNA Methylation in Cancer Cells

Numerous studies have been conducted in recent years showing that changes in 5mC patterns can discriminate the cancer cells. Except for CpG-rich regions, CpGs in the genome are 80% methylated, and the level of CpG methylation in cancer is around 40-60% on average (Hansen et al., 2011). Three important pathways have been classified that CpG methylation may contribute to the oncogenic profile: hypomethylation of the cancer genome, focal hypermethylation at TSG promoters, and direct mutagenesis in 5mC-comprising sequences through deamination, UV irradiation, or exposure to other carcinogens. (Baylin and Jones, 2011).

The mechanism that causes changes in the DNA methylation profile in the cancer epigenome is not yet understood. Alteration of the DNA methylation profile in the cancer epigenome may occur with the disordered loss of function of DNA methyltransferase proteins or activation of ten-eleven translocation family members (Baylin and Jones, 2011). Reduction or deletion of DNA methyltransferase results in increased mutation rates, tumor induction, and aneuploidies. DNA hypomethylation has an effective role in improving chromosomal fragibility (Ehrlich and Lacey, 2012).

Approximately 60% of all gene promoters have unmethylated CpG islands in adult cell renewal systems or normal development. The expression state of CGI genes is ready to be activated in open chromatin states due to the lack of methylation (Baylin and Jones, 2011; Shen and Laird, 2013). Hypomethylation occurs throughout the genome and is usually detected in repetitive regions of the DNA (Pfeifer, 2018).

DNA methylation patterns can be changed by altered activity or expression of epigenetic regulators for example TET (Baxter et al., 2014). Mutations in TET enzymes can be related to a DNA hypermethylation, related to the IDH1 and IDH2 isocitrate dehydrogenase enzymes. These enzymes produced α – ketoglutarate, which is a cofactor for the TET hydroxylases. As a result of mutations in IDH1/2, 2-hydroxyglutarate is formed from α - ketoglutarate. An increased DNA hypermethylation frequency is common in leukemias and brain tumors. (Baylin and Jones, 2011).

Loss of DNA methylation is mostly related to the dysfunction of TET2 methylcytosine dioxygenase. The TET2 mutation is found in about 15% of myeloid cancers, which causes hydroxylation disruption. The function of TET2 produced by mutant IDH1 is also inhibited in acute myeloid leukemias. 5-hydroxy methylcytosine levels and TET expression have been reported to decrease in liver and breast cancers (Baxter et al., 2014).

Role of Histone Modifications in Cancer Cells

Chromatin remodelling comprises several histone modifications such as methylation, phosphorylation, and acetylation (Jenuwein, 2001). The prominent N-terminal amino acid tails of H3 and H4 core histones are active cites for elaborate posttranslational modifications, involving acetylation, methylation, phosphorylation, ADP ribosylation, ubiquitination, and sumoylation (Peterson and Laniel, 2004; Shilatifard, 2006). The acetylation sites are H3K9, H3K18, H3K23and H3K14, and H4K5, H4K12, H4K8, and H4K16 (Kouzarides, 2007). The methylation sites are H3K4, H3K36, H3K9, H3K27, H3K79, and H4K20 (Lachner, 2003). The phosphorylation site is H3S10 (Berger, 2002). An ubiquitination site is designated in H2A, H2B (Jason et al., 2002). The misregulation of the histone demethylases (HDMs) and the histone methyltransferases (HMTs) have related to some types of cancer including lung, brain, prostate, and breast (Chen et al., 2010; Varambally et al., 2002; Kleer, et al., 2003). The HDMs and HTMs have an important role in regulating of lysine residues' (K4, K27, K9, K36) methylation status in histone H3. Histone modification patterns have an important role in the diagnosis of many types of cancers. H3K9ac, H3K9me3, and H4K16ac levels are usually reduced in non-small cell lung cancer (Song et al., 2012). Lower levels of H3K18ac and H3K4me2 were associated with a poor prognosis in prostate cancer. Loss of H3K9me3 has been detected in the promoter regions of acute myeloid leukemia genes. The prognosis patient with acute myeloid leukemia can be predicted by the global H3K9me3 patterns. These cancers have amplifications, somatic mutations, and deletions that cause changes in the activities of HDMs and HMTs (Baxter et al., 2014).

Nucleosome Remodeling in Cancer Cells

Nucleosome remodeling ATPases interact with histones and DNA altering DNA-histone interactions in the target nucleosome. When these bind and hydrolyze ATP, they experience conformational changes. Their efforts can guide complete or the movement of histone octamers in DNA, incomplete fragmentation of the nucleosome, nucleosome assembly, or the exchange of histones for variants.

In all areas of genome function, remodeling processes come into play. Nucleosome remodeling is integrated with other mechanisms, for example, RNA metabolism or histone modifications to assemble epigenetic states (Becker and Workman et al., 2013). Modification of the DNA and histone proteins strongly influences the regulation of chromatin structure. It could be said that active genes are associated with methylation of hte H3K4 and acetylation of H3 and H4 histones (Barth and Imhof, 2010). Chromatin modification has been found to be sensitive to the metabolic condition of the cell and the environment. There is also evidence in studies that some DNA and histone modifications are hereditary. In addition, defection of chromatin signaling pathways underlies a widespread of disorders and diseases (Ilango et al., 2020).

Many enzymes have been described as acetylate, deacetylate, phosphorylate, methylate, demethylate, sumoylate histones, or ubiquitinate. These genes, which have a role in epigenetic mechanisms, have been determined to be mutated in many cancers. As a result of this mutation in epigenetic modifications, gene expression patterns can be affected and contribute to tumor development indirectly. It also shows that epigenetic modifiers can be used as new targets for therapy.

DNMT3a mutations were detected in 22% of acute myeloid leukemia (AML) cases. Moreover, these mutations are associated with a poor outcome of AML cases (T. J. Ley et al., 2010). Similarly, methylcytosine dioxygenase TET2 mutations are found in approximately 15% of myeloid cancers (Moran-Crusio et al., 2011). The UTX (H3K27 demethylase) is mutated in several human cancers, and cancer in which it is most mutated is multiple myeloma (~10%) (Van Haaften, et al., 2009). The gene mutations which change the structure of chromatin suggest that the disturbance of epigenetic balance has an extremely significant role in the triggering of cancers (Baxter et al., 2014).

Micro RNAs (miRNAs) in Cancer Cells

Many studies have indicated that miRNAs have key roles in principle of biological processes, for example, cell proliferation development, fat metabolism, apoptosis, stress resistance, haematopoiesis, neural development, tumourigenesis, and death (Osaki et al., 2008). Accumulating studies demonstrate the significance of miRNAs in cancer. Despite their tight regulation in normal tissues and during development, studies show that miRNAs are misregulated in cancer. Overexpressed miRNAs in cancer can act as oncogenes, and downexpressed miRNAs in normal tissue may show tumor suppressive activity (Zhang et al., 2007). Downregulation of tumor suppressor miRNAs may lead to tumorigenesis by increasing the translation of oncogenes and thus the expression of oncogenic proteins. Besides upregulation of oncogenic miRNAs may lead to tumor formation by blocking tumor suppressor genes. The studies have shown that epigenetic modifications, including histone modification and DNA methylation, regulate both the expression of protein-coding genes and miRNAs such as miR34a, miR9, miR124, miR148, miR137, miR203, and let7a.

The expression of significant epigenetic regulators is mediated by some other subset of miRNAs involving polycomb group genes, histone deacetylases, and DNA methyltransferases. This network between miRNAs and epigenetic mechanisms influences the whole gene expression profile.

When this network is misregulated, normal physiological and biochemical functions are destroyed and contribute to several disease processes (Iswariya et al., 2011). The studies have demonstrated the role of miRNAs in the hallmarks of cancer (F. Sato et al., 2011). For example, the miR-16 and miR-15 were identified that are largely deleted in chronic lymphocytic leukemia. These miRNAs lead to aberrant anti-apoptotic genes expression (Calin et al., 2002).

Studies have shown that while the miR-9 locus is hypermethylated in carcinomas of the neck, colon, and lung, miR-9 is over-expressed in brain carcinomas (Nass et al., 2009). Furthermore, a study has demonstrated that CpG island methylation of miR-9 gene is quite high in gastric cancer (Li et al., 2014). In addition, the locus of miR-9-1 is extremely methylated both in the intra-ductal component of invasive ductal carcinoma of breast and invasive ductal carcinoma (Lehmann et al., 2008).

The production of several proteins related to apoptosis and cell cycle progression is regulated by miR-34a. MiR-34a is frequently inactivated in various malignancies (Lodygin, et al., 2008). A recent study demonstrated that miR-34a expression is epigenetically silenced in human cholangiocarcinoma cells and that miR-34a acts as a tumor suppressor (Kwon et al., 2017). MiR-34b/c hypermethylation is quite common in the late clinical stages of soft tissue sarcomas (Xie, et al., 2015). MiR-137 downregulation has been detected in some cancers caused by methylation of the CpG island (Deng et al., 2011; Balaguer et al., 2010; Zhao, et al., 2012). Evidences have demonstrated that miR-137 ectopic expression dramatically lowered the levels of Cdc42 and Cdk6 and cause to cell cycle arrest in the G1 phase in lung cancer cells (Zhu et al., 2012).

Studies have shown that miR-148/152 family members are tumor suppressor genes and oncogenes. Studies have demonstrated upregulation of the miR-148a leading to poor survival in the plasma of multiple myeloma (Huang et al., 2012). MiR-148b has also been shown to be upregulated in hepatocellular carcinoma (Xia, et al., 2014). The researchers have demonstrated the anti-tumor effect of miR-148a particularly in breast cancer (Neuzillet et al., 2015). Inactivation of the miR-148 family by DNA methylation leads to induced TGFβ signaling. The TGFβ signaling pathway have an important role in carcinogenesis by leading to metastasis and tumor growth and is the target of miR-148 family members (Neuzillet et al., 2015).

MiR-124 is the most common miRNA in the brain. Abberrant expression of miR-124 leads to malignancies associated with the central nervous system (Karsy et al., 2012). Recent studies suggest that miR-124 acts as a tumor suppressor. It may be effective in the treatment of human glioblastomas by targeting STAT3 (Li et al., 2016). Furthermore, studies have shown that induction of DNMT by hepatitis C virus in HCV-associated intrahepatic cholangiocarcinoma leads to the suppression of miR-124 (Zeng et al., 2012). In addition, MiR-124-1 hypermethylation was observed to be more frequent in non-Hodgkin lymphomas.

MiR-200 is recognized as a suppressor of metastasis and a cell's epithelial-to-mesenchymal transition (Liu et al., 2008). Evidences suggest that in various cancers it has been described that ZEB1 is involved in EMT. Studies have determined that overexpression of miR-200 inhibits ZEB1-mediated metastasis in colorectal cancer cells. Indeed, miR-200 silencing has been demonstrated to result in CpG island hypermethylation, switching between EMT and vice versa leading to tumorigenesis (Biswas and Rao et al., 2017).

Conclusion

Malignant cells arise through a multistep process in which genetic and epigenetic changes accumulate in healthy cells. The accumulation of epigenetic lesions changes the structure and function of chromatin, leading to unrestricted and uncontrolled cell growth. In addition, studies have recommended that epigenetic changes may have a more prominent role in tumor development.

Epigenetic modifications alter the methylation patterns of cytosines in DNA, the nucleosome positioning along DNA, and the modification of DNA-binding proteins. Acquisition of these epigenetic modifications in the genome, which affects gene expression, leads to tumorigenesis. These epigenetic modifications have been detected in both hematological malignancies and solid tumors, and the importance of epigenetic modifications in cancer cells has been determined in different types of cancer.

Epigenetic alterations have an important role in the development and progression of various types of cancer. With the increasing availability of technologies to study the epigenetic mechanisms, novel epigenetic alterations that are specific to cell-type will lead to a deeper understanding of the characteristics of tumors and thus help to treat cancers using combinations of epigenetic therapies with conventional chemotherapy.

References

Balaguer F., Link A., Lozano J. J., Cuatrecasas M., Nagasaka T., Boland C. R. and Goel A (2010). Epigenetic Silencing of miR-137 Is an Early Event in Colorectal Carcinogenesis. *Cancer Research*, 70(16):6609-6618.

Barth T K and Imhof A (2010). Fast signals and slow marks: the dynamics of histone modifications. *Trends in Biochemical Science*, 35(11):618-626.

Baxter E, Windloch K, Gannon F and Lee S J (2014). Epigenetic regulation in cancer progression. *Cell Biosciences*, 4:45-65.

Baylin S B and Jones P A (2011). A decade of exploring the cancer epigenome - biological and translational implications. *Nature Review Cancer*, 11(10):726-734.

Becker P B and Workman J L (2013). Nucleosome Remodeling and Epigenetics. *Cold Spring Harbor Perspectives in Biology,* 5(9):a017905-a017905.

Berger S L (2002). Histone modifications in transcriptional regulation. *Current Opinion Genetics Development*, 12(2):142-148.

Biswas S and Rao C M (2017). Epigenetics in cancer: Fundamentals and Beyond. *Pharmacology & Therapeutics*, 173:118-134.

Calin G A, Dumitru C D, Shimizu M, Bichi R, Zupo S, Noch E and Croce C M (2002). Nonlinear partial differential equations and applications: Frequent deletions and down-regulation of micro-RNA genes miR15 and miR16 at 13q14 in chronic lymphocytic leukemia. *Proceeding National Academy of Science*, 99(24):15524-15529.

Chen M W, Hua K T, Kao H J, Chi C C, Wei L H G, Johansson and Kuo M L (2010). H3K9 Histone Methyltransferase G9a Promotes Lung Cancer Invasion and Metastasis by Silencing the Cell Adhesion Molecule Ep-CAM. *Cancer Research*, 70(20):7830-7840.

Dawson M A, and Kouzarides T (2012). Cancer Epigenetics: From Mechanism to Therapy, *Cell*, 150(1):12-27.

Deng Y, Deng H, Bi F, Liu J, Bemis L T, Norris D and Zhang Q (2011). MicroRNA-137 Targets Carboxylterminal Binding Protein 1 in Melanoma Cell Lines. *International Journal of Biological Science*, 7(1):133-137.

Down, T. A., Rakyan, V. K., Turner, D. J., Flicek, P., Li, H., Kulesha, E., Gräf, S., Johnson, N., Herrero, J., Tomazou, E. M., Thorne, N. P., Bäckdahl, L., Herberth, M., Howe, K. L., Jackson, D. K., Miretti, M. M., Marioni, J. C., Birney, E., Hubbard, T. J. P., … Beck, S. (2008). A Bayesian deconvolution strategy for immunoprecipitation-based DNA methylome analysis. *Nature Biotechnology*, 26:779–885.

Eckhardt, F., Lewin, J., Cortese, R., Rakyan, V. K., Attwood, J., Burger, M., Burton, J., Cox, T. V., Davies, R., Down, T. A., Haefliger, C., Horton, R., Howe, K., Jackson, D. K., Kunde, J., Koenig, C., Liddle, J., Niblett, D., Otto, T., … Beck, S, (2006). DNA methylation profiling of human chromosomes 6, 20 and 22. *Nature Genetics,* 38:1378–1385.

Ehrlich M and Lacey M (2013). DNA Hypomethylation and Hemimethylation in Cancer. *Advances in Experimental Medicine and Biology*, 754:31-56.

Esteller M (2006). The necessity of a human epigenome project. *Carcinogenesis,* 27(6):1121–1125.

Flicek P, Aken B L, Ballester B, Beal K, Bragin E, Brent S, Chen Y, Clapham P, Coates G, Fairley S, Fitzgerald S, Fernandez-Banet J, et al., (2010). Ensembl's 10th year. *Nucleic Acids Research*, 38:D557–D562.

Gagliano T, Brancolini C (2021). Targeting histone deacetylases for combination therapies in neuroendocrine tumors. *Cancer Gene Therapy*, 28:547–550.

Hanahan D and Weinberg R A (2011). Hallmarks of Cancer: The Next Generation. *Cell*, 144(5):646-674.

Hansen K D, Timp W, Bravo H C, Sabunciyan S, Langmead B, McDonald O G and Feinberg A P (2011). Increased methylation variation in epigenetic domains across cancer types. *Nature Genetics*, 43(8):768-775.

Huang J, Yu J, Li J, Liu Y and Zhong R (2012). Circulating microRNA expression is associated with genetic subtype and survival of multiple myeloma. *Medical Oncology*, 29(4):2402-2408.

Ilango S, Paital B, Jayachandran P, Padma PR, Nirmaladevi R (2020). Epigenetic alterations in cancer. *Frontiers in Bioscience*, 25:1058-1109.

Iswariya G T, Paital B, Padma P R and Nirmaladevi R (2019). MicroRNAs: Epigenetic players in cancer and aging. *Frontiers in Bioscience*, 11:9-9.

Jason L J M, Moore S C, Lewis J D, and Lindsey G and Ausió J (2002). Histone ubiquitination: a tagging tail unfolds? *BioEssay*, 24(2):166-174.

Jenuwein T (2001). Translating the Histone Code. *Science,* 293(5532):1074-1080.

Jiang C and Pugh B F (2009). Nucleosome positioning and gene regulation: advances through genomics. *Nature Reviews Genetics*, 10(3):161-172.

Jones P A and Baylin S B (2007). The Epigenomics of Cancer. *Cell*, 128(4):683-692.

Jones P A, Ohtani H, Chakravarthy A, De Carvalho DD (2019). Epigenetic therapy in immune-oncology. *Nature Reviews Cancer,* 19:151–161.

Karsy M, Arslan E and Moy F (2012). Current Progress on Understanding MicroRNAs in Glioblastoma Multiforme. *Gene Cancer*, 3(1):3-15.

Kim J K, Samaranayake M and Pradhan S (2008). Epigenetic mechanisms in mammals. *Cellular Molecular Life Science*, 66(4):596-612.

Kleer C G, Cao Q, Varambally S, Shen R, Ota I, Tomlins S A and Chinnaiyan A M (2003). EZH2 is a marker of aggressive breast cancer and promotes neoplastic transformation of breast epithelial cells. *Proceedings of the National Academy of Sciences*, 100(20):11606-11611.

Kouzarides T (2007). Chromatin Modifications and Their Function. *Cell*, 128(4):693-705.

Kwon H, Song K, Han C, Zhang J, Ungerleider N, Yao L, and Wu T (2017). Epigenetic silencing of microRNA-34a in human cholangiocarcinoma cells via DNA methylation and EZH2: Impact on regulation of Notch pathway. *The American Journal of Pathology*, 187(10):2288-2299.

Lachner M (2003). An epigenetic road map for histone lysine methylation. *Journal of Cell Science*, 116(11):2117-2124.

Lechner M, Boshoff C and Beck S (2010). Cancer Epigenome, *Advances in Genetics,* 70:247-76.

Lehmann U, Hasemeier B, Christgen M, Müller M D, Römermann, Länger F and Kreipe H (2008). Epigenetic inactivation of microRNA genehsa-mir- 9-1in human breast cancer. *Journal of Pathology*, 214(1):17-24.

Ley T J, Ding T L, Walter M J, McLellan M D, Lamprecht T, Larson D E and Wilson R K. (2010). DNMT3A Mutations in Acute Myeloid Leukemia. *The New England Journal of Medicine*, 363(25):2424-2433.

Li W, Huang H, Su J, Ji X, Zhang X, Zhang Z and Wang H (2016). miR-124 Acts as a Tumor Suppressor in Glioblastoma via the Inhibition of Signal Transducer and Activator of Transcription 3. *Mol Neurobiol*, 54(4):2555-2561.

Li Y, Xu Z, Li B, Zhang Z, Luo H, Wang Y, Wu X (2014).Epigenetic silencing of miRNA-9 is correlated with promoterproximal CpG island hypermethylation in gastric cancer *in vitro* and *in vivo*. *International Journal of Oncology*, 45(6):2576-2586.

Liu Y, El-Naggar S, Darling D S, Higashi Y and Dean D C (2008). Zeb1 links epithelial-mesenchymal transition and cellular senescence. *Development*, 135(3):579-588.

Lodygin D, Tarasov V, Epanchintsev A, Berking C, Knyazeva T, Körner H and Hermeking H (2008). Inactivation of miR-34a by aberrant CpG methylation in multiple types of cancer. *Cell Cycle*, 7(16):2591-2600.

Moran-Crusio K, Reavie L, Shih A, Abdel-Wahab O, Ndiaye-Lobry D, Lobry C and Levine R L (2011). Tet2 Loss Leads to Increased Hematopoietic Stem Cell Self-Renewal and Myeloid Transformation. *Cancer Cell*, 20(1):11-24.

Nass D, Rosenwald S, Meiri E, Gilad S, Tabibian-Keissar H, Schlosberg A and Rosenfeld N (2009). MiR-92b and miR-9/9* Are Specifically Expressed in Brain Primary Tumors and Can Be Used to Differentiate Primary from Metastatic Brain Tumors. *Brain Pathology*, 19(3):375-383.

Neuzillet C, Tijeras-Raballand A, Cohen R, Cros J, Faivre S, Raymond E and de Gramont A (2015). Targeting the TGFβ pathway for cancer therapy. *Pharmacology & Therapeutics*, 147:22-31.

Osaki M, Takeshita F and Ochiya T (2008). MicroRNAs as biomarkers and therapeutic drugs in human cancer. *Biomarkers*, 13(7-8):658-670.

Peterson C L and Laniel M A (2004). Histones and histone modifications. *Current Biology*, 14(14):546-551.

Pfeifer G (2018). Defining Driver DNA Methylation Changes in Human Cancer. *International Journal of Molecular Science*, 19(4):1166.

Rakyan V K, Hildmann T, Novik K L, Lewin J, Tost J, Cox A V, Andrews T D, Howe K L, Otto T, Olek A, Fischer J, Gut I G, et al. (2004). DNA methylation profiling of the human major histocompatibility complex: A pilot study for the human epigenome project. *PLoS Biology*, 2(12):e405.

Rauscher F J 3rd (2005). It is time for a Human Epigenome Project. *Cancer Research*. 65(24):11229.

Sato F, Tsuchiya S, Meltzer SJ and Shimizu K (2011). MicroRNAs and epigenetics. *The FEBS Journal*, 278(10):1598-1609.

Sharma S, Kelly T K and Jones P A, (2009). Epigenetics in cancer. *Carcinogen*, 31(1):27-36.

Shen H and Laird P W (2013). Interplay between the Cancer Genome and Epigenome. *Cell*, 153(1):38-55.

Shilatifard A (2006). Chromatin Modifications by Methylation and Ubiquitination: Implications in the Regulation of Gene Expression. *Annual Review Biochemistry*, 75(1):243-269.

Song J S, Kim Y S, Kim D K, Park S I, and Jang S J (2012). Global histone modification pattern associated with recurrence and disease-free survival in non-small cell lung cancer patients. *Pathology International*, 62(3):182-190.

Toh T B, Lim J J, Chow E K (2017). Epigenetics in cancer stem cells. *Molecular Cancer*, 16(1):29.

Ushijima T & Asada K (2010). Aberrant DNA methylation in contrast with mutations. *Cancer Science*, 101(2):300-305.

Van Haaften G, Dalgliesh G L, Davies H, Chen L, Bignell G, Greenman C and Teague J (2009). Somatic mutations of the histone H3K27 demethylase gene UTX in human cancer. *Nature Genetics*, 41(5):521-523.

Varambally S, Dhanasekaran S M, Zhou M, Barrette T R, Kumar-Sinha C, Sanda M G and Chinnaiyan A M (2002). The polycomb group protein EZH2 is involved in progression of prostate cancer. *Nature*, 419(6907):624-629.

Xia J, Guo X, Yan J and Deng K (2014). The role of miR-148a in gastric cancer. Journal of *Cancer Res Clinical Oncology*, 140(9):1451-1456.

Xie Y, Zong P, Wang W, Liu D, Li B, Wang Y and Li F (2015). Hypermethylation of potential tumor suppressor miR-34b/c is correlated with late clinical stage in patients with soft tissue sarcomas. *Experimental and Molecular Pathology*, 98(3):446-454.

Zeng B, Li Z, Chen R, Guo N, Zhou J, Zhou Q and Gong Y (2012). Epigenetic regulation of miR-124 by Hepatitis C Virus core protein promotes migration and invasion of intrahepatic cholangiocarcinoma cells by targeting SMYD3. *FEBS Letters*, 586(19):3271- 3278.

Zhang B, Pan X, Cobb G P and Anderson TA (2007). MicroRNAs as oncogenes and tumor suppressors. *Developmental Biology*, 302(1):1-12.

Zhao Y, Li Y, Lou G, Zhao L, Xu Z, Zhang Y & He F (2012). MiR-137 Targets Estrogen-Related Receptor Alpha and Impairs the Proliferative and Migratory Capacity of Breast Cancer Cells. *PLoS ONE*, 7(6):e39102.

Zhu X, Li Y, Shen H, Li H, Long L, Hui L & Xu W (2012). MiR-137 inhibits the proliferation of lung cancer cells by targeting Cdc42 and Cdk6. *FEBS Letters*, 587(1):73-81.

Chapter 7

Epigenetics and Microbiota

Özlem Aldemir*, **MD**
Department of Infectious Diseases and Clinical Microbiology,
Sivas Medicana Hospital, Sivas, Turkey

Abstract

The human is a superorganism called the holobiont, which consists of human cells and a larger proportion of microbial cells. Microbiota is the ecological communities of microorganisms that live in a particular environment. It is known that the human microbiota, especially the gut microbiota, is known to affect the physiology and pathology of the host through various mechanisms. For example, the intestinal microflora regulates many epigenetic pathways, such as modifications to DNA or histones, their metabolites, and noncoding RNAs. Epigenetic factors are also known to regulate the gut microbiota within the host by various mechanisms.

Keywords: epigenetics, genetics, microbiota

Introduction

The human body contains trillions of microorganisms, including bacteria, viruses, eukaryotes, archaea, and fungi (Marchesi & Ravel, 2015). In humans, the gut microbiota has the most species and the most significant number of microorganisms compared to other body parts (Quigley, 2013). The gastrointestinal tract microbiota is known to have a significant impact on the human body, on metabolic processes, and therefore on human health. The composition and function of the gut microbiota vary depending on many factors. The collective genome content of the microbiota, or microbial metagenome, has been called the microbiome, but the microbiome and microbiota are used interchangeably today (Lederberg & McCray, 2001). While the human genome effectively decides which microorganisms will comprise our microbiota, the microbiome is also influential in the study and evolution of the human genome. The microbiota can show its effect on the human genome through epigenetic mechanisms.

* Corresponding Author's E-mail: ozlem_gulgec@hotmail.com.

In: Epigenetics: Beyond the Genetics and Medicine
Editors: Sevgi Durna Daştan and Nazan Yurtcu
ISBN: 979-8-88697-228-3

The Human Microbiota

Multicellular organisms exist as meta-organisms consisting of the macroscopic host and its symbiotic, commensal microbiota. The microorganisms that colonize humans are more numerous than host cells, with a cell composition of about 100 trillion. It seems that the microbiota has a greater complexity compared to the human genome (Ley RE et al., 2006). These complex communities of microorganisms, including bacteria, fungi, protozoa, and viruses, have a fundamental role in the overall control of host physiology. The microbiota has many functions such as energy and nutrient production specific to the host, storage of fat, maintaining the synthesis of carbohydrates, short-chain fatty acids, amino acids, and different types of vitamins, protection from infections, maintenance of the intestinal barrier, immunomodulation, and contribution to mental and behavioral characteristics (Martin & Kochhar, 2015). It has been described that there is a symbiosis between the microbiota and the human body in general. The microbiota is thought to be the human's most prominent external endocrine organ (Zhu et al., 2010).

The composition and function of the microbiota vary depending on the mode of delivery, age, host genetics, diet, and antibiotics used. Maternal factors can influence the composition and development of the infant's gut microbiota before birth. Maternal diet, obesity, smoking status during pregnancy, and antibiotic agents are among these factors (Vandenplas et al., 2020). The full or early pregnancy may change the infant microbiota during the developmental stage. The most severe changes in the microbiota occur in infancy and early childhood. The mode of birth (vaginal or cesarean section) is considered an essential factor that strongly influences the microbiota composition. In the case of cesarean birth, it has been reported that the microbiota is based on microbial communities characteristically located on the whole human skin instead of vaginal and fecal bacteria from the mother, and cesarean birth causes a significant reduction of bifidobacteria. It has been shown that babies born by vaginal delivery have a microbiota similar to their mother's vagina (Biasucci et al., 2008). What the baby is fed in the early stages of life is another critical factor in developing the microbiota. Breast milk, which is the most potent nutrient that regulates the formation of the intestinal microbiota in infants, is a synbiotic food containing prebiotics (breast milk oligosaccharides) and probiotics (Bifidobacterium, Lactobacillus). Oligosaccharides, lysosomes, lactoferrin, antibodies, and cytokines in breast milk are known to increase the number of Bifidobacterium in the intestine. Clostridium difficile, Escherichia coli, Bacteroides fragilis, and lactobacilli are more infants fed only with formula food (Coppa et al., 2004; Vandenplas et al., 2020). In addition to the beginning of life, the microbiota also undergoes significant changes during old age. However, these changes are unclear due to the various physiological changes experienced by the elderly. These include lifestyle changes, healthy behavior, increased infection rates, inflammatory, and metabolic diseases, and, therefore the need for more medication (Ottman et al., 2012). Diet is one of the factors that most affect the intestinal microbiota. The effect of diet on the microbiota begins quickly and is the most practical known method of microbiota modulation. Antibiotics make short- and long-term changes. These effects may be permanent in some people. Non-steroidal anti-inflammatory drugs and proton pump inhibitors (PPI) are other factors that affect the microbiota (Karakan, 2018).

The Gut Microbiota

The microbiota colonizes the skin, respiratory tract, digestive and reproductive system, and other parts connected with the external environment. The colon and rectum contain the most significant number and variety of microbiota in the body (Hillman et al., 2017). The density of bacterial cells in the colon is estimated to be between 10^{11} and 10^{12} per milliliter. Viruses, fungi, archaea, and protists, whose activities are less well known, are also found in the intestinal flora. The gut microbiome encodes more than 3 million genes that produce thousands of metabolites, while the human genome consists of approximately 23,000 genes (Rinninella et al., 2019). In the research, it has been shown that there are more than 1000 phylotypes in the gastrointestinal tract microbiota. The gut microbiota consists mainly of 6 phyla: Bacteroidetes, Firmicutes, Proteobacteria, Actinobacteria, Verrucomicrobia, and Fusobacteria. Firmicutes and Bacteroidetes comprise 90% of the gut microbiota. The Firmicutes phylum consists of more than two hundred different genera such as Lactobacillus, Bacillus, Clostridium, Enterococcus, and Ruminicoccus. Bacteroidetes consists of the dominant genera such as Prevotella and Bacteroides, while Actinobacteria comprise a lesser part of the intestinal microbiota, and Bifidobacterium is the dominant genus (Arumugam et al., 2011). The microbiota is said to be unique to each individual. However, it is known to always fulfill the same physiological functions with positive properties for the host. The gut microbiota regulates many physiological processes through interactions with the host, such as nutrient digestion, nutrient intake and metabolism, synthesis of vitamins and bile acids, modulation of innate and adaptive immunity, controlling epithelial cell proliferation and differentiation, and preventing the spread of pathogenic microorganisms by colonizing mucosal surfaces (Cuevas-Sierra et al., 2019; Gomaa, 2020). The gut microbiome has a role in shaping the host's gene expression as well as its metabolic functions. The bacteria that comprise the gut microbiota can affect host metabolism by inducing epigenetic changes of essential genes that mediate the initiation and progression of diseases. Based on this, it has been emphasized that intestinal dysbiosis, known as the deterioration of intestinal microbial balance, may be associated with the recent increase in pathological conditions such as metabolic diseases such as obesity, and diabetes, inflammatory bowel disease, rheumatoid arthritis, liver diseases and cancer (Yuille et al., 2018).

Epigenetics and Microbiota

The concept of "epigenetics" was first introduced by Conrad Waddington in the 1950s and was used to describe studies that examined "causal interactions between genes that comprise the phenotype and their products" (Waddington, 1968). Epigenetics is a hereditary and reversible feature that can change gene expression without changing the sequence and structure of DNA (Sharma et al., 2020). Epigenetic modifications, which represent a fundamental mechanism by which mammalian cells can adapt their transcriptional programs to environmental events, include various mechanisms such as post-transcriptional histone modification, DNA methylation, chromatin remodeling, regulation of gene expression by miRNA and long non-coding RNAs (lncRNA) (Allis & Jenuwein, 2016; El-Sayed et al., 2021).

The human genome comprises billions of nucleotides and heterochromatin, an inactivated region that does not allow gene transcription, and euchromatin, an active region that allows specific genes to be transcribed. These regions, which can contain various genes, determine the transcriptional activity of the cell. The activity of these regions results in whether the gene associated with structural changes in chromatin is expressed, and whether this gene results is up-regulated, or down-regulated. Studies emphasize that epigenetic mechanisms have critical importance in terms of structural differentiations in chromatin and, as a result, changes in gene expression (Haggarty, 2006; Schones & Zhao, 2008; Takahashi, 2014). Epigenetic mechanisms are affected by many factors. The microbiota affects epigenetic mechanisms in two ways: 1- By changing the substrate pool used in epigenetic mechanisms, 2- By changing the activation of enzymes involved in epigenetic reactions with the various metabolites they produce (Hullar & Fu, 2014).

DNA Methylation and Microbiota

DNA methylation is the most common and studied modification at the DNA level. DNA modification occurs by covalent attachment of a methyl group with the enzyme DNA methyltransferase (DNMT) to the cytosine (C) base at the 5' position of a cytidine preceding guanosine (G). S-Adenosyl Methionine (SAM) is used as the methyl donor. DNA methylation typically occurs in CG dinucleotide sequences (Waterland & Michels, 2007). The regions where CpG dinucleotides frequently cluster, called CpG islets (CG-rich region), are functionally important as they are associated with about half of the promoter regions of the human genome. CpG dinucleotides independent of islets are mostly methylated, while promoter-related genes are typically unmethylated, and this balance is achieved by enzymatic methylation and demethylation reactions (Takahashi, 2014).

Epigenetic-modifying enzymes require a variety of substrates to catalyze changes in chromatin. Most of these donor substrates are provided by the intrinsic pathways of the host. The importance of microbiota is increasing day by day as an additional source in the synthesis of epigenetic substrates, molecules involved in the regulation of epigenetic enzyme activity, and co-factors. There are many essential micronutrients involved in the process of DNA methylation that have been shown to be associated with the gut microbiota. For example, the gut microbiota produces B vitamins (B2, B12, B6) and folate, donating methyl groups for DNA or histone methylation, and participating in the host's one-carbon metabolism as co-factors. These vitamins are well known to be susceptible to dietary intervention and intestinal dysbiosis (Walker et al., 2011; Kau et al., 2012). In addition, folic acid has a vital role in the production of S-Adenosylmethionine (SAM), which is the primary methyl donor substrate for DNA and histone methylation (Rossi et al., 2011). In addition to dietary intake, many commensal microorganisms, especially the probiotic Lactobacillus and Bifidobacterium, have been shown to be essential in folate production (Kok et al., 2018). Based on this, it is known that changes in microbiota composition can affect SAM availability and ultimately alter the histone or DNA methylation status in the host.

Short-chain fatty acids (SCFAs) form another critical group of molecules that mediate the regulation of host homeostasis by influencing epigenetic pathways. SCFAs, synthesized in the intestine by the fermentation of indigestible carbohydrates of the certain microorganisms, are essential energy sources for the intestinal microbiota (Y. Wu et al., 2021). SCFAs contribute to cellular levels of acetyl coenzyme A, affecting intermediates of the tricarboxylic acid cycle (TCA) such as α-ketoglutarate, fumarate, and succinate, which modulates the enzymatic activity of ten-eleven translocation (TET) dioxygenases involved in DNA methylation (Miro-Blanch & Yanes, 2019). In addition, butyrate has been shown to affect the DNA methylation process by inducing phosphorylation of the MAP kinase pathway. Stimulation of MAP kinase decreased DNMT1 regulation, resulting in the demethylation of RARB2, p16, and p21, known as tumor suppressor genes (Sarkar et al., 2011). Studies have shown that microbe-free mice have lower intestinal and peripheral SCFA concentrations compared to conventional mice (Sivaprakasam et al., 2018).

The gut microbiota has an essential role in the epigenetic mechanisms that regulate inflammatory responses. TLR4 recognizes important lipopolysaccharide (LPS) antigens on the cell wall of gram-negative bacteria and stimulates the innate immune system response. The intestinal microbiota has been shown to decrease TLR4 transcription by increasing methylation in the TLR4 encoded gene. Thus, resistance against LPS bacteria is formed in the colon. The maintenance of intestinal homeostasis and regulation of the intestinal mucosal immune system can be achieved by suppressing the TLR4 gene in intestinal epithelial cells through DNA methylation (Takahashi et al., 2011).

Histone Modifications and Microbiota

Histones are essential proteins that package the eukaryotic genome in the nucleosome, chromatin, and chromosome state. H1, H2A, H2B, H3, and H4 are histone proteins. Post-translational modifications of histones are crucial for both dynamic and permanent regulation of the genome. Histone modifications affect the accessibility of transcriptional regulatory factors to DNA by creating changes in the structure of the chromatin. Histone modifications are reversible. Modifications occur at the N-terminal end of histones, and these modifications are phosphorylation, acetylation, methylation, and ubiquitination. There are many enzymes involved in histone modification, and there are many co-factors involved in the function of these enzymes. Iodine, cobalt, selenium, and zinc are minerals that act as cofactors for enzymes involved in epigenetic regulation, and the gut microbiota has a role in the uptake and secretion of these minerals. Moreover, the gut microbiota produces various enzymes such as methyltransferases, acetyltransferases, deacetylases, BirA protein ligase, phosphotransferases, kinases, and synthetases (Paul et al., 2015; Taylor & Young, 2021).

It is well known that histone lysine acetylation is essential in the epigenetic regulation of gene expression in eukaryotic cells. In general, histone acetylation activates the expression of genes, while histone deacetylation suppresses gene expression. Histone acetylation modifications are controlled by the balance between histone acetyltransferase (HAT) and histone deacetylase (HDAC). HATs catalyze the acetyl group from acetyl-CoA and transfer it to the amino group found in lysine deposits, forming N-acetyl lysine, which induces the euchromatin structure. In contrast, HDACs catalyze deacetylation by hydrolysis of acetyl groups from lysine residues, causing transcriptional repression and formation of heterochromatin (Guo et al., 2018).

The gut microbiota, with its diversity and wide metabolic capacity, are known to represent a major metabolic reservoir for the production of various molecules that have significant effects on HDAC and HAT activity. For example, epicatechin and epigallocatechin-3-gallate (EGCG), which can be broken down and metabolized by the gut microbiota, can act as HAT inhibitors (Choi et al., 2009; Lee et al., 2012). Similarly, it has been shown that isothiocyanate and allyl compounds of short-chain fatty acids are the mechanisms thought to initiate beneficial effects of the intestinal microbiota in the host and are the main fermentation products that inhibit HDAC activity (Rungapamestry et al., 2008; Ciarlo et al., 2016). One of the critical pathways by which SCFA regulates T cell function is HDAC inhibition. SCFA regulates Th1, Th17, and Treg formation in different cytokine environments (Sun et al., 2017). Butyrate is the main SCFA taken up by intestinal epithelial cells. Butyrate has been shown to induce histone acetylation of Foxp3 and promote Treg differentiation, which acts as an essential anti-inflammatory effector (Haase et al., 2018). Butyrate also suppresses nuclear factor kB (NF-kB) activation by inhibiting HDAC and thus has an important role in the inflammatory response. SCFA, which also inhibits intestinal macrophage production of proinflammatory cytokines by inhibiting HDAC, induces intestinal IgA production by B cells (Sun et al., 2017). An actual example of the effect of commensal bacteria on histone modifications is Bacteroides vulgatus. Bacteroides vulgatus can induce acetylation of histone H3 and does so through an inflammatory signaling cascade. In addition, B. vulgatus induces inhibition of NF-kB transcriptional activity. It also induces transforming growth factor-b1 (TGF-b1) signaling and TGF-b1 induces histone H3 deacetylation in IL-6 gene promoters. As a result, it inhibits intestinal inflammation by suppressing IL-6 expression (Haller et al., 2003). Similarly, Bifidobacterium breve and Lactobacillus rhamnosus GG, which inhibit LPS-induced IL-17 and IL-23 expression, have been shown to inhibit this by suppressing histone acetylation (Ghadimi et al., 2012). The microbial flora also regulates MHC gene expression such as MHC class II to affect immune homeostasis. It can do this by coordinating the activity of enzymes that acetylate histones (J. Wu et al., 2022). Therefore, HDAC inhibitors have taken their place as potential therapeutics in various stages of clinical trials. Microbial-derived HDAC inhibitors (HDACi) are evaluated in various studies to treat inflammatory and degenerative disorders, especially cancer (Yuille et al., 2018).

Noncoding RNA and Microbiota

In addition to chromatin remodeling via histone modification and DNA methylation, noncoding RNAs also have important roles in epigenetic regulation. Non-Coding RNAs (ncRNA), which are RNA transcripts that are not translated into proteins, have an epigenetic effect that inhibits the expression of target mRNA at the post-transcriptional level. According to their size, they can be classified as small ncRNAs (<200–300 bp) (including microRNA (miRNA)), long ncRNAs (lncRNAs; >200–300 bp), piwi interacting RNAs (piRNAs), and short interfering RNAs (siRNAs) (Röther & Meister, 2011; Dempsey et al., 2018).

The role of the gut microbiome in lncRNA gene regulation in the host is being understood more and more and the number of studies revealing this is increasing. A study comparing gut epithelial tissues from germ-free and gnotobiotic mice to identify microbiota-regulated lncRNA showed that six lncRNAs were up-regulated, supporting that it can distinguish mice by unique microbial compositions. Furthermore, these microbiota-derived lncRNAs were overexpressed in the thymus and spleen, supporting that they may also have a role in host immune regulation (Liang et al., 2015). For evaluating lncRNA expression, different tissue types such as colon, ileum, jejunum, duodenum, liver, adipose tissue, and skeletal muscles were evaluated instead of epithelial tissues, and tissue-specific modulation of lncRNAs was demonstrated in response to the microbiota in these peripheral tissues. Most of the lncRNAs found to be regulated by the gut microbiome are in the jejunum (Dempsey et al., 2018). This result showed that the microbiota has a vital role in the regulation of the expression of lncRNAs in the gut and immune organs, and metabolic tissues.

MiRNAs, which are important in different stages of the regulation of many physiological or pathological events (such as cell differentiation, cell proliferation, tumor development), can also regulate intestinal epithelial cells dependent on the commensal microbiota, which are known to regulate intestinal homeostasis and dysbiosis (Tsuchiya et al., 2006; Ohland & MacNaughton, 2010). Paneth and goblet cells from intestinal epithelial cells (IECs) have been shown to be the primary source of miRNAs in the intestinal lumen. The miRNA secreted from different cells then participates in shaping the gut microbiota. It is known that miRNAs expressed by the host, which affect the growth of microbial communities and regulate the transcription of microbial genes, can also be affected by the microbiota through microbiota-mediated metabolites that affect the host physiology (Y. Wu et al., 2021). Host epigenetic effects vary according to different gut microbiota species.

Recent studies have revealed that the relationship between circulating miRNA and the gut microbiota is essential in insulin resistance and obesity. MiR-21-5p, miR-185-5p, and miR-130b-3p, which were reported to control obesity-related pathologies, were found to have a negative correlation with Bacteroides eggerthii. It has also been shown that the excess of B. intestinihominis is inversely related to the expressions of miR-103'a-3p, miR-107, miR-142-5p, miR-222-3p. These miRNAs are known to regulate genes involved in metabolic pathways such as insulin signaling, fatty acid degradation, and glycerol lipid metabolism (Assmann et al., 2020).The microbiota, which is known to have a regulatory effect on host miRNA expression, down-regulates the expression of miR-107 in macrophages and dendritic cells and regulates immune hemostasis by affecting NF-κB and MyD88 pathways (Xue et al., 2014). The miRNA sequence in cells has been shown to change with the development of Helicobacter pylori, Salmonella enterica, and Mycobacterium tuberculosis infection. Mir-let-7f targets TNFAIP3, a negative regulator of the NF-κB pathway, which activates the host immune response and reduces microbial survival and is downregulated in Mycobacterium tuberculosis infections (Kumar et al., 2015; Y. Wu et al., 2021). MiRNAs have an essential role in the host response against both pathogenic bacteria and non-pathogenic members of the microbiota.

Conclusion

The microbiota is one of the main factors involved in epigenomic regulation in the host. The human genome is also effective in the formation of the microbiota. It has been shown that the epigenetic changes provided by the commensal microorganisms of the host have a significant effect on the regulation of life development, homeostasis, disease development, and course, starting from the in utero period. It is known that the disruption of the microbiota-host relationship with epigenetic misregulation is associated with various pathologies, including inflammatory bowel diseases, degenerative diseases, autoimmune diseases, and colorectal cancer. It is known that epigenetic changes can be reversible, and it is thought that this may benefit the development, progression or prevention of other metabolic diseases and cancer, especially obesity.

References

Allis, C. D., & Jenuwein, T. (2016). The molecular hallmarks of epigenetic control. *Nature Reviews Genetics*, *17*(8), 487–500. https://doi.org/10.1038/nrg.2016.59.

Arumugam, M., Raes, J., Pelletier, E., Paslier, D. le, Yamada, T., Mende, D. R., Fernandes, G. R., Tap, J., Bruls, T., Batto, J. M., Bertalan, M., Borruel, N., Casellas, F., Fernandez, L., Gautier, L., Hansen, T., Hattori, M., Hayashi, T., Kleerebezem, M., … Zeller, G. (2011). Enterotypes of the human gut microbiome. *Nature*, *473*(7346), 174–180. https://doi.org/10.1038/nature09944.

Assmann, T. S., Cuevas-Sierra, A., Riezu-Boj, J. I., Milagro, F. I., & Martínez, J. A. (2020). Comprehensive analysis reveals novel interactions between circulating micrornas and gut microbiota composition in human obesity. *International Journal of Molecular Sciences*, *21*(24), 1–17. https://doi.org/10.3390/ijms21249509.

Biasucci, G., Benenati, B., Morelli, L., Bessi, E., & Boehm, G. (2008). Cesarean delivery may affect the early biodiversity of intestinal bacteria. *Journal of Nutrition*, *138*(9), 1796–1800. https://doi.org/10.1093/jn/138.9.1796s.

Choi, K. C., Myung, G. J., Lee, Y. H., Joo, C. Y., Seung, H. K., Kang, H. B., Kim, M. J., Cha, J. H., Young, J. K., Woo, J. J., Jae, M. L., & Yoon, H. G. (2009). Epigallocatechin-3-gallate, a histone acetyltransferase inhibitor, inhibits EBV-induced B lymphocyte transformation via suppression of RelA acetylation. *Cancer Research*, *69*(2), 583–592. https://doi.org/10.1158/0008-5472.CAN-08-2442.

Ciarlo, E., Heinonen, T., Herderschee, J., Fenwick, C., Mombelli, M., le Roy, D., & Roger, T. (2016). Impact of the microbial derived short chain fatty acid propionate on host susceptibility to bacterial and fungal infections in vivo. *Scientific Reports*, *6*(37944), 1–15. https://doi.org/10.1038/srep37944.

Coppa, G. v., Bruni, S., Morelli, L., Soldi, S., & Gabrielli, O. (2004). The first prebiotics in humans: human milk oligosaccharides. *Journal of Clinical Gastroenterology*, *38*(6 Suppl), 80–83. https://doi.org/10.1097/01.mcg.0000128926.14285.25.

Cuevas-Sierra, A., Ramos-Lopez, O., Riezu-Boj, J. I., Milagro, F. I., & Martinez, J. A. (2019). Diet, Gut Microbiota, and Obesity: Links with Host Genetics and Epigenetics and Potential Applications. *Advances in Nutrition*, *10*, 17–30. https://doi.org/10.1093/advances/nmy078.

Dempsey, J., Zhang, A., & Cui, J. Y. (2018). Coordinate regulation of long non-coding RNAs and protein-coding genes in germ-free mice. *BMC Genomics*, *19*(1), 1–24. https://doi.org/10.1186/s12864-018-5235-3.

El-Sayed, A., Aleya, L., & Kamel, M. (2021). Microbiota and epigenetics: promising therapeutic approaches? *Environmental Science and Pollution Research*, *28*(36), 49343. – 49361. https://doi.org/10.1007/s11356-021-15623-6.

Ghadimi, D., Helwig, U., Schrezenmeir, J., Heller, K. J., & de Vrese, M. (2012). Epigenetic imprinting by commensal probiotics inhibits the IL-23/IL-17 axis in an in vitro model of the intestinal mucosal immune system. *Journal of Leukocyte Biology*, *92*(4), 895–911. https://doi.org/10.1189/jlb.0611286.

Gomaa, E. Z. (2020). Human gut microbiota/microbiome in health and diseases: a review. *Antonie van Leeuwenhoek, International Journal of General and Molecular Microbiology*, *113*(12), 2019–2040. https://doi.org/10.1007/s10482-020-01474-7.

Guo, P., Chen, W., Li, H., Li, M., & Li, L. (2018). The Histone Acetylation Modifications of Breast Cancer and their Therapeutic Implications. In *Pathology and Oncology Research* (Vol. 24, Issue 4, pp. 807–813). https://doi.org/10.1007/s12253-018-0433-5.

Haase, S., Haghikia, A., Wilck, N., Müller, D. N., & Linker, R. A. (2018). Impacts of microbiome metabolites on immune regulation and autoimmunity. In *Immunology* (Vol. 154, Issue 2, pp. 230–238). https://doi.org/10.1111/imm.12933.

Haggarty P. Epigenetics. In *"Modern Nutrition in Health and Disease"*. (eds) Shils ME, Shike M, Ross AC, Caballero B, Cousins RJ. 11th ed. Baltimore, Lippincott Williams & Wilkins. 2006;534-539..

Haller, D., Holt, L., Kim, S. C., Schwabe, R. F., Sartor, R. B., & Jobin, C. (2003). Transforming growth factor-β1 inhibits non-pathogenic Gram-negative bacteria-induced NF-κB recruitment to the interleukin-6 gene promoter in intestinal epithelial cells through modulation of histone acetylation. *Journal of Biological Chemistry*, *278*(26), 23851–23860. https://doi.org/10.1074/jbc.M300075200.

Hillman, E. T., Lu, H., Yao, T., & Nakatsu, C. H. (2017). Microbial ecology along the gastrointestinal tract. *Microbes and Environments*, *32*(4), 300–313. https://doi.org/10.1264/jsme2.ME17017.

Hullar, M. A. J., & Fu, B. C. (2014). Diet, the gut microbiome, and epigenetics. *Cancer Journal (United States)*, *20*(3), 170–175. https://doi.org/10.1097/PPO.0000000000000053.

Karakan, T. (2018). Factors Affecting Microbiota. *Turkey Clinics*, 1–4..

Kau, A. L., Ahern, P. P., Griffin, N. W., Goodman, A. L., & Jeffrey, I. (2012). Human nutrition, the gut microbiome, and immune system: envisioning the future. *Nature*, *474*(7351), 327–336..

Kok, D. E., Steegenga, W. T., & McKay, J. A. (2018). Folate and epigenetics: Why we should not forget bacterial biosynthesis. *Epigenomics*, *10*(9), 1147–1150. https://doi.org/10.2217/epi-2018-0117.

Kumar, M., Sahu, S. K., Kumar, R., Subuddhi, A., Maji, R. K., Jana, K., Gupta, P., Raffetseder, J., Lerm, M., Ghosh, Z., van Loo, G., Beyaert, R., Gupta, U. D., Kundu, M., & Basu, J. (2015). MicroRNA let-7 modulates the immune response to mycobacterium tuberculosis infection via control of A20, an inhibitor of the NF-κB pathway. *Cell Host and Microbe*, *17*(3), 345–356. https://doi.org/10.1016/j.chom.2015.01.007.

Lederberg, J., & McCray, A. T. (2001). "Ome Sweet Omics": a genealogical treasury of words. *The Scientist*, *15*(7), 8–8.

Lee, Y. H., Kwak, J., Choi, H. K., Choi, K. C., Kim, S., Lee, J., Jun, W., Park, H. J., & Yoon, H. G. (2012). EGCG suppresses prostate cancer cell growth modulating acetylation of androgen receptor by anti-histone acetyltransferase activity. *International Journal of Molecular Medicine*, *30*(1), 69–74. https://doi.org/10.3892/ijmm.2012.966.

Ley R. E., Peterson D. A., & Gordon J. I. (2006). Ecological and evolutionary forces shaping microbial diversity in the human gut. *Cell*, *124*(4), 837–848.

Liang, L., Ai, L., Qian, J., Fang, J. Y., & Xu, J. (2015). Long noncoding RNA expression profiles in gut tissues constitute molecular signatures that reflect the types of microbes. *Scientific Reports*, *5*, 1–8. https://doi.org/10.1038/srep11763.

Marchesi, J. R., & Ravel, J. (2015). The vocabulary of microbiome research: a proposal. *Microbiome*, *3*(1), 1–3. https://doi.org/10.1186/s40168-015-0094-5.

Martin FP, & Kochhar S. (2015). Introduction to Metabonomics in Systems Biology Research. In *Metabonomics and Gut Microbiota in Nutrition and Disease* (pp. 10–12). Springer, London..

Miro-Blanch, J., & Yanes, O. (2019). Epigenetic regulation at the interplay between gut microbiota and host metabolism. *Frontiers in Genetics*, *10*(JUL), 1–9. https://doi.org/10.3389/fgene.2019.00638.

Ohland, C. L., & MacNaughton, W. K. (2010). Probiotic bacteria and intestinal epithelial barrier function. *American Journal of Physiology - Gastrointestinal and Liver Physiology*, *298*(6), 807–819. https://doi.org/10.1152/ajpgi.00243.2009.

Ottman, N., Smidt, H., de Vos, W. M., & Belzer, C. (2012). The function of our microbiota: who is out there and what do they do? *Frontiers in Cellular and Infection Microbiology*, *2*(104), 1–11. https://doi.org/10.3389/fcimb.2012.00104.

Paul, B., Barnes, S., Demark-Wahnefried, W., Morrow, C., Salvador, C., Skibola, C., & Tollefsbol, T. O. (2015). Influences of diet and the gut microbiome on epigenetic modulation in cancer and other diseases. *Clinical Epigenetics*, *7*(1), 1–11. https://doi.org/10.1186/s13148-015-0144-7.

Quigley, E. M. M. (2013). Gut bacteria in health and disease. *Gastroenterology and Hepatology*, *9*(9), 560–569.

Rinninella, E., Raoul, P., Cintoni, M., Franceschi, F., Miggiano, G. A. D., Gasbarrini, A., & Mele, M. C. (2019). What is the healthy gut microbiota composition? A changing ecosystem across age, environment, diet, and diseases. *Microorganisms*, *7*(1), 1–22. https://doi.org/10.3390/microorganisms7010014.

Rossi, M., Amaretti, A., & Raimondi, S. (2011). Folate production by probiotic bacteria. *Nutrients*, *3*(1), 118–134. https://doi.org/10.3390/nu3010118.

Röther, S., & Meister, G. (2011). Small RNAs derived from longer non-coding RNAs. In *Biochimie* (Vol. 93, Issue 11, pp. 1905–1915). https://doi.org/10.1016/j.biochi.2011.07.032.

Rungapamestry, V., Rabot, S., Fuller, Z., Ratcliffe, B., & Duncan, A. J. (2008). Influence of cooking duration of cabbage and presence of colonic microbiota on the excretion of N-acetylcysteine conjugates of allyl isothiocyanate and bioactivity of phase 2 enzymes in F344 rats. *British Journal of Nutrition*, *99*(4), 773–781. https://doi.org/10.1017/S0007114507841134.

Sarkar, S., Abujamra, A. L., Loew, J. E., Forman, L. W., Perrine, S. P., & Faller, D. v. (2011). Histone deacetylase inhibitors reverse CpG methylation by regulating DNMT1 through ERK signaling. *Anticancer Research*, *31*(9), 2723–2732..

Schones, D. E., & Zhao, K. (2008). Genome-wide approaches to studying chromatin modifications. *Nature Reviews Genetics*, *9*(3), 179–191. https://doi.org/10.1038/nrg2270.

Sharma, M., Li, Y., Stoll, M. L., & Tollefsbol, T. O. (2020). The Epigenetic Connection Between the Gut Microbiome in Obesity and Diabetes. *Frontiers in Genetics*, *10*(1329), 1–15. https://doi.org/10.3389/fgene.2019.01329.

Sivaprakasam, S., Bhutia, Y. D., Yang, S., & Ganapathy, V. (2018). Short-chain fatty acid transporters: Role in colonic homeostasis. *Comprehensive Physiology*, *8*(1), 299–314. https://doi.org/10.1002/cphy.c170014.

Sun, M., Wu, W., Liu, Z., & Cong, Y. (2017). Microbiota metabolite short chain fatty acids, GPCR, and inflammatory bowel diseases. In *Journal of Gastroenterology* (Vol. 52, Issue 1, pp. 1–8). Springer Tokyo. https://doi.org/10.1007/s00535-016-1242-9.

Takahashi, K. (2014). Influence of bacteria on epigenetic gene control. *Cellular and Molecular Life Sciences*, *71*(6), 1045–1054. https://doi.org/10.1007/s00018-013-1487-x.

Takahashi, K., Sugi, Y., Nakano, K., Tsuda, M., Kurihara, K., Hosono, A., & Shuichi, K. (2011). Epigenetic control of the host gene by commensal bacteria in large intestinal epithelial cells. *Journal of Biological Chemistry*, *286*(41), 35755–35762. https://doi.org/10.1074/jbc.M111.271007.

Taylor, B. C., & Young, N. L. (2021). Combinations of histone post-Translational modifications. *Biochemical Journal*, *478*(3), 511–532. https://doi.org/10.1042/BCJ20200170.

Tsuchiya, S., Okuno, Y., & Tsujimoto, G. (2006). MicroRNA: Biogenetic and functional mechanisms and involvements in cell differentiation and cancer. *Journal of Pharmacological Sciences*, *101*(4), 267–270. https://doi.org/10.1254/jphs.CPJ06013X.

Vandenplas, Y., Carnielli, V. P., Ksiazyk, J., Luna, M. S., Migacheva, N., Mosselmans, J. M., Picaud, J. C., Possner, M., Singhal, A., & Wabitsch, M. (2020). Factors affecting early-life intestinal microbiota development. *Nutrition*, *78*, 1–7. https://doi.org/10.1016/j.nut.2020.110812.

Waddington C. H. The basic ideas of biolog. In *Towards a Theoretical Biology.* (ed.) CH Waddington. Vol.1. 1st ed. Edinburgh, Edinburgh University Press. 1968; 1–32.

Walker, A. K., Jacobs, R. L., Watts, J. L., Rottiers, V., Jiang, K., Finnegan, D. M., Shioda, T., Hansen, M., Yang, F., Niebergall, L. J., Vance, D. E., Tzoneva, M., Hart, A. C., & Näär, A. M. (2011). A conserved SREBP-1/phosphatidylcholine feedback circuit regulates lipogenesis in metazoans. *Cell*, *147*(4), 840–852. https://doi.org/10.1016/j.cell.2011.09.045.

Waterland, R. A., & Michels, K. B. (2007). Epigenetic epidemiology of the developmental origins hypothesis. *Annual Review of Nutrition*, *27*, 363–388. https://doi.org/10.1146/annurev.nutr.27.061406.093705.

Wu, J., Zhao, Y., Wang, X., Kong, L., Johnston, L. J., Lu, L., & Ma, X. (2022). Dietary nutrients shape gut microbes and intestinal mucosa via epigenetic modifications. In *Critical Reviews in Food Science and Nutrition* (Vol. 62, Issue 3, pp. 783–797). https://doi.org/10.1080/10408398.2020.1828813.

Wu, Y., Wang, C. Z., Wan, J. Y., Yao, H., & Yuan, C. S. (2021). Dissecting the interplay mechanism between epigenetics and gut microbiota: Health maintenance and disease prevention. In *International Journal of Molecular Sciences* (Vol. 22, Issue 13, pp. 1–26). https://doi.org/10.3390/ijms22136933.

Xue, X., Cao, A. T., Cao, X., Yao, S., Carlsen, E. D., Soong, L., Liu, C. G., Liu, X., Liu, Z., Duck, L. W., Elson, C. O., & Cong, Y. (2014). Downregulation of microRNA-107 in intestinal CD11c+ myeloid cells in response to microbiota and proinflammatory cytokines increases IL-23p19 expression. *European Journal of Immunology*, *44*(3), 673–682. https://doi.org/10.1002/eji.201343717.

Yuille, S., Reichardt, N., Panda, S., Dunbar, H., & Mulder, I. E. (2018). Human gut bacteria as potent class I histone deacetylase inhibitors in vitro through production of butyric acid and valeric acid. *PLoS ONE*, *13*(7), 1–12. https://doi.org/10.1371/journal.pone.0201073.

Zhu, B., Wang, X., & Li, L. (2010). Human gut microbiome: The second genome of human body. *Protein and Cell*, *1*(8), 718–725. https://doi.org/10.1007/s13238-010-0093-z.

Chapter 8

The Role of Non-Coding RNAs in Epigenetic Mechanisms

Gözde Öztan*, PhD
Department of Medicine, Istanbul University, Istanbul, Turkey

Abstract

The study of epigenetics examines how genetic changes in gene expression are transmitted from one generation to another and are not caused by changes in the DNA sequence. A key role played by epigenetic mechanisms is thought to be in cellular growth, differentiation, and autoimmune diseases. There are several epigenetic mechanisms, including DNA methylation, histone modifications, and non-coding RNA regulation.

Transcripts that do not have protein-coding capacity in our genome are defined as non-coding RNA (ncRNA). The post-transcriptional regulation of genes is greatly influenced by non-coding RNAs. These ncRNAs are composed of small non-coding RNAs (sncRNA) and long non-coding RNAs (lncRNA) according to their length. Epigenetic mechanisms (genetic imprinting and dosage compensation) have been found to regulate the expression of lncRNAs. The function of centromeres is regulated by sncRNAs, which are involved in gene expression, chromatin organization, and modification.

In this chapter, the potential epigenetic mechanisms of ncRNAs and their associated cellular processes are presented. The importance of non-coding RNAs in the etiology of diseases has been revealed in recent genetic studies. Non-coding RNAs have been shown to have functions ranging from control of gene expression, epigenetic mechanisms, and signal transduction. In particular, it has been determined that some piRNAs, miRNAs, and siRNAs function in common pathways and are involved in regulatory mechanisms.

Keywords: epigenetics, non-coding RNA, gene expression, genetic mechanisms

Introduction

Non-Coding RNAs (ncRNAs)

Higher organisms have DNA as their genetic material, and after DNA is translated into RNA, RNA transforms the genetic code into proteins. RNA consists of mRNA that can be translated into protein, along with non-coding RNA (ncRNA), which cannot be translated into protein.

* Corresponding Author's E-mail: gozdeoztan@yahoo.com.

In: Epigenetics: Beyond the Genetics and Medicine
Editors: Sevgi Durna Daştan and Nazan Yurtcu
ISBN: 979-8-88697-228-3

The numbers of non-coding RNA genes are not the same among species, and the complexity of organism does not appear to be correlated with the abundance of ncRNA gene. The existence of ncRNAs implies their potential importance. Approximately 80% of mammalian genome DNA is actively transcribed and elaborately regulated, most of which are ncRNA's, according to systematic annotated and functionally characterized genes (Li & Liu, 2019).

There are different categories of ncRNA depending on their length. In a lncRNA (long non-coding RNAs), the RNA sequences are longer than 200 nucleotides and their loci may exist in any part of the genome, either inside other genes, opposite strands, intergenic or introns regions. Non-coding RNAs (sncRNAs) are thought to consist of a heterogeneous group of molecules that includes microRNAs (miRNAs), PIWI-interacting RNAs (piRNAs), and short interfering RNAs (siRNAs) (Figure 1). Various cell types and tissues contain ncRNAs capable of transporting glycans to sialine in the cell membrane (Burgosa et al., 2021).

An important role for ncRNAs, particularly small ncRNAs, is to regulate gene expression, especially through epigenetic controls. Chromatin remodeling, RNA-associated gene silencing, chromosome inactivation, genomic imprinting, and paramutation occur through epigenetic mechanisms. Mammalian cells have been shown to suppress transcription through siRNA-mediated DNA methylation and histone methylation in the promoter region. The formation of chromatin structure is a complex process that requires multiple epigenetic factors. The role of non-coding RNAs in epigenetic regulation of eukaryotic chromatin is becoming increasingly apparent (Zhou et al., 2010).

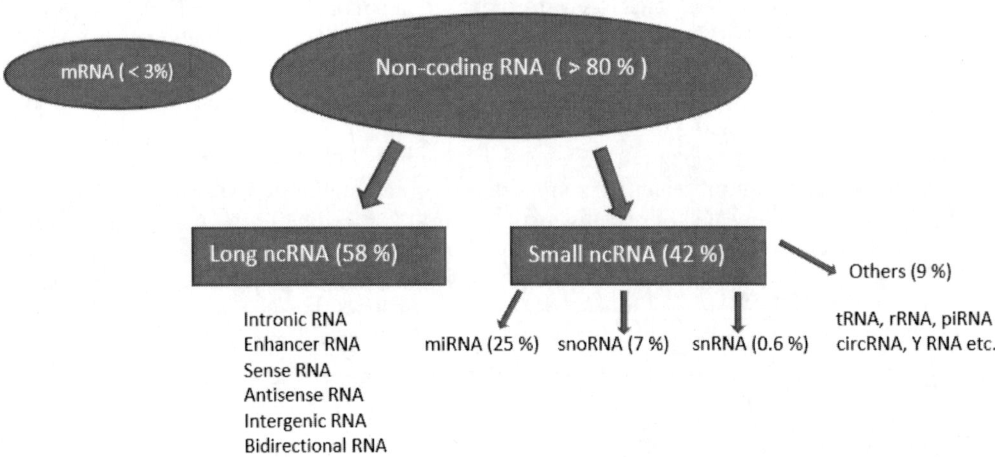

Figure 1. RNA types and relative abundances in cells: ncRNA, non-coding RNA; miRNA, microRNA; snoRNA, small nucleolar RNA; transfer RNA; rRNA, ribosomal RNA; piRNA, PIWI-interacting RNA; circRNA, circular RNA; snRNA, small nuclear RNA; tRNA, Y RNA (Burgosa et al., 2021).

RNA interference (RNAi) occurs when non-coding RNA interferes with gene transcription. RNAi may impair the function of the suppressor of antisense non-coding RNAs, resulting in the failure to direct epigenetic silencing complexes to a specific location by suppressing antisense non-coding RNAs. Several antisense non-coding RNAs have been identified in bidirectionally transcribed genes, most of which are tumor suppressors. A substantial amount of sequence overlap is found among the sense mRNA and antisense non-coding RNA in the 3' UTR region of genes that have been reported to demonstrate bidirectional transcription (Morris, 2009).

MicroRNAs (miRNAs)

MiRNAs are non-coding RNAs (ncRNAs) with an approximate length of 20-22 nt, which regulate gene expression post-transcriptionally (Coelho-Lima & Spyridopoulos, 2018). Many biological processes are regulated by miRNA Primary precursors of most of those genes are transcribed by RNA polymerase II. Pri-miRNAs are converted into precursor miRNAs (pre-miRNAs) by the microprocessor, a complex protein made up of DROSHA and DGCR8 involved in ribonuclease activity (Burgosa et al., 2021). A mature miRNA partially binds to the 3′ UTR of a mRNA to modulate gene expression by repressing translation or degrading mRNA (Figure 2). In the genome, miRNA-coding sequences are transcribed by RNA polymerase II, which formulates primary miRNA transcripts (pri-miRNAs), which are found in intragenic or intergenic regions. A multi-protein complex of microprocessor containing DiGeorge syndrome critical region 8 (DGCR8) and Drosha cleaves the pri-miRNA into smaller hairpin structures of ~70-100 nucleotides, termed precursor miRNAs.

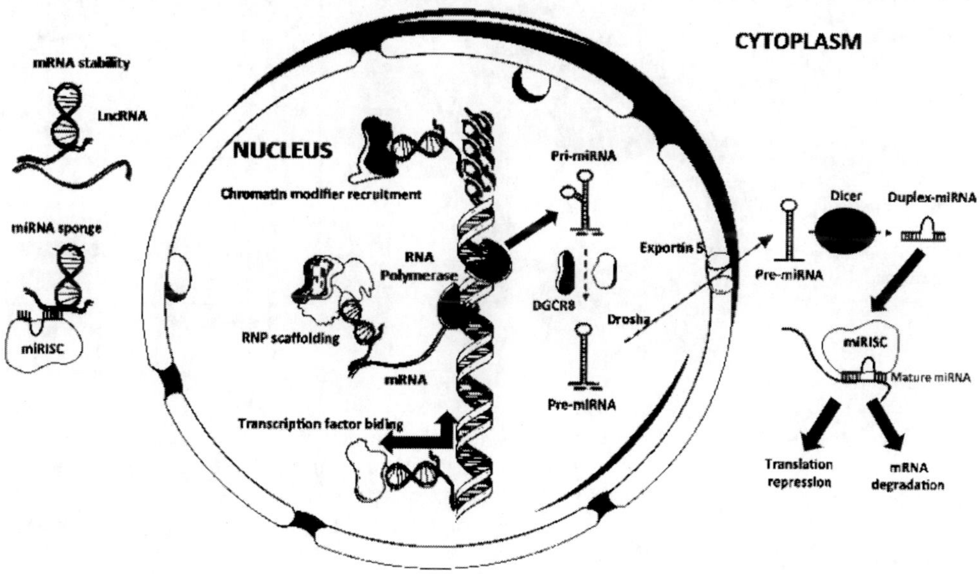

Figure 2. The function of microRNA and lncRNA. As RNA Polymerase II transcribes microRNAs from intragenic or intergenic regions of the genome, multiple hairpin transcripts are created known as primary miRNAs (Pri-miRNA). Drosha and DGCR8 are involved in the processing of pri-miRNAs to create precursor miRNAs (pre-miRNAs). The pre-miRNAs are exported to the cytoplasm by Exportin 5, which is responsible for assembling miRNA transcripts (Coelho-Lima & Spyridopoulos, 2018).

As the mature miRNA binds to the target mRNA transcript, it is incorporated into the miRNA-induced silencing complex (miRISC) (Coelho-Lima & Spyridopoulos, 2018). Several expression profiling studies have indicated that miRNAs are important for gonadal development (Burgosa et al., 2021).

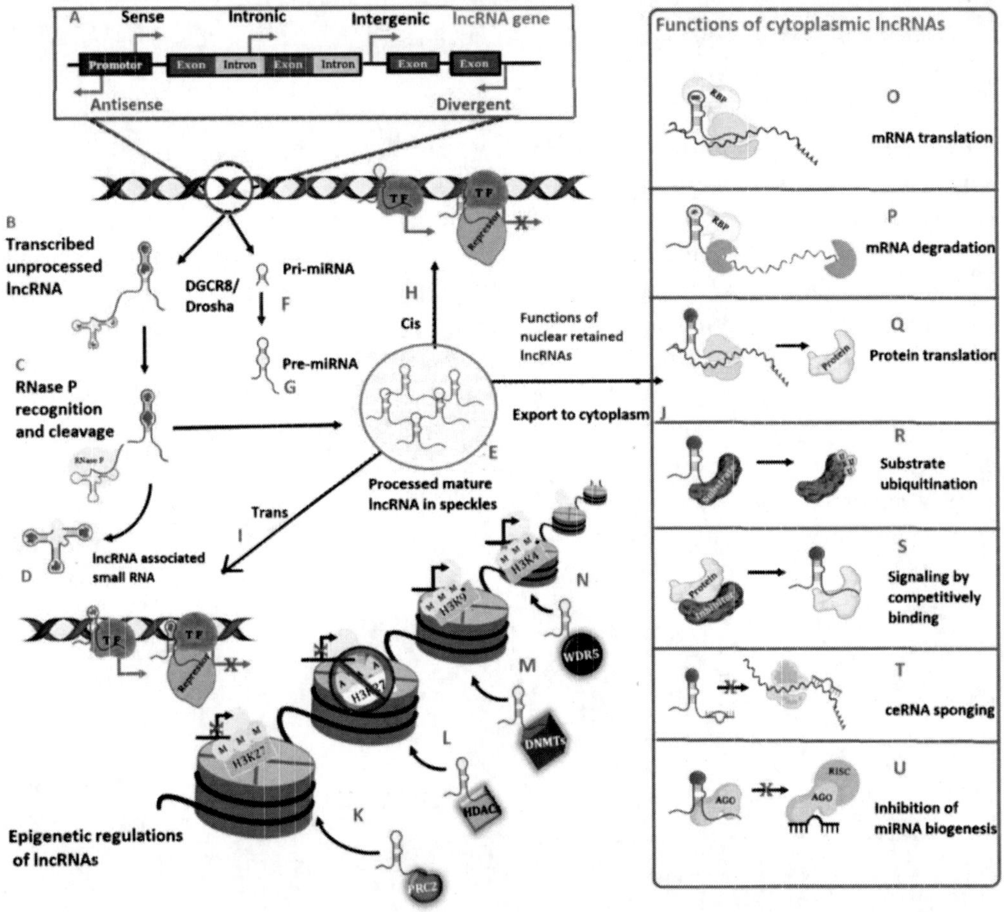

Figure 3. The biogenesis and functions of lncRNA. (A) There are five classes of heterogeneous transcriptions over 200 nucleotides, depending on their genomic localization: sense, antisense, intronic, intergenic, and divergent. (B) These categories of lncRNA are transcribed by RNA polymerase II from the gene for each lncRNA. (C) A poly A-tail and flanking motif region of the mature RNA is processed by RNase P due to its presence of t-RNA-like structures at its 3' end. (D) The 5' end of the lncRNA is exported to the cytoplasm following the action of RNase Z and CCA addition. (E) In nuclear speckles, matured lncRNA can be found either in the nuclear nucleus or in the cytoplasm, depending on where it functions. (F) As well as lncRNAs, some small RNAs are transcribed from lncRNAs, such as pri-miRNAs. (G) A pri-miRNA is converted by the DGCR8 and Drosha complex to a pre-miRNA. (H) Transcripts can be found in the same gene or (I) in different distantly located genes or chromosomes. (J) Typically, nuclear pores are the means by which cytoplasmic transcripts are transported to the cytoplasm (Jayasuriya et al., 2022).

Many cellular processes during pregnancy are regulated by miRNAs, including placental development, endometrial receptivity, angiogenesis, and immune cells. MicroRNAs regulate the immune balance between a mother and her children, as well as helping placenta development and pregnancy success. RNA can be silenced by miRNA similarly to siRNA, The short hairpins of miRNA are derived from the self-folding areas of RNA transcripts. They cleave mRNA targets with a complementary base sequence as part of their molecular mechanism. Additionally, translational repression occurs as a result of an imperfect base sequence (Frías-Lasserre & Villagra, 2017).

Long Non-Coding RNAs (lncRNAs)

The term "long non-coding RNA" (lncRNA) refers to ncRNAs longer than 200 nucleotides, and they are classified according to their length, genomic localization or molecular function. The non-coding RNAs find their origins in the introns of protein-coding genes (intronic lncRNAs), intergenic regions (LincRNAs, long intervening non-coding RNAs), and antisense strands of a gene (antisense lncRNAs), or are synthesized by back-splicing of exons (circular RNAs). Functioning lncRNAs differ from microRNAs in that they are located both in the nucleus and cytoplasm, enabling them to generate effects at the epigenetic, transcriptional, translational, and post-translational levels (Figure 3). A lncRNA regulates transcription of genes by binding to transcription factors, stimulating or inhibiting transcription (Coelho-Lima & Spyridopoulos, 2018).

Multiple diseases are caused by epigenetic modifications and transcriptional and post-transcriptional processes regulated by long non-coding RNAs. In recent studies, researchers have discovered that long non-coding RNAs have an important role in modulating the type of programmed cell death known as pyroptosis, which has a significant role in the development of many diseases. The lncRNAs act on proteins related to the pyroptosis signaling pathway directly or indirectly to influence diseases such as cardio-vascular diseases, kidney diseases, and immune diseases (He et al., 2020).

LncRNAs are transcripts that contain longer and fewer exons. lncRNAs have a 3'-polyadenylated tail and a 5'-methyl-guanosine cap, similar to mRNAs, making them unique. LncRNA interacts with DNA, RNA, and transcriptional molecules in the context of various biological processes, including modifications of histones, DNA methylation, chromatin remodeling, gene expression, gene silencing, heat shock response, and embryogenesis. These lncRNAs regulate gene transcription by binding to RNA-DNA, RNA-RNA, RNA-protein (Jayasuriya et al., 2022).

PIWI-Interacting RNAs (piRNAs)

PIWI interacting RNAs (piRNAs) have a length of 21-35 nucleotides that regulate gene expression, silence transposons, and inhibit viral infection in animals. Precursors of piRNA are synthesized at genomic loci called piRNA clusters. A piRNA directs its target RNA to be cleaved, promotes the assambly of heterochromatin, and methylates DNA. PiRNAs are 2′-O-methyl-modified 3′ termini and regulate PIWI-clade Argonautes rather than AGO-clade proteins, which are components of the miRNA and siRNA pathways (Ozata et al., 2019).

These piRNAs have a vital role in animal gametogenesis, reproductive function, control of endogenous genes expression, and fight against viruses. Since old transposons decay and new transposon invasions lead to new piRNAs that protect germline genomes, transposon silencing piRNAs diverge. Three types of piRNAs are produced by specific mammalian species:

transposon-silencing piRNAs, pachytene piRNAs, and 3' untranslated region piRNAs (Wu & Zamore, 2021).

The piRNA molecule can be found in various genomic sequences, including exons, introns, and repetitive sequences. Primary and secondary amplification have an important role in the biogenesis of piRNAs. RNA polymerase II, the Rhino-Deadlock-Cutoff complex, Moonshiner, TBP-related factor 2, three prime repair exonucleases, and U2AF-associated protein are some of the proteins involved in the transcription of piRNA precursors. RNA polymerase II first associates with piRNA clusters and is then recruited by the RDC complex to initiate transcription. Pre-piRNAs are incorporated into PIWI proteins, trimmed with Nibbler, and methylated by Hen1. The AGO3 and Aubergine (Aub) proteins catalyze the primary piRNAs, and a subsequent secondary amplification produces mature piRNAs. AUB contains piRNAs that recognize and cleave complementary RNAs. This process creates a new piRNA that is loaded into AGO3 and induces the degradation of complementary RNA (Cai et al., 2022).

Importance of ncRNAs in Epigenetic Mechanisms

An epigenetic change is an inheritable variation of the epigenotype of cells which does not alter the primary structure of DNA. Epigenetics is the study of how genes grow, which is linked to paramutation, metastable epialleles, DNA methylation, and chromatin remodeling, which require various types of ncRNAs (Frías-Lasserre & Villagra, 2017). Furthermore, there is emerging evidence that long non-coding RNAs can regulate biological processes by interacting with chromatin. A critical epigenetic factor is DNA methylation at promoters of protein-coding genes. Until now, there have been only a small number of examples of lncRNA regulating promoter methylation of targets genes, which led us to focus our attention more intently on these possibilities. The DNA demethylation and chromatin structure of enhancer regions with distant CpGs influence gene activity and transcription (Yang et al., 2021).

The researchers discovered the ability of polycomb proteins (PcG) to cause heritable gene silencing specifically through mediating X-inactivation in D. melanogaster. The targeting of PcG proteins to coding regions is largely caused by lncRNAs. The gene expression of this class of transcripts is also regulated by several epigenetic enzymes, as well as interacting with PcG protein complexes. Fendrr, an lncRNA that participates in cardiac development, modulates the promoter occupancy of the H3K4 methyltransferases TrxG/MLL and PRC2 by directly binding and/or binding to their promoters. Additionally to regulating gene expression via histone modification, it appears that lncRNAs also contribute to DNA methylation-mediated gene silencing. The transcription of 50-200 nucleotide short RNAs has been identified in H3K27me3-rich PRC2 target genes that are silenced by cell type. By interacting with PRC2, these short RNAs regulate chromatin repression in cis and stabilize the complex near transcription sites by stabilizing stem-loop structures (Peschansky & Wahlestedt, 2014).

The antisense unspliced lncRNA has been proposed to be epigenetically repressive of the RASSF1A tumor suppressor gene. ANRASSF1 specifically represses RASSF1 expression by covering up the antisense transcript in locations specific to RASSF1. PRC2 binds to the RASSF1A promoter through ANRASSF1, resulting in a decrease in RASSF1A expression as well as an increase in cell proliferation. In vitro and in vivo, loc285194 has been shown to be a target of p53 transcription, and ectopic expression inhibits tumor cell growth (Cao, 2014).

Gene regulation is accomplished by short double-stranded RNAs called ncRNAs that bind to either the coding sequences or the promoter sequences of an mRNA as part of the RNAi mechanism. The binding process disrupts normal mRNA processing, which in turn suppresses mRNA expression. These short ncRNAs regulate chromatin-mediated gene silencing and DNA rearrangement, which are important cellular processes. It is evident that ncRNAs have a role in epigenetic imprinting. There is an imprinted cluster of genes controlled by a region, the imprint control element (ICE), that contains parental information regarding DNA methylation. The genes regulated by ICE include insulin-like growth factor 2 (Igf2), insulin-like growth factor 2 receptors (Igf2r), potassium voltage-gated channels (KCNQ1), and guanine nucleotide binding protein* stimulating factor (Gnas) (Collins et al., 2011).

Role of ncRNAs in Cancer

A combination of genetic and epigenetic changes promotes cancer development. Tumor suppressor genes are inactivated by the genetic mechanism, while oncogenes and epigenetic factors are responsible for their transcriptional regulation. There are several cancer-causing mechanisms that result in 'epimutations' caused by abnormal histone modifications and DNA hypermethylation and hypomethylation events throughout the genome. A chromatin conformation associated with hypomethylation allows transcription factors to access genetic information. ncRNAs and epigenetics are important in the whole process of tumorigenesis. Tumor suppressor and oncogenic ncRNAs are epigenetically deregulated. Cancer cells exhibit genome-wide hypomethylation of DNA, including genomic regions containing ncRNA (Ferreira & Esteller, 2018).

In addition to its well-known role in malignancies, XIST has been researched in a variety of malignancies and has been found to participate in several of them. One of the most studied long non-coding RNAs, XIST has also been found in several human tumors. Human cancers overexpressing XIST are more likely to have an advanced cancer stage, lymph node or distant metastasis, and a poor outcome. Non-small-cell lung cancer (NSCLC), nasopharyngeal and hepatocellular carcinoma, osteosarcoma, gastric, colorectal, pancreatic, and bladder cancers increase the expression of this protein, which acts as an oncogene and promotes cell proliferation and migration. A large number of solid tumours, such as hepatocellular cancer and bladder cancer, have aberrant expression of lncRNA H19. The long-noncoding RNA HOTAIR has a role in gene silencing by interacting with two chromatin-modifying complexes and has a variety of functions in cancer development. In many different CpG regions throughout the genome, the DNMT1-associated lncRNA (DACOR1) is known to be directly involved in the demethylation of CpG regions by directing DNMT1 methylation patterns, and it is suppressed in colon cancer (Pedroso Ayub et al., 2019).

A few long non-codingRNAs have been proven to serve as biomarkers for cancer diagnosis. PCA3 has been found in urine samples from prostate cancer patients, and HULC in blood samples from patients with hepatocellular cancer (Vadaie & Morris, 2013). S lncRNAs have an integral role in the development of multiple myeloma (MM), according to studies. Hypermethylated MEG3 promoters with differentially methylated regions are present in all MM patients with a high risk classification. MALAT1 lncRNA is upregulated in MM, while OIP5-AS1 lncRNA is downregulated. A dysregulation of miRNA expression coupled with epigenetic abnormalities is associated with the development and prognosis of MM. As a regulator of proliferation and growth, miRNA-15a and miRNA-16 inhibit the serine/threonine protein kinase AKT3, ribosomal protein S6, MAP kinases, and nuclear factor-kappaB activator MAP3KIP3 in MM cells (Cui Ayub et al., 2019).

The importance of IncRNAs as emerging key players in cellular homeostasis draws our attention to the important role of miRNAs and lncRNAs in the development and progression of pancreatic cancer. Researchers suggest that pancreatic cancer may be associated with different levels of ncRNA expression, which may provide a therapeutic approach. Downregulated miRNA targets can result in excessive cell growth, abnormal differentiation, and tumorigenesis when the miRNA target genes are expressed. Overexpressed miRNAs can cause the transcription of target genes that function as tumor suppressors to be reduced, promoting the growth and development of tumors. The levels of miR-15b and miR-16 in the body are downregulated under hypoxic conditions, decreasing their inhibitory effects on VEGF and promoting tumor angiogenesis. A number of miRNAs, including miR-10b and miR-373, participate in tumor metastasis (Tang et al., 2014).

The Function of ncRNAs in Other Diseases

A chronic inflammatory autoimmune disease, rheumatoid arthritis (RA) is driven by genetic, environmental, and epigenetic factors. The epigenetic machinery is directed by lncRNAs which act in concert with other epigenetic factors and genes to effectively modify chromatin and gene expression. A study has determined that RP11-498C9.15 may have an important role in the pathogenesis of RA through its modulation of microRNAs and gene expression (Dolcino et al., 2019).

In cardiac fibrosis, extracellular matrix proteins accumulate abnormally in the interstitial space. Studies have shown that considerable numbers of ncRNAs, including miRNAs and lncRNAs regulate pathological fibrosis. In cardiac fibrosis, miRNAs regulate the expression of a large number of genes post-transcriptionally - they act as RNA molecules that regulate gene expression. The lncRNAs act as regulators of cellular differentiation and proliferation and may also have fibrosis-suppressive properties (Tao et al., 2015).

The risk of developing diabetic kidney disease (DKD), a common complication of diabetes mellitus, is genetic and environmental. The gene expression of genes associated with DKD is influenced by epigenetic modifications, such as DNA methylation, chromatin histone modifications, and non-coding RNAs. The metabolic memory process may also account for the persistence of genes and phenotypes related to DKD that were induced by prior glycaemic experience. The detection of epigenetic changes at an early stage of DKD can prevent advanced renal disease by allowing timely diagnosis and treatment (Kato & Natarajan, 2019).

As a result of liver injury or inflammation, liver fibrosis occurs as an inappropriate repair procedure is performed. The lncRNAs that induce liver fibrosis are usually overexpressed or upregulated in liver tissues with fibrosis. The lncRNAs activate hematopoietic stem cells (HSCs) and promote the expression of ECM proteins. These lncRNAs also act through the TGF pathway. IGFBPrP1 (Insulin like growth factor binding protein related protein 1) promotes liver fibrosis by interacting with TGF signaling. Atg9a and NEAT1 regulate HSC activation and autophagy, which is induced by IGFBPrP1. Overexpression of miR122 inhibits NEAT1 overexpression and its downstream effects on liver fibrosis further after KLF6 elimination (Ganguly & Chakrabarti, 2021).

Conclusion

It is a central dogma of molecular biology that DNA is converted into RNA and RNA is translated into proteins. Approximately 50% of the transcriptome is not protein-coding and belongs to a class of regulatory molecules responsible for fine-tuning gene expression (Harries, 2012). NcRNAs are categorized into two categories: regulatory ncRNAs and infrastructure ncRNAs. In addition to ribosomal ncRNAs, small nuclear RNAs and small nucleolar RNAs constitute constitutively expressed infrastructural ncRNAs. The regulatory ncRNAs can be categorized into siRNAs, and lncRNAs, miRNAs, and piRNAs (Kaikkonen et al., 2011).

The role of small regulatory RNAs (microRNAs and siRNAs) is well defined, whereas lncRNAs (long non-coding RNAs) are less well understood. A large number of lncRNAs in eukaryotic genomes regulate their target genes by influencing their epigenetic regulation, chromatin state, mRNA processing, and translation capacity (Harries, 2012). Non-coding RNAs can also regulate post-transcriptional processing, including splicing, transport, translation, and degradation. PTGS is most clearly defined as the siRNA-mediated post-transcriptional gene silencing (RNAi) mediated by miRNAs and siRNAs. As siRNAs silence genes from which they originate, miRNAs regulate genes (Kaikkonen et al., 2011).

During cell division, disruption of epigenetic systems can lead to genomic instability and cell death, as centromere organization ensures proper chromosome segregation. Gene regulation pathways, which regulate the expression of many proteins and transcripts that impact genome stability, may also include epigenetic mechanisms. The stability of genomes is significantly affected by DNA modifications, histone variants, chromatin structure, and non-coding RNAs. The stability of genome is ensured by epigenetic mechanisms that regulate centromeres and telomeres. The role of non-coding RNAs in centromere function and genome stability is another way for epigenetic mechanisms to influence these processes (Feng & Riddle, 2020).

The human genome contains a set of non-coding RNAs that are expressed differently and have altered genomic structure during cancer development. Various types of non-coding RNAs (ncRNAs) are involved in regulating protein coding gene expression in cancer, including small non-coding RNAs and long non-coding RNAs. MiRNAs have been associated with cancer through genomic alterations and dysregulated expression in many tumor types. In both mouse models and cell culture studies, mir17-92, the first oncogenic miRNA, has shown significant oncogenic activity. MiRNAs influence multiple molecular pathways during tumorgenesis, and abnormal alterations in their levels and activities can lead to aberrant gene dosages, which can ultimately lead to aberrant outcomes (Xue & He, 2014).

In this chapter, the effects and functions of non-coding RNAs in cells through epigenetic mechanisms were investigated. It is possible to uncover the information and functions of non-coding RNAs using gene and genome scanning technologies to determine their functions. In conclusion, by identifying the regulatory mechanisms via non-coding RNAs, it seems possible to detect the interactions of these ncRNAs with normal cells and disease states. LncRNAs have an important role in many cancers and can therefore be used as biomarkers to predict recurrence and prognosis. Also, like protein-coding genes and miRNAs, lincRNAs can be used as biomarkers in cancer.

References

Burgosa, M., Rafael Jiméneza, A. H., Barrionuevo, F. J. (2021). Non-Coding RNAs: lncRNAs, miRNAs, and piRNAs in Sexual Development. *Sexual Development,* 15, 335-350. https://doi.org/10.1159/000519237.

Cai, A., Hu, Y., Zhou, Z., Qi, Q., Wu, Y., Dong, P., Chen, L., Wang, F. (2022). PIWI-Interacting RNAs (piRNAs): Promising Applications as Emerging Biomarkers for Digestive System Cancer. *Frontiers in Molecular Biosciences.* 9, 848105. https://doi.org/10.3389/fmolb.2022.848105.

Cao, J. (2014). The functional role of long non-coding RNAs and epigenetics. *Biological Procedures Online,* 16, 11. https://doi.org/10.1186/1480-9222-16-11.

Coelho-Lima, J., & Spyridopoulos, I. (2018). Non-coding RNA regulation of T cell biology: Implications for age-associated cardiovascular diseases. *Experimental Gerontology,* 109, 38-46. https://doi.org/10.1016/j.exger.2017.06.014.

Collins, L. J., Schönfeld, B., Chen, X. S. The Epigenetics of Non-coding RNA. (2011). *Handbook of Epigenetics.* (pp. 49-61). https://doi.org/10.1016/B978-0-12-375709-8.00004-6.

Cui, Y. S., Song, Y. P., Fang, B. J. (2019). The role of long non-coding RNAs in multiple myeloma. *European Journal of Haematology,* 103, 3-9. https://doi.org/10.1111/ejh.13237.

Dolcino, M., Tinazzi, E., Puccetti, A., Lunardi, C. (2019). Long Non-Coding RNAs Target Pathogenetically Relevant Genes and Pathways in Rheumatoid Arthritis. *Cells,* 8, 816. https://doi.org/10.3390/cells808 0816.

Feng, J. X. & Riddle, N. C. (2020). Epigenetics and genome stability. *Mammalian Genome,* 31, 181-195. https://doi.org/10.1007/s00335-020-09836-2.

Ferreira, H. J. & Esteller, M. (2018). Non-coding RNAs, epigenetics, and cancer: tying it all together. *Cancer and Metastasis Reviews,* 37, 55-73. https://doi.org/10.1007/s10555-017-9715-8.

Frías-Lasserre, D. & Villagra, C. A. (2017). The Importance of ncRNAs as Epigenetic Mechanisms in Phenotypic Variation and Organic Evolution. *Frontiers in Microbiology,* 8, 2483. https://doi.org/10.33 89/fmicb.2017.02483.

Ganguly, N. & Chakrabarti, S. (2021). Role of long non-coding RNAs and related epigenetic mechanisms in liver fibrosis (Review). *International Journal of Molecular Medicine,* 47, 04856. https://doi.org/10.38 92/ijmm.2021.4856.

Harries, L. W. (2012). Long non-coding RNAs and human disease. *Biochemical Society Transactions,* 40, 902-6. https://doi.org/10.1042/BST20120020.

He, D., Zheng, J., Hu, J., Chen, J., Wei, X. (2020). Long non-coding RNAs and pyroptosis. *Clinica Chimica Acta,* 504, 201-208. https://doi.org/10.1016/j.cca.2019.11.035.

Jayasuriya, R., Ganesan, K., Xu, B., Ramkumar, K. M. (2022). Emerging role of long non-coding RNAs in endothelial dysfunction and their molecular mechanisms. *Biomedicine & Pharmacotherapy,* 145, 112421. https://doi.org/10.1016/j.biopha.2021.112421.

Kaikkonen, M. U., Lam, M. T. Y., Glass, C. K. (2011). Non-coding RNAs as regulators of gene expression and epigenetics. *Cardiovascular Research,* 90, 430-440. https://doi.org/10.1093/cvr/cvr097.

Kato, M. & Natarajan, R. (2019). Epigenetics and epigenomics in diabetic kidney disease and metabolic memory. *Nature Reviews Nephrology,* 15, 327-345. https://doi.org/10.1038/s41581-019-0135-6.

Li, J. & Liu, C. (2019). Coding or Noncoding, the Converging Concepts of RNAs. *Frontiers in Genetics,* 10, 496. https://doi.org/10.3389/fgene.2019.00496.

Morris, K. V. (2009). Non-coding RNAs, epigenetic memory and the passage of information to progeny. *RNA Biology,* 6, 242-247. https://doi.org/10.4161/rna.6.3.8353.

Ozata, D. M., Gainetdinov, I., Zoch, A., O'Carroll, D., Zamore, P. D. (2019). PIWI- interacting RNAs: small RNAs with big functions. *Nature Reviews Genetics,* 20, 89-108. https://doi.org/10.1038/s41576-018-0073-3.

Pedroso Ayub, A. L., D'Angelo Papaiz, D., da Silva Soares, R., Jasiulionis, M. G. (2019). The Function of lncRNAs as Epigenetic Regulators. *Non-Coding RNAs.* (pp.1-20). IntechOpen. https://doi.org/10.5772/intechopen.88071.

Peschansky, V. J. & Wahlestedt, C. (2014). Non-coding RNAs as direct and indirect modulators of epigenetic regulation. *Epigenetics.* 9, 3-12. https://doi.org/10.4161/epi.27473.

Tang, Y. T., Xu, X. H., Yang, X. D., Hao, J., Cao, H., Zhu, W., Zhang, S. Y., Cao. J. P. (2014). Role of non-coding RNAs in pancreatic cancer: The bane of the microworld. *World Journal of Gastroenterology,* 20, 9405-9417. https://doi.org/10.3748/wjg.v20.i28.9405.

Tao, H., Yang, J. J., Shi, K. H. (2015). Non-coding RNAs as direct and indirect modulators of epigenetic mechanism regulation of cardiac fibrosis. *Expert Opinion on Therapeutic Targets,* 19, 707-16. https://doi.org/10.1517/14728222.2014.1001740.

Vadaie, N. & Morris, K. V. (2013). Long antisense non-coding RNAs and the epigenetic regulation of gene expression. *BioMol Concepts,* 4, 411-415. https://doi.org/10.1515/bmc-2013-0014.

Wu, P. H., & Zamore, P. D. (2021). Defining the functions of PIWI-interacting RNAs. *Nature Reviews Molecular Cell Biology,* 22, 239-240. https://doi.org/10.1038/s41580-021-00336-y.

Xue, B. & He, L. (2014). An expanding universe of the non-coding genome in cancer biology. *Carcinogenesis,* 35, 1209-1216. https://doi.org/10.1093/carcin/bgu099.

Yang, Z., Xu, F., Wang, H., Teschendorff, A. E., Xie, F., He, Y. (2021). Pan-cancer characterization of long non-coding RNA and DNA methylation mediated transcriptional dysregulation. *EBioMedicine,* 68, 103399. https://doi.org/10.1016/j.ebiom.2021.103399.

Zhou, H., Hu, H., Lai, M. (2010). Non-coding RNAs and their epigenetic regulatory mechanisms. *Biology of the Cell,* 102, 645-655. https://doi.org/10.1042/BC20100029.

Chapter 9

General Overview of the Current Methodology in Epigenetics Research

Buket Er Urganci*

Department of Medical Biology, University of Pamukkale, Denizli, Turkey

Abstract

Epigenetics generally describes inherited DNA methylation, histone modifications, and chromatin-based events including chromatin structure that regulate gene expression. In the field of epigenetics, microRNAs have also been shown to have a role in epigenetic regulation. While DNA methylation and histone modifications add a new dimension to gene regulation at the transcriptional level, miRNAs are involved in the regulation at the post-transcriptional level. Analysis of histone modifications is done by chromatin immunoprecipitation (ChIP) and 3C Chromosome conformation capture. There are many methods used for DNA methylation analysis. These methods are hybridization (Southern blot and microarray), restriction enzyme PCR, methylation-sensitive single-nucleotide primer extension, cutting with methylation-sensitive restriction enzymes, bisulfite genomic DNA sequence analysis techniques and epigenetic MR. This chapter offers a reference of various techniques for epigenetic analysis.

Keywords: epigenetics, DNA methylation, histone modification, small RNAs, bisulfite, ChIP, RNAi

Introduction

The concept of 'epigenetics' was made known by Conrad Waddington in 1942 and was defined as 'the processes at the stage of the transformation of genotype into the phenotype' (D'Addario et al., 2013). In 1999, Jones et al., proposed the concept of modern epigenetics (Li et al., 2012). Today, while all macromolecular structures are determined by the genome nucleotide sequences, the mechanism that determines gene expression, which can be inherited and can be transferred from cell to cell, is called the epigenetic code. In the creation of this code, the DNA sequence is not changed in any way. Here, epigenetic regulation lets on cells to recall their gene expression profiles during successive cell divisions without changing the DNA sequence (Sashida and Iwama, 2012).

---

* Corresponding Author's E-mail: aber@pau.edu.tr.

In: Epigenetics: Beyond the Genetics and Medicine
Editors: Sevgi Durna Daştan and Nazan Yurtcu
ISBN: 979-8-88697-228-3

Epigenetics generally describes inherited DNA methylation, histone modifications, and chromatin-based events including chromatin structure that regulate gene expression. In the field of epigenetics, microRNAs (miRNAs) have also been shown to have a role in epigenetic regulation (Sashida and Iwama, 2012). While DNA methylation and histone modifications add a new dimension to gene regulation at the transcriptional level, miRNAs are involved in the regulation at the post-transcriptional level. Accordingly, epigenetic mechanisms are grouped under three main headings:

- Transcriptional
  - Histone modifications
  - DNA methylation
- Post-Transcriptional
  - RNA-induced silencing

As a result of these mechanisms working together, hereditary changes occur in gene expression. An error in any of the mechanisms causes the expression of genes to be excessively increased or suppressed, leading to epigenetic diseases.

Histone Modifications

Histone modifications work in conjunction with DNA methylation to regulate gene expression. Modifications change the chromatin structure by affecting the electrostatic charge of histones, and histone-DNA can control many biological events such as DNA packaging, replication, repair, and control of gene expression by affecting the histone-histone relationship (Chen et al., 2017). Histone modifications cause changes in gene expression by changing the accessibility of regulatory factors to DNA and the DNA binding capacity of histones (Güneş and Kulaç, 2012).

Covalent changes in amino acids in the tail regions of central histone proteins constitute the epigenetic code (D'Addario et al., 2013). As a result of these changes, differences in chromosome structure are observed as an active, open structure called euchromatin or an inactive heterochromatin structure. Histone changes can be listed as acetylation, methylation, phosphorylation (Li et al., 2012) ubiquitination, and ADP-ribosylation of glutamic acids (D'Addario et al., 2013). Methylation, phosphorylation, acetylation, and ubiquination are the leading modifications of lysine and serine residues in histone tails (Güneş and Kulaç, 2012).

Gene expression regulated by histone modifications with two mechanisms: remodeling of chromatin by activating ATPases and disruption of contact between nucleosomes. Histone acetyltransferases (HATs) catalyze the acetylation of lysine terminal tail amino acids and cause disruption of contact between nucleosomes. The essential charge on lysine was neutralized by acetylation and allowed the stabilization of chromatin with its affinity for negatively charged DNA. DNA is more accessible to the transcriptional machinery under a loose chromatin state, and therefore has activated expression. By removal of histone acetyl groups with deacetylases, the process can be reversed (Barski et al., 2007).

Analysis of histone modifications is done by chromatin immunoprecipitation (ChIP) and 3C Chromosome conformation capture.

Chromatin Immunopresipitation (ChIP)

ChIP is widely used to determine the chromatin status of the cell. By providing cross-linking of DNA and associated proteins by chemical treatment, DNA-protein complexes are immunoprecipitated with an antibody suitable for the histone modification sought. When this method is applied with microarray chips, fast and healthy analyzes can be made, and it is called "ChIP on chip." The method provides flexibility to the practitioner, and histone modifications in desired regions can be examined using specific or more general antibodies (Barski et al., 2007).

To study histone modifications at the true genome level, other high-throughput methods were combined with chromatin immunoprecipitation, namely: next generation sequencing (ChIP-Seq), PET: paired end-ditag sequencing (ChIP-PET), SAGE: serial analysis of gene expression (ChIP-SAGE). ChIP-seq has a similar procedure as chromatin immunoprecipitation; DNA fragments are directly sequenced using next-generation parallel resequencing, instead of amplification of purified DNA and hybridization to a microarray. It has been determined to be an efficient method for analyzing protein target sites and histone modification patterns, presenting higher resolution (Barski et al., 2007).

Table 1. Advantages and Disadvantages of ChIP-chip vs ChIP-seq

	Advantages	Disadvantages
ChIP-chip	– Examining histone changes at the genome level – Less complex bioinformatically and analytically	– Requires knowing the sequence of the region to be designed as a probe, high signal-to-noise ratio – Limited dynamic range
ChIP-seq	– Quantification of signal from ChIP is dependent on counting of sequence reads – Larger dynamic working range – Allows multiplexing of samples for next-generation sequencing for barcoding purposes	– Difficulty in ordering the sequences obtained in short reading of the repeated regions – More difficult bioinformatically and analytically

3C Chromosome Conformation Capture

Long-range enhancer interactions and regulation of promoter regions are also important in epigenetics. The 3C (Chromatin Conformation Capture) and then 4C (Circular Chromosome Conformation Capture) methods have provided important information to understand the interactions of the promoter region and the enhancer region in three dimensions. In these methods, the cross-linking of DNA segments is ensured by adding formaldehyde. Afterward, by adding restriction enzymes, the cross-linking DNA is separated from the non-cross-linking DNA. Ligation of relevant DNA fragments is achieved using very low concentrations of DNA. The high temperature reverses cross-link formation and inhibits specific restriction. After the formation of linear DNA fragments with the same ending, the restriction enzyme is added for the second time. After self-circulation of the DNA fragments is ensured, primers are designed against the outer restriction region of the simple sequence created, and they are not bound to other proteins or fragments. The 4C library is analyzed by the multiNA microchip electrophoresis system (Van de Werken et al., 2012).

DNA Methylation

DNA methylation is the most common epigenetic event that occurs in the mammalian genome (Li et al., 2012). It was first described in 1948. It is an important mechanism of transcriptional control.

DNA methylation is an epigenetic mechanism that directly affects DNA (Chen et al., 2017). Among all epigenetic mechanisms, DNA methylation, which is the most studied and understood, is an enzymatic change and the conversion of cytosines to 5'-methyl cytosine (20). S-adenosyl methionine (SAM) is catalyzed by transferring the methyl group from guanine (G) to cytosine (C) located before it, and 5-methyl cytosine (5mC) is formed (Chen et al., 2017; Güneş and Kulaç, 2012; Dalton and Bellacosa, 2012). 5mC; It is named the fifth base after A, T, G, C (Chen et al., 2011). The formation of 5mC is a covalent chemical modification (Chen et al., 2017; D'Addario et al., 2013). SAM and DNA DNMT have an important role in DNA methylation (D'Addario et al., 2013; Li et al., 2012). DNMT family members use SAM and DNA as co-substrates. Only methyl donors and cofactors provide the methyl groups required for all methylation reactions.

DNA methylation in the CpG islands, which functions as a mechanism for the control of specific gene expression in adult tissues, is mainly caused by the restriction of two small gene families. Female X chromosome inactivation is associated with widespread methylation of CpG islands on the inactive X chromosome. Inactivation of the unexpressed allele in imprinted genes where the gene allele is only paternally or maternally involved is associated with methylation in the gene's promoter (Hackett and Surani, 2013). Although most genes are associated with CpG islands in normal tissues, these islands remain unmethylated regardless of whether genes are expressed or not. This contrasts with human cancer cell lines in which methylation in CpG islands increases.

There are many methods used for DNA methylation analysis (Chen et al., 2017; Kulis and Esteller, 2010). These methods are hybridization (Southern blot and microarray), restriction enzyme PCR, methylation-sensitive single-nucleotide primer extension, cutting with methylation-sensitive restriction enzymes, and bisulfite genomic DNA sequence analysis techniques (Kulis and Esteller, 2010).

Southern Blot

It is a technique that is frequently used in DNA methylation analysis. Genomic DNA is cut with methylation-specific and non-methylation-specific endonucleases specific for the same sequence (such as HpaI and MspII, Sma I-Xmal) (Li et al., 2012). While these enzymes break the unmethylated chromosomes into small pieces, the methylated DNA escapes this trimming. These fragments are then tested by PCR or Southern blot (Li et al., 2012). Restriction fragments separated on agarose gel during Southern blotting. The fragments are transferred to a membrane and target sequence-specific probe hybridization occurs. The presence of bands whose sizes are estimated by autoradiography is shown. Large amounts of high molecular weight DNA are required for the Southern hybridization method.

Microarray

First, Huang et al., developed a microarray-based technique by combining it with a methylation-specific restriction enzyme, and with this technique, thousands of CpG islets were visualized simultaneously. This method is used to identify unknown methylation hotspots or to detect methylated CpG islands in the genome. Multi-PCR is performed after DNA modification with bisulfite. The primers used are specific to the bisulfite modified yarn. Thus, erroneous results arising from incomplete bisulfite modification are prevented (Li and Tollefsbol, 2021).

Restriction Enzyme PCR

In the restriction enzyme PCR method, genomic DNA is bound with methylation-specific and non-methylation-specific restriction enzymes, and digested DNA is amplified using target site primers. The size of the amplified DNA can be estimated if the target sequence contains methylated CpG domains. Possible amplification will not occur if the methylation region of the target DNA sequence is ignored with the use of non-methylation-specific endonucleases prior to PCR. In this method, enzyme digestion must be carried out completely. Unsatisfactory results will be obtained if there are CpG sites in the methylated and unmethylated target region. However, this technique is very important in monitoring DNA methylation in the target sequence (Kulis and Esteller, 2010).

Methylation-Specific PCR (MSP)

Methylation-Specific PCR (MSP) was first described in 1996 by Herman et al. (Chen et al., 2017). MSP is one of the most used methods in DNA methylation analysis. It is a specific and sensitive method for methylation (Chen et al., 2017). After bisulfite treatment, it is made by exploiting the existing sequence differences between methylated and unmethylated DNA (Kulis and Esteller, 2010). In MSP, the DNA to be used as a template is modified by bisulfite treatment (Chen et al., 2017). Cytosines deaminate in uracil (Chen et al., 2017) and cytosines replicate like thymine during PCR (Chen et al., 2017). Two PCR reactions are performed for each DNA sample (Chen et al., 2017). The placement of the primers is particularly in sequences containing either methylated (C) or modified (T) domains. After PCR, the amplified DNA is obtained with the specific primer pair for methylated or unmethylated sequences. MSP is a fast and high-quality method used to detect the presence of methylation in a DNA region (Kulis and Esteller, 2010).

This sensitive and easy-to-use method can analyze a limited number of CpG dinucleotides. In addition, this method cannot provide complete information about the methylation status of a single CpG site (Brakensiek et al., 2007).

Careful selection of primers is very important for this method because the false positive results can be obtained with both methyl and unmethyl primer pairs. Incomplete bisulfite modification of genomic DNA can cause false positives for methylated cytosine (Kulis and Esteller, 2010).

Methylation-Sensitive Single-Nucleotide Primer Extension

Methylation-sensitive single-nucleotide primer extension was represented by Kuppuswamy et al., and is used to identify mutations in abnormal alleles (Kulis and Esteller, 2010). The amplified DNA is used as a template for the methylation-sensitive single-nucleotide primer extension reaction, after bisulfite application and amplification of the target sequence with primers specific for the modified DNA. The primers used in the single nucleotide extension reaction are designed according to the binding site that recognizes the methylation site only one nucleotide before. Purified amplified DNA is incubated with DNA polymerase and radioactive dTTP or dCTP. At the methylated target site, a cytosine (C) is joined during nucleotide elongation. If there is no methylation at the site, thymine (T) is combined instead of cytosine. Complete modification of DNA and primer design are important for obtaining good results in the analysis.

Bisulfite DNA Sequence Analysis

The gold standard for studying DNA methylation is the modification of the conversion of cytosine to uracil by bisulfite treatment, followed by the detection of changes in the sequence by PCR and DNA sequence analysis (Chen et al., 2017, Hackett and Surani, 2013).

Bisulfite modification is used to detect all methylated and non-methylated CpG islands in the genome (Chen et al., 2017). Bisulfite DNA sequencing has led to the development of new techniques for analyzing the methylation states of genes for 5-methylcytosine containing DNA sequences. This method was first developed by Frommer et al. in 1992. The purpose of bisulfite DNA sequence analysis is based on the determination of 5-methylcytosine in genomic DNA (Kulis and Esteller, 2010). Sodium bisulfite deaminates cytosine localized in single-stranded DNA. In this reaction, DNA is first converted to a single-stranded form by denaturation. Then, respectively; Cytosine is converted to cytosine sulfonate by bisulfite reaction, to uracil sulfonate by hydrolytic deamination, and to uracil by alkaline desulfonation. Thus, all cytosines are converted to uracil, but 'methylated cytosine' remains as cytosine (Chen et al., 2017; Hackett and Surani, 2013; Kulis and Esteller, 2010).

There are important points to be considered in the bisulfite modification process. For example, reversion of the reaction to an alkaline environment causes the degradation of sodium bisulfite. In addition, if the incubation period with bisulfite is long, 60% of the purine bases and phosphodiester bonds in the DNA molecule are damaged, and pyrimidine bases are destroyed (Chen et al., 2017).

Different methods are used for the analysis of methylated and unmethylated DNA after bisulfite chemical modification. These are qualitative (MSP, etc.) and quantitative [Bisulfite genomic sequencing, COBRA (Combined Bisulfite Restriction Analysis), etc.] methylation analysis methods (Chen et al., 2017).

In bisulfite modified DNA, two different sets of methylation-specific primers are used to separate methylated DNA from unmethylated DNA. While the methylated primer contains CG due to methylation, the non-methylated primer contains TG, although it is located in the same DNA region (Chen et al., 2017).

The product after bisulfite PCR can be analyzed in two different ways. The first of these is the post-cutting analysis of the PCR product obtained using restriction enzymes. In this method, using an enzyme such as BstUI that recognizes the CGCG sequence, the pattern depending on the change in these sequences (if there is methylation, the sequence is preserved, if there is no methylation, it turns into TGTG and the cut region is lost) is examined after electrophoresis. This technique is called COBRA (Chen et al., 2017; Kulis and Esteller, 2010). Another method that gives more sensitive results is the bisulfite PCR product bisulfite DNA sequence analysis. The result of the analysis obtained is compared with the reference DNA sequence and quantitatively the methylation analysis is performed (Chen et al., 2017).

The most important and most common epigenetic mechanism for hypermethylation-related silencing of tumor suppressor genes in human tumorigenesis has been analyzed. These techniques are hampered by limitations to the analysis of this abnormality, such as the absence of quantification in the methylation state and the limited number of analyzable CpG sites. Pyrosequencing is useful for the analysis of genes with heterogeneous methylation patterns and is a technique that overcomes these limitations. Initial reports established the reliability of this technique, showing exact quantification of the methylation level in a single CpG site (Brakensiek et al., 2007).

Epigenetic MR

Scientists and engineers working in the biomedical field are working on animal models of various methods that can reveal gene expression in the brain. Since these methods are generally invasive, they cannot be applied to humans. Non-invasive experiments with optical techniques such as fMRI and PET are generally limited to a few genes and do not provide comprehensive information about human gene expression. However, it has been demonstrated that DNA methylation in the brain can be visualized with a new technique applied by the University of Illinois Urbana-Champaign on newborn pigs (Lam et al., 2002).

Lam, et al., call this new technique epigenetic MRI (eMRI). The basis of this method is the labeling of this molecule in the DNA helix by crossing the blood-brain barrier in newborn pigs fed with foods enriched with a special amino acid (^{13}C-Met), and then imaging with Carbon-13 nuclear magnetic resonance (^{13}C NMR) and magnetic resonance spectroscopy (MRS) (2022). The researchers state that the epigenetic MR method has some advantages and disadvantages, as with any imaging technique.

Advantages of the Epigenetic MR Method

- The fact that both the DNA labeling method (^{13}C-Met enriched foods) and the imaging method (^{13}C NMR and MRS) are non-invasive, so they can be applied on humans.
- Ability to measure DNA methylation, which regulates gene expression, in vivo.
- Being able to give information about a general gene activity in the brain.

Disadvantages of the Epigenetic MRI

Carbon-13 nuclear magnetic resonance imaging is a technique with low sensitivity. However, in the study, this problem was tried to be solved by using a good labeling method, a high-tech imaging device, and advanced signal processing methods.

13C-Met may be involved in DNA methylation as well as RNA and other protein methylation. Researchers say that this change in RNA occurs faster than DNA and that the rate of incidence is much lower; however, more work needs to be done in this area.

RNA-Induced Silencing

RNAi technology has made the greatest advances in studying the function of genes in recent years. It not only helps us in the treatment of diseases but also helps us to understand the functions of genes whose functions we do not know. It is promising in the treatment of diseases by preventing the development and formation of many diseases by stopping gene expression.

It has been suggested that some specific non-coding RNA and siRNAs are triggers for the initiation of histone modifications and DNA methylation. It is thought that by contributing to the formation of the heterochromatin region, it causes hereditary silencing (Chen et al., 2017). In recent years, some small RNA molecules, called non-coding RNA, have been shown to be involved in the epigenetic process (D'Addario et al., 2013; Chen et al., 2011). When non-coding RNAs are examined, in addition to functionally important ones such as tRNA and rRNA, siRNAs, piRNAs, and microRNAs can be demonstrated (Sweatt et al., 2013; Nestler, 2014).

For example, miRNA, which is known as RNA interference, is responsible for posttranscriptional and posttranslational silencing, and XIST RNA, which is responsible for X chromosome inactivation, are examples of this process. An X chromosome is randomly selected during early embryogenesis and undergoes heterochromatinization, thereby inactivating the X chromosome (Xi). Xist is called an X inactivation specific transcript gene, and its antisense gene Tsix helps control inactivation (Bateson et al., 2004). In Xi, Xist RNA coats the chromosome to suppress Tsix expression, and Tsix RNA on active X stops Xist RNA. Inactivation of the X chromosome is sustained by histone acetylation and DNA methylation. Xist is not methylated in Xi while hypermethylated on active X. Moreover, Xi is hypermethylated in the CpG islands and gene promoter regions. It is released in the hypoacetylation of histone H4. The interaction between histone methylation and acetylation, DNA methylation is complete, and Xist RNA remains prominent (Petronis, 2004; Skinner et al., 2009).

Conclusion

Epigenetic data are candidates for many new contributions to the genomic sciences. Epigenetic information is multiplex in nature, as a single gene can carry hundreds of methylated cytosines and dozens of histone modifications. Second, epigenetic information is quantitative, unlike sequence information, which is discrete. Partial methylation may be observed at certain tissue-specific loci and there may be differences in the intensity of methylation observed. It may also contribute to understand the function of regulatory sequences in the mammalian genome.

Indeed, non-coding sequences are much larger than coding sequences in the genomes of many complex organisms and are thought to have a role in regulation. Finally, the topological conformation of DNA in the nucleus is thought to be epigenetically controlled, and recent studies have shown that this regulation has a very important role in gene regulation. Large-scale epigenomic approaches enable the necessary experiments to be made for new information with technological developments.

References

Barski, A., Cuddapah, S., Cui, K., Roh, T. Y., Schones, D. E., Wang, Z., Wei, G., Chepelev, I., & Zhao, K. (2007). High-resolution profiling of histone methylations in the human genome. *Cell*, *129*(4), 823–837.

Bateson, P., Parker, D., Clutton-Brock, T., Deb, D., D'Udine, B., & Foley, R. A. (2004). Developmental Plasticity and Human Health. *Nature*, *430*, 419-421.

Brakensiek, K., Wingen, L. U., Länger, F., Kreipe, H., & Lehmann, U. (2007). Quantitative high-resolution CpG island mapping with Pyrosequencing reveals disease-specific methylation patterns of the CDKN2B gene in myelodysplastic syndrome and myeloid leukemia. *Clinical Chemistry*, *53*(1), 17–23.

Chen, H., Hardy, T. M., & Tollefsbol, T. O. (2011). Epigenomics of ovarian cancer and its chemoprevention. *Frontiers in Genetics*, *2*, 67.

Chen, Y., Hong, T., Wang, S., Mo, J., Tian, T., & Zhou, X. (2017). Epigenetic modification of nucleic acids: from basic studies to medical applications. *Chemical Society Reviews*, *46*(10), 2844–2872.

D'Addario, C., Di Francesco, A., Pucci, M., Finazzi Agrò, A., & Maccarrone, M. (2013). Epigenetic mechanisms and endocannabinoid signalling. *The FEBS Journal*, *280*(9), 1905–1917.

Dalton, S. R., & Bellacosa, A. (2012). DNA demethylation by TDG. *Epigenomics*, *4*(4), 459–467.

Güneş S, Kulaç T. (2013). The role of epigenetics in spermatogenesis *Turkish Journal of Urology*, *39*(3), 181-7.

Hackett, J. A., & Surani, M. A. (2013). DNA methylation dynamics during the mammalian life cycle. *Philosophical Transactions of the Royal Society of London. Series B, Biological Sciences*, *368*(1609), 20110328.

Kulis, M., & Esteller, M. (2010). DNA methylation and cancer. *Advances in Genetics*, *70*, 27–56.

Lam, F., Chu, J., Choi, J. S., Cao, C., Hitchens, T. K., Silverman, S. K., Liang, Z. P., Dilger, R. N., Robinson, G. E., & Li, K. C. (2022). Epigenetic MRI: Noninvasive imaging of DNA methylation in the brain. *Proceedings of the National Academy of Sciences of the United States of America*, *119*(10), e2119891119.

Li, S., & Tollefsbol, T. O. (2021). DNA methylation methods: Global DNA methylation and methylomic analyses. *Methods (San Diego, Calif.)*, *187*, 28–43.

Li, X. Q., Guo, Y. Y., & De, W. (2012). DNA methylation and microRNAs in cancer. *World Journal of Gastroenterology*, *18*(9), 882–888.

Nestler, E. J. (2014). Epigenetic mechanisms of drug addiction. *Neuropharmacology*, 76: 259-268.

Petronis, A. (2004). The origin of schizophrenia: Genetic thesis, epigenetic antithesis, and resolving synthesis. *Biol. Psychiat.,* 55(10): 965-970.

Sashida, G., & Iwama, A. (2012). Epigenetic regulation of hematopoiesis. *International Journal of Hematology*, *96*(4), 405–412.

Skinner, M. K. 2007. Epigenetic transgenerational toxicology and germ cell disease. *Int. J. Androl.*, *30*, 393-397.

Sweatt, J. D., Guzman-Karlsson, M. C., & Rahn, E. J. (2013). Cellular, molecular and epigenetic mechanisms in non-associative conditioning: implications for pain and memory. *Neurobiol. Learn. Mem.*, *105*, 133-150.

Van de Werken, H. J., de Vree, P. J., Splinter, E., Holwerda, S. J., Klous, P., de Wit, E., & de Laat, W. (2012). 4C technology: Protocols and data analysis. *Methods Enzymol.*, *513*, 89-112.

Chapter 10

Computational Modeling of Epigenetics

Mesude Avci*, **PhD**
Department of Chemical Engineering, Sivas Cumhuriyet University, Sivas, Turkey

Abstract

Epigenetics is a new critical field that has arisen to investigate the effect of elements apart from genes on the character and on the role of an organism. Using computational tools constitutes the core of this new research area and has critical roles because controlling the choice of basic tests, developing recent provable theories from precise examination of complicated genomic knowledge, which is not attainable utilizing classical methods, only possible with computational tools. Epigenomics connects conventional genomics with computer science, biochemistry, mathematics, chemistry, proteomics for the extensive investigation of hereditary diversities in phenotype, and gene activity or gene interpretation, which are not dependent on gene array. Moreover, it helps us to better understand transcriptional adjustment, nuclear arrangement, improvement, and illness. Here, current computational approaches to investigate epigenetic factors are explored. Essential data sources and bioinformatic apparatus in this fast-developing area have been evaluated.

Keywords: epigenetics, computational modeling, data sources, computational tools, bioinformatics

Introduction

Epigenetics is generally described as the examination of mitotically (epigenetic heritage happens among generations of cells) and/or meiotically (epigenetic heritage happens among generations of species) inherited diversity in gene functions which are not described and related clearly by alternation in DNA sequence (Russo et al., n.d.). The important purpose of epigenetics is to explain the regulation of gene expression by both genetic and non-genetic information jointly. So, non-genetic means to DNA are packaged inside the nucleus, whereas genetic information is coded in the DNA sequence.

Large volumes of data have been produced by resembling and decoding the genomes of model organisms to improve understanding of advancement and evolution for the explanation of disease, and natural selection. Besides, to extract any valuable information from the

* Corresponding Author's E-mail: mesude@cumhuriyet.edu.tr.

In: Epigenetics: Beyond the Genetics and Medicine
Editors: Sevgi Durna Daştan and Nazan Yurtcu
ISBN: 979-8-88697-228-3

genotypes and phenotypes interaction during development (Lim et al., 2010). Especially, a large amount of data helps research molecular evolution (Cutter & Ward, 2005), the evolution of DNA for particular illnesses (Eileithyia et al., 2005; Nishimura et al., 1999), and bio variety analysis (Smith & Donoghue, 2008). Although genomic research has been studied extensively, investigation of gene factors is inadequate to clarify inherited variations in phenotype and gene function (Lim et al., 2010).

The chemical modification process requires miscellaneous enzymes, which are related to the epigenetic structures (Basso et al., 2013; Petronis, 2010). Protein grouping, DNA methylation, and different covalent posttranscriptional histone modifications were more comprehensively studied (Alelú-Paz et al., 2012; Du et al., 2015; LeRoy et al., 2013). From these, histone modification directly affects chromatin structure and influences gene expression values. Besides, DNA methylation generally behaves as a procedure to shift the gene "off," because of an extra methyl group to a DNA strand. These alterations are molecule- as well as modification-specific. The diversity of histone variation (decoded from separate genes) is distinctively represented as "open" and "closed." Also, "compact" chromatin regions adds more level of complexity (Cedar & Bergman, 2009; Ioudinkova et al., 2012). Epigenetic symbols also express gene signatures where these are obtained and passed on to subsequent generations and also due to environmental factors such as diet and lifestyle (Bjornsson et al., 2007; Burggren, 2016; Falls et al., 1999).

Data Sources for Epigenetic Research

Scientific research, molecular datasets, and incident information include a large number of information suitable for epigenetic studies. Although a large amount of epigenetic information is available, the value of epigenetic study is mostly based on the capability to recover valuable information, which facilitates exploration of recent information, understanding of issues, and arrangement of tests (Krallinger & Valencia, 2005).

The primary source of data from these is the scientific literature, which provides a top-profile description of biological systems and procedures. For example, while the PubMed consist of more than 288,000 records for epigenetic research, the data is in the mode of unorganized content and difficult to extract biologically meaningful information.

The amount and capacity of molecular datasets are increasing regularly. The Nucleic Acids Research online Molecular Biology Database Collection characterizes a total of 1078 molecular collection of biology data as of 2009 (Galperin, 2008). Inside this database collection; 3 nucleotide sequence databases, 60 transcriptional regulatory sites datasets, 65 microarray information and genetic expression databases, and 114 human genes and diseases databases (Lim et al., 2010). Moreover, archives of the nucleotide sequence of different origins include the global shared GenBank (Benson et al., 2002), DNA Data Bank of Japan (DDBJ) (Tateno et al., 2002) and EMBL (Kanz et al., 2005).

Data sources for the insertion of methyl groups into the DNA molecule are valuable for investigating the covalent alteration of a cell's genetic onent. Some of the important sources of DNA methylation datasets consist of MethDB (Negre & Grunau, 2006), MethPrimerDB (Pattyn et al., 2006), and MethyLogiX. Compression and convenience of eukaryotic and possibly archael genetic DNA are studied in histone databases. The National Human Genome Research Institute (NHGRI)'s Histone Dataset (S. Sullivan et al., 2002; S. A. Sullivan et al.,

2000) is used for main data origin for histone and its proteins, which are responsible for folding. Miscellaneous cancers are correlated with random methylation arrangements, which are analyzed by cancer methylation databases. Information of gene methylation profiles of specific cancer types is included in important data sources for example, PubMeth (Ongenaert et al., 2008) and MeInfoText (Fang et al., 2008). Cell-, living thing-, and phase explicit gene interpretation behaviors are ready for use in online resources. The main archive for large-output gene interpretation information is The National Center for Biotechnology Information (NCBI)'s Gene Expression Omnibus (GEO) arrett et al., 2009). In addition, this database collects large output of practical genetic information for example, genetic duplication figure alterations, chromatin format, methylation condition, and replication element attachment. The Gene Expression Nervous System Atlas (GENSAT) (Heintz, 2004) supplies data related to the exact dispersion of particular genes and proteins during complete brain growth. Rat, mouse, and human stem cells and derivative information are clarified by Stem Base (Porter et al., 2007). The entire gene explanation figure in healthful people tissues (bone marrow, brain, heart, kidney, liver, lung, pancreas, prostate, skeletal muscle, spinal cord, spleen, and thymus) utilizing the Affymetrix Gene Chip HG-U95 set is included in the Gene Normal Tissue Expression (GeneNote) dataset (Shmueli et al., 2003). Mice blood cell interpretation portraits including progenitors and finally discriminated cells, acquired from batch examination and separate analysis, are specified in the Blood Express database (Miranda-Saavedra et al., 2009). More information sources can be reviewed in (Baxevanis, 2006).

Computational Tools for Epigenetic Research

In the literature, many computational, numerical and analytical approaches, varying from data mining, sequence analysis, molecular interactions, to complex system-level simulations are studied. Although there is not much improvement in this field, text mining of epigenetic information has been studied. Acquiring and investigating DNA methylation behaviors in different cancer types have been mainly studied currently (Fang et al., 2008; Ongenaert et al., 2008). Practical, fundamental, or developmental connections among DNA or protein arrangements are concluded using classical series examination apparatus, such as ClustalW (Thompson et al., 1994), BLAST software suite (Altschul et al., 1990), BLAT (BLAST-Like Alignment Tool) (Kent, 2002) and MEGA (Molecular Evolutionary Genetics Analysis) (Kumar et al., 2008). These methods are used in different applications and used in enhancing the actions of histone deacetylase blockages (Park & Lee, 2004), analogy modeling of DNA methyltransferases (Koudan et al., 2004), forecasting the alternate formation of histone deacetylases and used to homology examination of ortholog applications for the KEGG/GENES dataset (Itoh et al., 2005).

Computational Examination of DNA Methylation

DNA methylation has an extensive function in gene balance and cell elasticity (Adams, 1990). It contributes for usual cell improvement and several important operations for example X-chromosome deactivation (Kaslow & Migeon, 1987), carcinogenesis (Jones, 2002), genomic imprinting (Li et al., 1993), and maintenance of repetitive factors (Liang et al., 2002). DNA methylation primarily occurs when methyl groups from S-adenosyl-methionine are transferred to the 5 positions of the cytosine pyrimidine ring by the DNA methyltransferase (DNMT) or methylase catalyzer. DNMT1, 2, 3A, and 3B (Robertson et al., 1999; Xie et al., 1999) are the four effective DNA methyltransferases in mammals. Of these, the most frequently encountered DNA methyltransferases in mammals is the DNMT1 and it mostly methylates hemimethylated CpG dinucleotides. DNMT2 is analyzed as a DNA methyltransferases analog that adds methyl groups into cytosine-38 in the anticodon loop of aspartic acid transfer RNA instead of DNA (Goll et al., 2006). Moreover, de novo methyltransferases DNMT3A and DNMT3B function hemimethylated and unmethylated CpG sites (Robertson et al., 1999; Xie et al., 1999).

Distinct type of modelling and prediction of DNA methylation methods are studied. For example, particular lung cancer cell lines are analyzed by using linear discriminant analysis and artificial neural networks (ANN) (Marchevsky et al., 2004). Moreover, characterization of methylation behavior of all human autosomes has been studied by using support vector machines (SVM) (Das et al., 2006). Recently, the prediction of protein methylation sites are simplified by improvement of computational technologies such as support-vector networks (SVM), hidden Markov models (HMM), ANNs, naive bayes, logistic regression, K-nearest neighbors, and decision trees (Bhasin et al., 2005; Chen et al., 2006). Nevertheless, inadequate publicly available experimental data make model development for the application of these systems difficult. Since experimental data are the most easily available and the mechanism is the best understood, arginine and lysine methylations are the most studied areas by such systems (Chen et al., 2006). Histone H3K9/14 acetylation, polymerase II preinitiation complex binding, DNase I hypersensitivity, DNA methylation, histone H3K4 di- and trimethylation, and SP1 binding are incorporated by epigenome prediction pipeline (Bock et al., 2007). Now, significance of such computational tools remains unexplained, but when experimental data keep increasing, these computational technologies will be more explicit and more integrative applications are going to be available.

Computational Examination of Histone Alteration

Histones are the essential protein parts of chromatin. The main job of these is the availability and compaction of eukaryotic and archaeal genomic DNA (S. A. Sullivan et al., 2000). Moreover, they perform several post-transformations, for example sumoylation, chemical reaction of attachment of a phosphoryl group, methylation, adding ubiquitin, and acetylation (Nathan et al., 2003; S. Sullivan et al., 2002). The surface of the nucleosome and globular core region originate from amino-thermal regions, which are primarily responsible for covalent modifications of the histone proteins (Grant, 2001; Vaquero et al., 2003). Chromosome behavior is influenced by histone modification in two different processes (Iizuka & Smith, 2003). First, they may change their electrostatic properties and change the main component of chromosome construction or DNA attachment movement. Next, attachment areas of protein identification elements are developed by these to aid particular functional complexes joining to their appropriate action sites.

Using data processing for the simulation, prediction, and analysis of histone alterations in DNA arrays is getting increased interest. Different kinds of epigenetic modifications are investigated. For example, heredity and biostability of nucleosome modification based on epigenetic memory was examined by Sneppen and coworkers (Dodd et al., 2007). It was found that during modification reactions coordination of two or more modified nucleosomes are demanded, which provides robust biostability. In higher eukaryotic genomes, regulatory elements and histone marks are needed to be analyzed with the help of new technologies in comparative genomics. A study related to the gen analogy of chromatin arrangement in more advanced eukaryotes was studied by Schübeler and colleagues (Schübeler et al., 2004), and it was found that a dual arrangement of histone alterations between euchromatic genes (with active hyperacetylated in H3/4 and hypermethylated in H3 genes, and passive hypomethylated and deacetylated genomes at the identical places) occurs. The dispersion of lysine-9/14-diacetylated histone H3 in human peripheral T cells was demonstrated by a gen related outlining method (T.-Y. Roh et al., 2005). It was demonstrated that this mode of chromatin alteration is related to managerial factors related to gene interpretation and with active gene promoters. In the next study of the group, histone acetylation patterns were used to perform the genome-related structure of saved and non-saved booster (T. Roh et al., 2007).

Discovering acetylation, phosphorylation, methylation, and histone occupied in a DNA array using the arrangement of machine-learning algorithms has also been quite addressed (Kouskoumvekaki et al., 2008; Miranda-Saavedra & Barton, 2007; Won et al., 2008; Xu et al., 2008). ChIPon- chip and ChIP-seq datasets also contain some of these tools. ChIP fragment numbers were used at each genomic position to deduce the states of histone modification changes by using HMMs (Xu et al., 2008). Wavelet analysis incorporated with HMMs was used for finding dynamic and restraining histone alterations by applying picked P-on-chip data files from the ENCODE project (Thurman et al., 2007). The entire genes of greater complication organisms have large sets of protein sequences, in which those algorithms support the griding of histone points. Several structure-based techniques, such as homology modeling (Lin et al., 2008), measurable arrangement-action connection (QSAR) analysis (Dessalew, 2007; Juvale et al., 2006), and molecular advance methods (Angeles et al., n.d.), for the configuration of epigenetic avoidance were also explained. The practical explanations of epigenetic aspects have been used for the improvement of at least five computational methods (Kouskoumvekaki et al., 2008; Miranda-Saavedra & Barton, 2007). These tools will help us to understand epigenetic events in particular cell types and in an evolutionary text.

Conclusion

The effectiveness of that current information is handled, interpreted, discovered, and presented to scientists is needed to be improved to understand the entire assets of the informatics revolution. High performance methodologies produce a large quantity of research relevant to epigenetics that will help the future to switch against the computational epigenetics example. Along this switch, one critical problem is the efficient information operation and annotation. Now, a concentrating storage for epigenetic-related information is still inadequate and research on this area will considerably help computational studies on epigenetics. Adequate strategy of empirical information requires interpretation and normalization of data for different researches of different study organizations, which is another difficulty in the area of computational epigenetics.

Various attitudes of epigenetic alterations (Bhasin et al., 2005; Bock et al., 2007; Chen et al., 2006; Das et al., 2006; Marchevsky et al., 2004) and sickness (Bock et al., 2008; Eden et al., 2007; Keshet et al., 2006; Laird, 2005) have been modeled by computational algorithms yet. Cellular automata have also been studied for investigating different epigenetic modifications (Dodd et al., 2007). When the variety, number, and complication of sources and examination apparatus increase, the challenge is to combine the effectiveness and not the weakness of every application. Central (cloud) computing, cluster computing, and dispensed schemes for major epigenetic information examination, and griding will increase the interest in epigenetic modeling. High-throughput scientific research problem has been solved with the help of network science, which collects the sources of several computers in a system of connections (Talukdar et al., 2009). However, scalable resources on demand are presented by cloud computing technologies, which recently have arisen to integrate the pace of information products and push the pace of data examination and learning invention (Rosenthal et al., 2010). Better realization of epigenetic alterations at several layers of complication, from the intracellular molecular layer to the cellular and systems level, and beyond will be possible with the distinct bioinformatics and mathematical modeling paths, in mixture among progress in a computational framework. More importantly, when the computational investigation, recognition, and categorization of variations in epigenetic modifications are developed, epigenetic-related diseases will be known better and that will help to better forming of appropriate diagnostic, therapeutic, and prophylactic devices. Due to the fact that the nature of epigenetics is greatly combinatorial, an inspiring circumstance is the classification of people's genomes and epigenomes and the improvement of customized or exact medicines having lessened toxicity and fewer side effects. That will wide medicine for each specific person and a modern stage of "personal"-omics (Rosenthal et al., 2010).

References

Adams, R. L. (1990). DNA methylation. The effect of minor bases on DNA-protein interactions. *The Biochemical Journal*, *265*(2), 309–320. https://doi.org/10.1042/bj2650309.

Alelú-Paz, R., Ashour, N., González-Corpas, A., & Ropero, S. (2012). DNA methylation, histone modifications, and signal transduction pathways: a close relationship in malignant gliomas pathophysiology. *Journal of Signal Transduction*, *2012*, 956958. https://doi.org/10.1155/2012/956958.

Altschul, S. F., Gish, W., Miller, W., Myers, E. W., & Lipman, D. J. (1990). Basic local alignment search tool. *Journal of Molecular Biology*, *215*(3), 403–410. https://doi.org/10.1016/S0022-2836(05)80360-2.

Angeles, E., HugoVazquez-Valadez, V., Vazquez-Valadez, O., Velazquez-Sanchez, A. M., Ramirez, A., Martinez, L., Diaz-Barriga, S., Romero-Rojas, A., Cabrera, G., Lopez-Castanares, R., & Duenas-Gonzalez, A. (n.d.). Computational Studies of 1-Hydrazinophthalazine (Hydralazine) as Antineoplasic Agent. Docking Studies on Methyltransferase. In *Letters in Drug Design & Discovery* (Vol. 2, Issue 4, pp. 282–286). https://www.ingentaconnect.com/content/ben/lddd/2005/00000002/00000004/art00006.

Barrett, T., Troup, D. B., Wilhite, S. E., Ledoux, P., Rudnev, D., Evangelista, C., Kim, I. F., Soboleva, A., Tomashevsky, M., Marshall, K. A., Phillippy, K. H., Sherman, P. M., Muertter, R. N., & Edgar, R. (2009). NCBI GEO: archive for high-throughput functional genomic data. *Nucleic Acids Research*, *37*(Database issue), D885-90. https://doi.org/10.1093/nar/gkn764.

Basso, M., Sleiman, S., & Ratan, R. R. (2013). Looking above but not beyond the genome for therapeutics in neurology and psychiatry: epigenetic proteins and RNAs find a new focus. *Neurotherapeutics : The Journal of the American Society for Experimental NeuroTherapeutics*, *10*(4), 551–555. https://doi.org/10.1007/s13311-013-0225-2.

Baxevanis, A. D. (2006). The importance of biological databases in biological discovery. *Current Protocols in Bioinformatics*, *Chapter 1*, Unit 1.1. https://doi.org/10.1002/0471250953.bi0101s13.

Benson, D. A., Karsch-Mizrachi, I., Lipman, D. J., Ostell, J., Rapp, B. A., & Wheeler, D. L. (2002). GenBank. *Nucleic Acids Research*, *30*(1), 17–20. https://doi.org/10.1093/nar/30.1.17.

Bhasin, M., Zhang, H., Reinherz, E. L., & Reche, P. A. (2005). Prediction of methylated CpGs in DNA sequences using a support vector machine. *FEBS Letters*, *579*(20), 4302–4308. https://doi.org/10.1016/j.febslet.2005.07.002.

Bjornsson, H. T., Brown, L. J., Fallin, M. D., Rongione, M. A., Bibikova, M., Wickham, E., Fan, J.-B., & Feinberg, A. P. (2007). Epigenetic specificity of loss of imprinting of the IGF2 gene in Wilms tumors. *Journal of the National Cancer Institute*, *99*(16), 1270–1273. https://doi.org/10.1093/jnci/djm069.

Bock, C., Walter, J., Paulsen, M., & Lengauer, T. (2007). CpG island mapping by epigenome prediction. *PLoS Computational Biology*, *3*(6), e110–e110. https://doi.org/10.1371/journal.pcbi.0030110.

Bock, C., Walter, J., Paulsen, M., & Lengauer, T. (2008). Inter-individual variation of DNA methylation and its implications for large-scale epigenome mapping. *Nucleic Acids Research*, *36*(10), e55–e55. https://doi.org/10.1093/nar/gkn122.

Burggren, W. (2016). Epigenetic Inheritance and Its Role in Evolutionary Biology: Re-Evaluation and New Perspectives. *Biology*, *5*(2). https://doi.org/10.3390/biology5020024.

Cedar, H., & Bergman, Y. (2009). Linking DNA methylation and histone modification: patterns and paradigms. *Nature Reviews Genetics*, *10*(5), 295–304. https://doi.org/10.1038/nrg2540.

Chen, H., Xue, Y., Huang, N., Yao, X., & Sun, Z. (2006). MeMo: a web tool for prediction of protein methylation modifications. *Nucleic Acids Research*, *34*(Web Server issue), W249–W253. https://doi.org/10.1093/nar/gkl233.

Cutter, A. D., & Ward, S. (2005). Sexual and Temporal Dynamics of Molecular Evolution in C. elegans Development. *Molecular Biology and Evolution*, *22*(1), 178–188. https://doi.org/10.1093/molbev/msh267.

Das, R., Dimitrova, N., Xuan, Z., Rollins, R. A., Haghighi, F., Edwards, J. R., Ju, J., Bestor, T. H., & Zhang, M. Q. (2006). Computational prediction of methylation status in human genomic sequences. *Proceedings of the National Academy of Sciences of the United States of America*, *103*(28), 10713–10716. https://doi.org/10.1073/pnas.0602949103.

Dessalew, N. (2007). QSAR study on aminophenylbenzamides and acrylamides as histone deacetylase inhibitors: An insight into the structural basis of antiproliferative activity. *Medicinal Chemistry Research*, *16*(7), 449–460. https://doi.org/10.1007/s00044-007-9085-9.

Dodd, I. B., Micheelsen, M. A., Sneppen, K., & Thon, G. (2007). Theoretical analysis of epigenetic cell memory by nucleosome modification. *Cell*, *129*(4), 813–822. https://doi.org/10.1016/j.cell.2007.02.053.

Du, J., Johnson, L. M., Jacobsen, S. E., & Patel, D. J. (2015). DNA methylation pathways and their crosstalk with histone methylation. *Nature Reviews. Molecular Cell Biology*, *16*(9), 519–532. https://doi.org/10.1038/nrm4043.

Eden, E., Lipson, D., Yogev, S., & Yakhini, Z. (2007). Discovering motifs in ranked lists of DNA sequences. *PLoS Computational Biology*, *3*(3), e39–e39. https://doi.org/10.1371/journal.pcbi.0030039.

Eileithyia, S., Andrew, H., Stephen, H., & Philip, W. (2005). Disease-associated mutations cause premature oligomerization of myelin proteolipid protein in the endoplasmic reticulum. *Proceedings of the National Academy of Sciences*, *102*(12), 4342–4347. https://doi.org/10.1073/pnas.0407287102.

Falls, J. G., Pulford, D. J., Wylie, A. A., & Jirtle, R. L. (1999). Genomic imprinting: implications for human disease. *The American Journal of Pathology*, *154*(3), 635–647. https://doi.org/10.1016/S0002-9440(10)65309-6.

Fang, Y.-C., Huang, H.-C., & Juan, H.-F. (2008). MeInfoText: associated gene methylation and cancer information from text mining. *BMC Bioinformatics*, *9*, 22. https://doi.org/10.1186/1471-2105-9-22.

Galperin, M. Y. (2008). The Molecular Biology Database Collection: 2008 update. *Nucleic Acids Research*, *36*(suppl_1), D2–D4. https://doi.org/10.1093/nar/gkm1037.

Goll, M. G., Kirpekar, F., Maggert, K. A., Yoder, J. A., Hsieh, C.-L., Zhang, X., Golic, K. G., Jacobsen, S. E., & Bestor, T. H. (2006). Methylation of tRNAAsp by the DNA methyltransferase homolog Dnmt2. *Science (New York, N.Y.)*, *311*(5759), 395–398. https://doi.org/10.1126/science.1120976.

Grant, P. A. (2001). A tale of histone modifications. *Genome Biology*, *2*(4), REVIEWS0003–REVIEWS0003. https://doi.org/10.1186/gb-2001-2-4-reviews0003.

Heintz, N. (2004). Gene expression nervous system atlas (GENSAT). *Nature Neuroscience*, *7*(5), 483. https://doi.org/10.1038/nn0504-483.

Iizuka, M., & Smith, M. M. (2003). Functional consequences of histone modifications. *Current Opinion in Genetics & Development*, *13*(2), 154–160. https://doi.org/10.1016/s0959-437x(03)00020-0.

Ioudinkova, E. S., Barat, A., Pichugin, A., Markova, E., Sklyar, I., Pirozhkova, I., Robin, C., Lipinski, M., Ogryzko, V., Vassetzky, Y. S., & Razin, S. V. (2012). Distinct Distribution of Ectopically Expressed Histone Variants H2A.Bbd and MacroH2A in Open and Closed Chromatin Domains. *PLOS ONE*, *7*(10), e47157. https://doi.org/10.1371/journal.pone.0047157.

Itoh, M., Goto, S., Akutsu, T., & Kanehisa, M. (2005). Fast and accurate database homology search using upper bounds of local alignment scores. *Bioinformatics (Oxford, England)*, *21*(7), 912–921. https://doi.org/10.1093/bioinformatics/bti076.

Jones, P. A. (2002). DNA methylation and cancer. *Oncogene*, *21*(35), 5358–5360. https://doi.org/10.1038/sj.onc.1205597.

Juvale, D. C., Kulkarni, V. V, Deokar, H. S., Wagh, N. K., Padhye, S. B., & Kulkarni, V. M. (2006). 3D-QSAR of histone deacetylase inhibitors: hydroxamate analogues. *Organic & Biomolecular Chemistry*, *4*(15), 2858–2868. https://doi.org/10.1039/b606365a.

Kanz, C., Aldebert, P., Althorpe, N., Baker, W., Baldwin, A., Bates, K., Browne, P., van den Broek, A., Castro, M., Cochrane, G., Duggan, K., Eberhardt, R., Faruque, N., Gamble, J., Diez, F. G., Harte, N., Kulikova, T., Lin, Q., Lombard, V., … Apweiler, R. (2005). The EMBL Nucleotide Sequence Database. *Nucleic Acids Research*, *33*(suppl_1), D29–D33. https://doi.org/10.1093/nar/gki098.

Kaslow, D. C., & Migeon, B. R. (1987). DNA methylation stabilizes X chromosome inactivation in eutherians but not in marsupials: evidence for multistep maintenance of mammalian X dosage compensation. *Proceedings of the National Academy of Sciences of the United States of America*, *84*(17), 6210–6214. https://doi.org/10.1073/pnas.84.17.6210.

Kent, W. J. (2002). BLAT--the BLAST-like alignment tool. *Genome Research*, *12*(4), 656–664. https://doi.org/10.1101/gr.229202.

Keshet, I., Schlesinger, Y., Farkash, S., Rand, E., Hecht, M., Segal, E., Pikarski, E., Young, R. A., Niveleau, A., Cedar, H., & Simon, I. (2006). Evidence for an instructive mechanism of de novo methylation in cancer cells. *Nature Genetics*, *38*(2), 149–153. https://doi.org/10.1038/ng1719.

Koudan, E. V, Bujnicki, J. M., & Gromova, E. S. (2004). Homology modeling of the CG-specific DNA methyltransferase SssI and its complexes with DNA and AdoHcy. *Journal of Biomolecular Structure & Dynamics*, *22*(3), 339–345. https://doi.org/10.1080/07391102.2004.10507005.

Kouskoumvekaki, I., Hansen, N. T., Björkling, F., Vadlamudi, S. M., & Jónsdóttir, S. O. (2008). Prediction of pH-dependent aqueous solubility of Histone Deacetylase (HDAC) inhibitors. *SAR and QSAR in Environmental Research*, *19*(1–2), 167–177. https://doi.org/10.1080/10629360701843367.

Krallinger, M., & Valencia, A. (2005). Text-mining and information-retrieval services for molecular biology. *Genome Biology*, *6*(7), 224. https://doi.org/10.1186/gb-2005-6-7-224.

Kumar, S., Nei, M., Dudley, J., & Tamura, K. (2008). MEGA: a biologist-centric software for evolutionary analysis of DNA and protein sequences. *Briefings in Bioinformatics*, *9*(4), 299–306. https://doi.org/10.1093/bib/bbn017.

Laird, P. W. (2005). Cancer epigenetics. *Human Molecular Genetics*, *14 Spec No*, R65-76. https://doi.org/10.1093/hmg/ddi113.

LeRoy, G., DiMaggio, P. A., Chan, E. Y., Zee, B. M., Blanco, M. A., Bryant, B., Flaniken, I. Z., Liu, S., Kang, Y., Trojer, P., & Garcia, B. A. (2013). A quantitative atlas of histone modification signatures from human cancer cells. *Epigenetics & Chromatin*, *6*(1), 20. https://doi.org/10.1186/1756-8935-6-20.

Li, E., Beard, C., & Jaenisch, R. (1993). Role for DNA methylation in genomic imprinting. *Nature*, *366*(6453), 362–365. https://doi.org/10.1038/366362a0.

Liang, G., Chan, M. F., Tomigahara, Y., Tsai, Y. C., Gonzales, F. A., Li, E., Laird, P. W., & Jones, P. A. (2002). Cooperativity between DNA methyltransferases in the maintenance methylation of repetitive elements. *Molecular and Cellular Biology*, *22*(2), 480–491. https://doi.org/10.1128/MCB.22.2.480-491.2002.

Lim, S. J., Tan, T. W., & Tong, J. C. (2010). Computational Epigenetics: the new scientific paradigm. *Bioinformation*, *4*(7), 331–337. https://doi.org/10.6026/97320630004331.

Lin, Y.-C., Lin, J.-H., Chou, C.-W., Chang, Y.-F., Yeh, S.-H., & Chen, C.-C. (2008). Statins increase p21 through inhibition of histone deacetylase activity and release of promoter-associated HDAC1/2. *Cancer Research*, *68*(7), 2375–2383. https://doi.org/10.1158/0008-5472.CAN-07-5807.

Marchevsky, A. M., Tsou, J. A., & Laird-Offringa, I. A. (2004). Classification of individual lung cancer cell lines based on DNA methylation markers: use of linear discriminant analysis and artificial neural networks. *The Journal of Molecular Diagnostics : JMD*, *6*(1), 28–36. https://doi.org/10.1016/S1525-1578(10)60488-6.

Miranda-Saavedra, D., & Barton, G. J. (2007). Classification and functional annotation of eukaryotic protein kinases. *Proteins*, *68*(4), 893–914. https://doi.org/10.1002/prot.21444.

Miranda-Saavedra, D., De, S., Trotter, M. W., Teichmann, S. A., & Göttgens, B. (2009). BloodExpress: a database of gene expression in mouse haematopoiesis. *Nucleic Acids Research*, *37*(Database issue), D873–D879. https://doi.org/10.1093/nar/gkn854.

Nathan, D., Sterner, D. E., & Berger, S. L. (2003). Histone modifications: Now summoning sumoylation. *Proceedings of the National Academy of Sciences of the United States of America*, *100*(23), 13118–13120. https://doi.org/10.1073/pnas.2436173100.

Negre, V., & Grunau, C. (2006). The MethDB DAS Server: Adding an Epigenetic Information Layer to the Human Genome. *Epigenetics*, *1*(2), 101–105. https://doi.org/10.4161/epi.1.2.2765.

Nishimura, M., Yu, G., Levesque, G., Zhang, D. M., Ruel, L., Chen, F., Milman, P., Holmes, E., Liang, Y., Kawarai, T., Jo, E., Supala, A., Rogaeva, E., Xu, D.-M., Janus, C., Levesque, L., Bi, Q., Duthie, M., Rozmahel, R., … St George–Hyslop, P. (1999). Presenilin mutations associated with Alzheimer disease cause defective intracellular trafficking of β-catenin,a component of the presenilin protein complex. *Nature Medicine*, *5*(2), 164–169. https://doi.org/10.1038/5526.

Ongenaert, M., Van Neste, L., De Meyer, T., Menschaert, G., Bekaert, S., & Van Criekinge, W. (2008). PubMeth: a cancer methylation database combining text-mining and expert annotation. *Nucleic Acids Research*, *36*(Database issue), D842-6. https://doi.org/10.1093/nar/gkm788.

Park, H., & Lee, S. (2004). Homology modeling, force field design, and free energy simulation studies to optimize the activities of histone deacetylase inhibitors. *Journal of Computer-Aided Molecular Design*, *18*(6), 375–388. https://doi.org/10.1007/s10822-004-2283-3.

Pattyn, F., Hoebeeck, J., Robbrecht, P., Michels, E., De Paepe, A., Bottu, G., Coornaert, D., Herzog, R., Speleman, F., & Vandesompele, J. (2006). methBLAST and methPrimerDB: web-tools for PCR based methylation analysis. *BMC Bioinformatics*, *7*(1), 496. https://doi.org/10.1186/1471-2105-7-496.

Petronis, A. (2010). Epigenetics as a unifying principle in the aetiology of complex traits and diseases. *Nature*, *465*(7299), 721–727. https://doi.org/10.1038/nature09230.

Porter, C. J., Palidwor, G. A., Sandie, R., Krzyzanowski, P. M., Muro, E. M., Perez-Iratxeta, C., & Andrade-Navarro, M. A. (2007). StemBase: a resource for the analysis of stem cell gene expression data. *Methods in Molecular Biology (Clifton, N.J.)*, *407*, 137–148. https://doi.org/10.1007/978-1-59745-536-7_11.

Robertson, K. D., Uzvolgyi, E., Liang, G., Talmadge, C., Sumegi, J., Gonzales, F. A., & Jones, P. A. (1999). The human DNA methyltransferases (DNMTs) 1, 3a and 3b: coordinate mRNA expression in normal tissues and overexpression in tumors. *Nucleic Acids Research*, *27*(11), 2291–2298. https://doi.org/10.1093/nar/27.11.2291.

Roh, T., Wei, G., Farrell, C. M., & Zhao, K. (2007). Genome-wide prediction of conserved and nonconserved enhancers by histone acetylation patterns. *Genome Research*, *17*(1), 74–81. https://doi.org/10.1101/gr.5767907.

Roh, T. Y., Cuddapah, S., & Zhao, K. (2005). Active chromatin domains are defined by acetylation islands revealed by genome-wide mapping. *Genes & Development*, *19*(5), 542–552. https://doi.org/10.1101/gad.1272505.

Rosenthal, A., Mork, P., Li, M. H., Stanford, J., Koester, D., & Reynolds, P. (2010). Cloud computing: a new business paradigm for biomedical information sharing. *Journal of Biomedical Informatics*, *43*(2), 342–353. https://doi.org/10.1016/j.jbi.2009.08.014.

Russo, V. E. A., Martienssen, R. A., & Riggs, A. D. (n.d.). Epigenetic mechanisms of gene regulation. 1996. *Plainview, NY: Cold Spring Harbor Laboratory Press, Xii.*

Schübeler, D., MacAlpine, D. M., Scalzo, D., Wirbelauer, C., Kooperberg, C., van Leeuwen, F., Gottschling, D. E., O'Neill, L. P., Turner, B. M., Delrow, J., Bell, S. P., & Groudine, M. (2004). The histone modification pattern of active genes revealed through genome-wide chromatin analysis of a higher eukaryote. *Genes & Development*, *18*(11), 1263–1271. https://doi.org/10.1101/gad.1198204.

Shmueli, O., Horn-Saban, S., Chalifa-Caspi, V., Shmoish, M., Ophir, R., Benjamin-Rodrig, H., Safran, M., Domany, E., & Lancet, D. (2003). GeneNote: whole genome expression profiles in normal human tissues. *Comptes Rendus Biologies*, *326*(10–11), 1067–1072. https://doi.org/10.1016/j.crvi.2003.09.012.

Smith, S. A., & Donoghue, M. J. (2008). Rates of molecular evolution are linked to life history in flowering plants. *Science (New York, N.Y.)*, *322*(5898), 86–89. https://doi.org/10.1126/science.1163197.

Sullivan, S. A., Aravind, L., Makalowska, I., Baxevanis, A. D., & Landsman, D. (2000). The histone database: a comprehensive WWW resource for histones and histone fold-containing proteins. *Nucleic Acids Research*, *28*(1), 320–322. https://doi.org/10.1093/nar/28.1.320.

Sullivan, S., Sink, D. W., Trout, K. L., Makalowska, I., Taylor, P. M., Baxevanis, A. D., & Landsman, D. (2002). The Histone Database. *Nucleic Acids Research*, *30*(1), 341–342. https://doi.org/10.1093/nar/30.1.341.

Talukdar, V., Konar, A., Datta, A., & Choudhury, A. R. (2009). Changing from computing grid to knowledge grid in life-science grid. *Biotechnology Journal*, *4*(9), 1244–1252. https://doi.org/10.1002/biot.200800073.

Tateno, Y., Imanishi, T., Miyazaki, S., Fukami-Kobayashi, K., Saitou, N., Sugawara, H., & Gojobori, T. (2002). DNA Data Bank of Japan (DDBJ) for genome scale research in life science. *Nucleic Acids Research*, *30*(1), 27–30. https://doi.org/10.1093/nar/30.1.27.

Thompson, J. D., Higgins, D. G., & Gibson, T. J. (1994). CLUSTAL W: improving the sensitivity of progressive multiple sequence alignment through sequence weighting, position-specific gap penalties and weight matrix choice. *Nucleic Acids Research*, *22*(22), 4673–4680. https://doi.org/10.1093/nar/22.22.4673.

Thurman, R. E., Day, N., Noble, W. S., & Stamatoyannopoulos, J. A. (2007). Identification of higher-order functional domains in the human ENCODE regions. *Genome Research*, *17*(6), 917–927. https://doi.org/10.1101/gr.6081407.

Vaquero, A., Loyola, A., & Reinberg, D. (2003). The constantly changing face of chromatin. *Science of Aging Knowledge Environment : SAGE KE*, *2003*(14), RE4. https://doi.org/10.1126/sageke.2003.14.re4.

Won, K.-J., Chepelev, I., Ren, B., & Wang, W. (2008). Prediction of regulatory elements in mammalian genomes using chromatin signatures. *BMC Bioinformatics*, *9*, 547. https://doi.org/10.1186/1471-2105-9-547.

Xie, S., Wang, Z., Okano, M., Nogami, M., Li, Y., He, W. W., Okumura, K., & Li, E. (1999). Cloning, expression and chromosome locations of the human DNMT3 gene family. *Gene*, *236*(1), 87–95. https://doi.org/10.1016/s0378-1119(99)00252-8.

Xu, H., Wei, C. L., Lin, F., & Sung, W.-K. (2008). An HMM approach to genome-wide identification of differential histone modification sites from ChIP-seq data. *Bioinformatics (Oxford, England)*, *24*(20), 2344–2349. https://doi.org/10.1093/bioinformatics/btn402.

Chapter 11

The Role of Epigenetics in Aging

Yusuf Muhammed Durna, MD
and Dilek Arslan Ateşşahin*, PhD
Department of Otolaryngology and Head and Neck Surgery,
Private Practice, Istanbul, Turkey
Department of Plant and Animal Production,
Baskil Vocational School, Firat University, Elazığ, Turkey

Abstract

Aging is a multifactorial process happening with many biological, biochemical, and physiological changes. There are a lot of theories to explain the nature of aging. There are also many data supporting the relationships between epigenetic modifications and the aging process. Nucleosomal remodeling is frequently stressed by numerous research due to its critical nature in cellular senescence and aging. Different mechanisms are postulated for nucleosomal remodeling, which include (1) modification of nucleosome residency by histone loss, (2) alteration of nucleosome affinity to either DNA or histones induced by histone protein variants, and (3) ATP-dependent nucleosome relocation to modify recruitment of transcriptional factors and other modifiers. Recent advances have revealed aging-related genes that have modifying properties for histone repositioning, which supports the fact that both aging and senescence are directly related to the disruption of heterochromatin and euchromatin ratios in the chromatin landscape. Thus, leading to the dissolution of the clear distinctions between chromatin regions in cellular senescence, which is more pronounced in the aging process. This dissolution correlates with the downregulation of genes in the senescence that are normally in an active state before the senescence period. However, conflicting results are present in terms of the genome-wide heterochromatin association with the aging and senescence processes. Therefore, specific analyses are necessary of which genomic regions, related loci, and gene expressions are affected. This review will try to describe the intricate associations between cellular senescence and known epigenetic mechanisms, e.g., chromatin remodeling and restructuring. Also, the currently established properties of the aging process with epigenetic mechanisms are described using different models for the aging phenomenon.

Keywords: aging, epigenetics, epigenomics, gene expression, histone modifications, nucleosomal complex, senescence

---

* Corresponding Author's E-mail: datessahin@firat.edu.tr.

In: Epigenetics: Beyond the Genetics and Medicine
Editors: Sevgi Durna Daştan and Nazan Yurtcu
ISBN: 979-8-88697-228-3

Abbreviations

SASP	Senescence-associated Secretory Phase
PTMs	Post-translational Modifications.

Introduction

Aging is an organism-level process, which is related to systems-wide pathologies through aggregated impairments from the cellular, tissue, and organ levels. An important lead in the process of aging or cell senescence is the increasing amounts of senescence in the tissue currently being affected, which is strongly linked to the development of the aging phenotype through the imbalance of cellular homeostasis (Couteau and Mallette, 2016; Munoz-Espin and Serrano, 2014). Research indicates that tissue degeneration is induced by the increasing amount of age-related senescent cells in several tissues, e.g., skin, liver, spleen, and lungs (Couteau and Mallette, 2016; Herbig et al., 2006; Jeyapalan et al., 2007; Wang et al., 2009). Organisms can initiate cellular senescence, which is a constant state of cell cycle stasis, to defend their integrity against a diverse array of offenses towards the physiological integrity, e.g., oxidative stress, oncogene activation, oncovirus infections, physical mutagenic factors, and telomere shortening (Guillaumet-Adkins et al., 2017). The constant state of cell cycle stasis can be defined by the metabolic activity and the morphological changes (flattening, multiple nucleations, pronounced nucleolus) of the cells, but these cells are kept impervious to the mitogenic triggers. One of the most comprehensively known markers for cellular senescence is the elevated activity of B-galactosidase, which is related to the increased lysosomal mass in the cell (Kurz et al., 2000). Cellular aging is also strongly associated with the increase in the heterochromatin ratios in the nuclear landscape, which is also involved in the recruitment of histone protein variants. Modifications of the chromatin structure initiate the other modulatory functions known as the SASP, which is related to the production of cytokines, growth factors, and matrix metalloproteinases (Couteau and Mallette, 2016; Coppe et al., 2010). It is now mostly agreed that aging-related diseases are the result of the lifelong aggregation of senescent cells in various tissues. Cellular aging works like a double-edged blade for the organisms, while it is a preservative of the integrity of the organism during the early phases of life, it will be baneful for the late-life, which is attributed to antagonistic pleiotropy (Couteau and Mallette, 2016). Young to adult organisms can eliminate the senescent aggregation by the immune system, which is known to decline in function with the age, and also the impairments in stress tolerance in organisms in late life are all postulated to be the reason why senescent cells cannot be eliminated effectively in late-life (Kang et al., 2011; Xue et al., 2007). Overall, the increase in senescent cells in a tissue gradually contributes to tissue dysfunctions and, consequently, to tissue degeneration. Numerous in vitro and in vivo models have been established for the determination of aging-related mechanisms (Couteau and Mallette, 2016, Bobak et al., 2022). With aging, there is an overall decrease in DNA methylation and promoter hypermethylation is detected in specific genes (Guillaumet-Adkins et al., 2017; Heyn et al., 2012; Gentilini et al., 2013). It has also been shown that hypermethylation of specific genes is very effective in apoptosis, development, differentiation (Salpea et al., 2012), and aging. Bocklandt et al., (2011) identified the epigenetic pattern of aging (Guillaumet-Adkins et al., 2017; Koch and Wagner,

2011). In addition, studies investigate and describe the use of certain cytosines to predict epigenetic age in specific tissues (Bocklandt et al., 2011; Weidner et al., 2014; Hannum et al., 2013). Also, several research using both methylation sequence and transcriptomic data analysis in many tissue types ensures the evidence that epigenetic regulation that is associated with proportionally oxidative stress triggered aging and is correlated with cellular senescence, analyzed by both epigenomic and transcriptomic based biological clocks (Bobak et al., 2022). This section has explained how the interrelated effects of epigenetic changes affect the aging process. In addition, it is aimed to help understand the molecular basis of aging and the effects of aging on the epigenetic machinery.

Theoretical Perspectives

The Aging and Chromatin Structure

Chromatin is the name of structure given to the equivalent conglomerate of DNA and histone proteins. The structure has dynamic nature to control and regulate gene expression through reversible mechanisms that make up the chromatin condensation, which include tail modifications of histone proteins, e.g., methylation and acetylation of lysine and arginine amino acids (Kouzarides 2007). DNA itself contributes to chromatin condensation by methylation of cytosine bases located on CpG islands. Investigations revealed a complicated network apparent between chromatin modifications and the aging process (Munoz-Espin and Serrano, 2014). Among the results, two of them are of particular notice; (1) global alteration of total gene expression profile (Lu et al., 2004); and (2) pronounced differences in epigenetic makeup observed in cellular senescence (Herbig et al., 2006; Narita et al., 2003; Zhang t al., 2005). Investigations postulated the epigenetic balance hypothesis to explain the age-dependent manner of chromatin modifications spanning entire chromosomes (Oberdoerffer and Sinclair, 2007). It should not go without saying that a fundamental schism still requires a decisive answer: Are chromatin modifications resulting from accumulated genomic damages or are chromatin modifications pre-programmed to trigger in age-dependent phases of cells (Couteau and Mallette, 2016).

The Nucleosome Structure and Aging

Chromatin is made up of nucleosomes, which are formations of DNA and core histone protein dimers. Enzymes that have chromatin remodeling capabilities form installations to modify nucleosome composition or its access to DNA, which enables other modifiers to bind to chromatin that ultimately regulate the gene expression. In terms of epigenetic regulation, the elevation in histone protein expression and nucleosome formation are stressed in aging. Initial investigations revealed a significant increase in genes expressing the histone proteins by transcriptomics in aged yeasts (Lesur and Campbell, 2004), whereas later studies contradict the initial findings by showing a significant reduction in certain histone proteins (H2A, H3, H4) in aged yeast cells compared to young yeast cells (Dang et al., 2009; Feser et al., 2010). A significant increase in gene expressions for H3 and H4 is agreed to prolong the reproductive period of yeast cells, but it is unclear if the same increase can be translated to nucleosome formations or preservation against histone variants (Feser et al., 2010; Feser and Tyler, 2011). Nucleosome positioning analysis revealed that particularly nucleosome-rich genomic regions become nucleosome-poor with aging to enable the expression of genes normally suppressed in young cells [42]. Among these genes are the retrotransposition genes, which translate into genomic corruption observed in aged yeast cells (Hu et al., 2014). One remarkable feature of histone loss is that it is potentially conserved in cellular senescence, as shown in aged human fibroblasts that have significantly lower (w50%) amounts of H3 and H4 histone proteins compared to young human fibroblasts (O'Sullivan et al., 2010). The established findings of aging are correlated with the increases in transcriptions of these genes, as well as those of DNA damage and metabolic disorders. Higher eukaryote organisms require a histone protein variant, H2AZ, for proper development (Faast et al., 2001). H2AZ is found primarily in heterochromatin regions (Rangasamy et al., 2003), but is also available in the remaining part of the genome, which may serve different purposes. Related to this, it is shown in cellular senescence that H2AZ accumulation is specifically prevented in the INK4 locus by a long non-coding RNA that binds to P400 installation, which is known to reserve H2AZ to chromatin (Couteau and Mallette, 2016; Lazorthes et al., 2015).

For decades, aging is related to DNA damage, which is supported by the fact that gH2AX foci have persevered in the genome of senescent cells; however, whether such DNA damage-related indicators are associated with aging, if any, is still dubious. It is presumed that gH2AX foci are removed from action following the initial DNA damage and remain persistent to ensure proper induction of the senescence process (Turinetto and Giachino, 2015). It is shown both in aged cells of higher eukaryote organisms and in senescent fibroblasts that the H3.3 histone protein variant, which is bereft of replication, replaces the canon H3 variants that are H3.1 and H3.2 (Rai and Adams, 2013). Concerning the deposition of the H3.3 variant on nucleosomes, one of the histone protein chaperons named HIRA, which is specialized for the H3.3 variant, is shown to be markedly elevated in fibroblasts of dermal tissue from old primates that strongly suggests the role of HIRA in histone protein variant accumulation in aging (Couteau and Mallette, 2016; Jeyapalan et al., 2007).

Aging-Related Post-Translational Modifications (PTMs) of Histone Proteins

Among the PTMs, histone acetylation and histone methylation are the most pronounced, and the enzymes responsible for these modifications are collectively known as chromatin modifiers. Histone acetylation is related to the increase in expression by their modification to make chromatin regions open to transcriptional factor binding. Therefore, to reveal the associations between chromatin restructuring and the aging process, localized and global variations in histone modifications with aging should be assessed. Towards this end, chromatin immunoprecipitation (ChIP) coupled with genome-wide association studies (GWAS) are necessary to perform. Research revealed a global reduction in histone acetylation of several lysine residues in histone tails of H3 and H4 histone proteins and revealed that the same residues were methylated instead (Chicas et al., 2012). One of the striking results is the potential of alleviating cognitive deterioration associated with advancing ages due to the hypoacetylated states of H4K12 and H4K9 variants with the use of histone deacetylase enzymes in certain animal models (Kilgore et al., 2010; Peleg et al., 2010; Zeng et al., 2011). Inducing the overexpression of Mof, a histone acetyltransferase enzyme, and repressing the histone deacetylase enzymes are shown in the murine HPGS model to prolong the expected lifespan while preventing age-related impairments (Couteau and Mallette, 2016).

Aging-Related Chromatin Modifier Expressions

While it is a fact that chromatin structural changes are directly associated with cellular senescence, the stream of molecular actions that end with changes is debatable. It is still blurry if the modifications of the epigenetic landscape are directly related to aging. Analysis of gene expression profiles of genes responsible for chromatin modifications both in senescent and aged cells is one of the possible ways to correlate coherent changes to aging. Transcriptome analysis conducted on a global scale failed to reveal any coherent changes directly associated with modifier expressions in senescent cells. On the other hand, localized histone modifications are agreed to be induced by aging. Research revealed that p16INK4A and p4/p19ARF, which are coded by INK4A/ARF located on chromosome 9 in humans, are associated with aging (Kim and Sharpless, 2006). In its hypophosphorylated form, p16INK4a, which is a cyclin-dependent kinase enzyme, is known to conserve pRB, and both p16INK4A and p4/p19ARF are considered aging markers for humans since they are markedly elevated in aged cells from different tissues (Couteau and Mallette, 2016; Krishnamurthy et al., 2004; Bobak et al., 2022).

Telomers in Regard to Aging

Telomers are, similar to other repeat sequences in the genome, positioned in the heterochromatin regions, and their integrity is ensured by the chromatin structure (Gonzalo et al., 2006). The subtelomeric regions of chromosomes are strikingly similar to the fundamental heterochromatin regions with the properties of having variants of H3K9me3 and H4K20me3, capability for HP1a binding, and hypermethylated DNA sequences. As shown in human fibroblasts, deacetylation of H3K9 variants in telomers by lysine deacetylase treatment leads to telomere impairment associated with precocious senescence and lifespan reduction, and inappropriate aged phenotype development (Michishita et al., 2008). On the other hand, it is shown that excessively shortened telomers exhibit subtelomeric deviations from the normal heterochromatin structure and hypomethylation of histone tails (Benetti et al., 2007). Near-senescent cells revealed a noteworthy trait of affecting H3 and H4 expression triggered by shortened telomers similar to accumulated DNA damage responses, which lead to global chromatin restructuring. Taking these into account, modifications in telomere structural integrity are accepted as the driving force behind the genome corruption related to advanced age. This is further explained by the fact that impairments in telomeric sequences initiate subtelomeric structure modifications and telomere dysfunctions from subtelomeric modifications. Overall, it is evident that critically short telomeres are responsible for the differentiations in the epigenetic frame that are obvious in both cellular senescence and aged cells (Couteau and Mallette, 2016).

Conclusion

The aging process is evident in all layers of epigenetic mechanisms, which include chromatin remodeling, histone modifications, and DNA methylation. While they are genome-wide, it is clear that certain changes are more site-specific for particular loci than general, and all changes are connecting numerous cellular pathways to lead to genome-wide loss of integrity and functioning. Apart from physiological aging, DNA damage such as a virus, environmental hazards, and genetic factors are initiating the aging-related epigenetic modifications. These modifications have their potential in personalized medicine as they can be used for the prediction of the true biological age of an organism and susceptibility to aging-related health conditions. Embryonic stem cells, among all others, solely can reset all kinds of epigenetic changes to maintain their pluripotency, and reinstall tissue-specific marks during cellular differentiation, which is true for induced pluripotent stem cells. Some of the aging-related chromatin modifications, at least in some aspects, are shown to be reversed or stopped by external intervention, which provides future directions for their use in epigenetic-based clinical manipulations for both treatment and prolonging the life expectancy.

References

Benetti, R. Garcia-Cao, M. and Blasco, M. A. (2007). Telomere length regulates the epigenetic status of mammalian telomeres and subtelomeres. *Nature Genetics,* 39(2), 243-250.

Bobak, C., Abhimanyu, Natarajan, H. Gandhi, T., Sandra L. Grimm, Tomoki Nishiguchi, Kent Koste, Santiago Carrero Longlax, Qiniso Dlamini, Jacquiline Kahari, Godwin Mtetwa, Jeffrey D. Cirillo, James O'Malley, Jane E. Hill, Cristian Coarfa, Andrew R. DiNardo (2022). Increased DNA methylation, cellular senescence and premature epigenetic aging in guinea pigs and humans with tuberculosis. *Aging,* 14 (5), 2174-2193.

Bocklandt, S. Lin, W. Sehl, M. E., Francisco J. Sánchez, Janet S. Sinsheimer, Steve Horvath, Eric Vilain (2011). Epigenetic predictor of age. *PloS One,* 6, e14821.

Chicas, A. Kapoor, A., Wang, X. Aksoy, O. Evertts, A. G. Zhang, M. Q., Benjamin A. Garcia, Emily Bernstein, Scott W. Lowe (2012). H3K4 demethylation by Jarid1a and Jarid1b contributes to retinoblastoma-mediated gene silencing during cellular senescence. *Proceedings of the National Academy of Science,* 109(23), 8971-8976.

Coppe, J. P. Desprez, P. Y. Krtolica, A. Campisi, J. (2010). The senescence-associated secretory phenotype: the dark side of tumor suppression. *Annual Review of Pathology,* 5, 99-118.

Couteau, F. and Mallette, F. A. (2016). Chromatin signaling in aging and cellular senescence. In: O. Binda and M. E. Fernandez-Zapico (Eds.) *Chromatin Signaling Diseases* (pp. 288-315). Elsevier, London, UK. ISBN: 978-0-12-802389-1.

Dang, W. Steffen, K. K. Perry, R. Dorsey, J. A. Johnson, F. B. Shilatifard, A., Matt Kaeberlein, Brian K. Kennedy & Shelley L. Berger (2009). Histone H4 lysine 16 acetylation regulates cellular lifespan. *Nature,* 459(7248), 802-807.

Faast, R. Thonglairoam, V. Schulz, T. C. Beall, J. Wells, J. R. Taylor, H. K. Matthaei, P. D. Rathjen, D. J. Tremethick, I. Lyons (2001). Histone variant H2A.Z is required for early mammalian development. *Current Biology,* 11(15), 1183-1187.

Feser, J. Truong, D. Das, C. Carson, J. J. Kieft, J. Harkness, T., Jessica K. Tyler (2010). Elevated histone expression promotes life span extension. *Molecular Cell,* 39(5), 724-735.

Feser, J. and Tyler, J. (2011). Chromatin structure as a mediator of aging. *FEBS Letters,* 585(13), 2041-2048.

Gentilini, D. Mari, D. Castaldi, D., Daniel Remondini, Giulia Ogliari, Rita Ostan, Laura Bucci, Silvia M Sirchia, Silvia Tabano, Francesco Cavagnini, Daniela Monti, Claudio Franceschi, Anna Maria Di Blasio, Giovanni Vitale (2013). Role of epigenetics in human aging and longevity: genome-wide DNA methylation profile in centenarians and centenarians' offspring. *Age (Dordrecht, Netherlands)*, 35(5), 1961-1973.

Gonzalo, S. Jaco, I., Fraga, M. F. Chen, T. Li, E. Esteller, M., María A. Blasco (2006). DNA methyltransferases control telomere length and telomere recombination in mammalian cells. *Nature Cell Biology*, 8(4), 416-424.

Guillaumet-Adkins, A. Yanez, Y. Peris-Diaz, M. D., Ines Calabria, Cora Palanca-Ballester and Juan Sandoval (2017). Epigenetics and oxidative stress in aging. *Oxidative Medicine and Cellular Longevity*, 9175806, 8.

Hannum, G. Guinney, J. Zhao, L. Li Zhang, Guy Hughes, Srini Vas Sadda, Brandy Klotzle, Marina Bibikova, Jian-Bing Fan, Yuan Gao, Rob Deconde, Menzies Chen, Indika Rajapakse, Stephen Friend, Trey Ideker and Kang Zhang. (2013). Genome-wide methylation profiles reveal quantitative views of human aging rates. *Molecular Cell*, 49, 359-367.

Herbig, U. Ferreira, M. Condel, L. Carey, D. Sedivy, J. M. (2006). Cellular senescence in aging primates. *Science*, 311(5765), 1257.

Heyn, H. Li, N. Ferreira, H. J., Sebastian Moran, David G. Pisano, Antonio Gomez, Javier Diez, Jose V. Sanchez-Mut, Fernando Setien, F. Javier Carmona, Annibale A. Puca, Sergi Sayols, Miguel A. Pujana, Jordi Serra-Musach, Isabel Iglesias-Platas, Francesc Formiga, Agustin F. Fernandez, Mario F. Fraga, Simon C. Heath, Alfonso Valencia, Ivo G. Gut, Jun Wang and Manel Esteller (2012). Distinct DNA methylomes of newborns and centenarians. *Proceedings of the National Academy of Sciences of the United States of America*, 109, 10522-10527.

Hu, Z. Chen, K. Xia, Z. Chavez, M. Pal, S. Seol, J. H., Chin-Chuan Chen, Wei Li, Jessica K. Tyler (2014). Nucleosome loss leads to global transcriptional up-regulation and genomic instability during yeast aging. *Genes Development*, 28(4), 396-408.

Jeyapalan, J. C. Ferreira, M. Sedivy, J. M. Herbig, U. (2007). Accumulation of senescent cells in mitotic tissue of aging primates. *Mechanisms of Ageing Development*, 128(1), 36-44.

Kang, T. W. Yevsa, T. Woller, N. Hoenicke, L. Wuestefeld, T. Dauch, D., Daniel Dauch, Anja Hohmeyer, Marcus Gereke, Ramona Rudalska, Anna Potapova, Marcus Iken, Mihael Vucur, Siegfried Weiss, Mathias Heikenwalder, Sadaf Khan, Jesus Gil, Dunja Bruder, Michael Manns, Peter Schirmacher, Frank Tacke, Michael Ott, Tom Luedde, Thomas Longerich, Stefan Kubicka & Lars Zender (2011). Senescence surveillance of pre-malignant hepatocytes limits liver cancer development. *Nature*, 479(7374), 547-551.

Kilgore, M. Miller, C. A. Fass, D. M. Hennig, K. M. Haggarty, S. J. Sweatt, J. D. and Gavin Rumbaugh (2010). Inhibitors of class 1 histone deacetylases reverse contextual mem ory deficits in a mouse model of Alzheimer's disease. *Neuropsychopharmacology*, 35(4), 870-880.

Kim, W. Y. Sharpless, N. E. (2006). The regulation of INK4/ARF in cancer and aging. *Cell*, 127(2), 265-275.

Koch, C. M. and Wagner, W. (2011). Epigenetic-aging-signature to determine age in different tissues. *Aging (Albany NY)*, 3, 1018-1027.

Kouzarides, T. (2007). Chromatin modifications and their function. *Cell*, 128(4), 693-705.

Krishnamurthy, J. Torrice, C. Ramsey, M. R. Kovalev, G. I. Al-Regaiey, K. Su, L. and Norman E. Sharpless (2004). Ink4a/Arf expression is a biomarker of aging. *Journal of Clinical Investigation*, 114(9), 1299-1307.

Krishnan, V. Chow, M. Z. Wang, Z. Zhang, L. Liu, B. Liu, X., Zhongjun Zhou (2011). Histone H4 lysine 16 hypoacetylation is associated with defective DNA repair and premature senescence in Zmpste24-deficient mice. *Proceedings of the National Academy of Science USA*, 108(30), 12325-12330.

Kurz, D. J. Decary, S. Hong, Y. Erusalimsky, J. D. (2000). Senescence-associated (beta)-galactosidase reflects an increase in lysosomal mass during repli cative ageing of human endothelial cells. *Journal of Cell Science*, 113(20), 3613-3622.

Lazorthes, S. Vallot, C. Briois, S. Aguirrebengoa, M. Thuret, J. Y. St Laurent, G., Claire Rougeulle, Philipp Kapranov, Carl Mann, Didier Trouche and Estelle Nicolas. (2015). A vlincRNA participates in senescence maintenance by relieving H2AZ-mediated repression at the INK4 locus. *Nature Communications*, 6, 5971.

Lesur, I. Campbell, J. L. (2004). The transcriptome of prematurely aging yeast cells is similar to that of telomerase-deficient cells. *Molecular Biology of the Cell*, 15(3), 1297-1312.

Lu, T. Pan, Y. Kao, S. Y. Li, C. Kohane, I. Chan, J. and Bruce A. Yankner. (2004). Gene regulation and DNA damage in the ageing human brain. *Nature*, 429(6994), 883-891.

Michishita, E. McCord, R. A. Berber, E. Kioi, M. Padilla-Nash, H. Damian, M. Peggie Cheung, Rika Kusumoto, Tiara L. A. Kawahara, J. Carl Barrett, Howard Y. Chang, Vilhelm A. Bohr, Thomas Ried, Or Gozani & Katrin F. Chua. (2008). SIRT6 is a histone H3 lysine 9 deacetylase that modulates telomeric chromatin. *Nature,* 452(7186), 492-496.

Munoz-Espin, D. Serrano, M. (2014). Cellular senescence: from physiology to pathology. *Nature Reviews Molecular Cell Biology,* 15(7), 482-496.

Narita, M. Nunez, S. Heard, E. Lin, A. W. Hearn, S. A. Spector, D. L. Gregory J. Hannon, and Scott W. Lowe (2003). Rb-mediated heterochromatin formation and silencing of E2F target genes during cellular senescence. *Cell,* 113(6), 703-716.

Oberdoerffer, P. Sinclair, D. A. (2007). The role of nuclear architecture in genomic instability and ageing. *Nature Reviews Molecular Cell Biology,* 8(9), 692-702.

O'Sullivan, R. J. Kubicek, S. Schreiber, S. L. Karlseder, J. (2010). Reduced histone biosynthesis and chromatin changes arising from a damage signal at telomeres. *Nature Structural and Molecular Biology,* 17(10), 1218-1225.

Peleg, S. Sananbenesi, F. Zovoilis, A. Burkhardt, S. Bahari-Javan, S. Agis-Balboa, R. C., Perla Cota, Jessica Lee Wittnam, Andreas Gogol-Doering, Lennart Opitz, Gabriella Salinas-Riester, Markus Dettenhofer, Hui Kang, Laurent Farinelli, Wei Chen, André Fischer (2010). Altered histone acetylation is associated with age dependent memory impairment in mice. *Science,* 328(5979), 753-756.

Rai, T. S. Adams, P. D. (2013). Lessons from senescence: chromatin maintenance in non-proliferating cells. *Biochimica et Biophysica Acta,* 1819(3-4), 322-331.

Rangasamy, D. Berven, L. Ridgway, P. Tremethick, D. J. (2003). Pericentric heterochromatin becomes enriched with H2A.Z during early mammalian development. *EMBO J,* 22(7), 1599-1607.

Salpea, P. Russanova, V. R. Hirai, T. H. Thomae G. Sourlingas, Kalliope E. Sekeri-Pataryas, Roberto Romero, Jonathan Epstein, and Bruce H. Howard (2012). Postnatal development- and age-related changes in DNA-methylation patterns in the human genome. *Nucleic Acids Research,* 40, 6477-6494.

Turinetto, V. Giachino, C. (2015). Multiple facets of histone variant H2AX: a DNA double-strand-break marker with several biological functions. *Nucleic Acids Research*, 43(5), 2489-2498.

Wang, C. Jurk, D. Maddick, M. Nelson, G. Martin-Ruiz, C. von Zglinicki, T. (2009). DNA damage response and cellular senescence in tissues of aging mice. *Aging Cell,* 8(3), 311-323.

Weidner, C. I. Lin, Q. Koch, C. M., Lewin Eisele, Fabian Beier, Patrick Ziegler, Dirk Olaf Bauerschlag, Karl-Heinz Jöckel, Raimund Erbel, Thomas Walter Mühleisen, Martin Zenke, Tim Henrik Brümmendorf & Wolfgang Wagner (2014). Aging of blood can be tracked by DNA methylation changes at just three CpG sites. *Genome Biology,* 15, R24.

Xue, W. Zender, L. Miething, C. Dickins, R. A. Hernando, E. Krizhanovsky, V., Carlos Cordon-Cardo, and Scott W. Lowe (2007). Senescence and tumour clearance is triggered by p53 restoration in murine liver carcinomas. *Nature*, 445(7128), 656-660.

Zeng, Y. Tan, M. Kohyama, J. Sneddon, M. Watson, J. B. Sun, Y. E., and C. W. Xie. (2011). Epigenetic enhancement of BDNF signaling rescues synaptic plasticity inaging. *Journal of Neuroscience,* 31(49), 17800-17810.

Zhang, R. Poustovoitov, M. V. Ye, X. Santos, H. A. Chen, W. Daganzo, S. M., Jan P. Erzberger, Ilya G. Serebriiskii, Adrian A. Canutescu, Roland L. Dunbrack, John R. Pehrson, James M. Berger, Paul D. Kaufman, Peter D. Adams (2005). Formation of MacroH2A-containing senescence-associated heterochromatin foci and senescence driven by ASF1a and HIRA. *Developmental Cell*, 8(1), 19-30.

Chapter 12

Epigenetics and Familial Mediterranean Fever

Ekin B. Doğancı*, MD

Department of Physical Medicine and Rehabilitation,
Department of Rheumatology, Sivas Cumhuriyet University, Sivas, Turkey

Abstract

FMF represents an autosomal recessive hereditary disease, which may have recurrent episodes of fever, serositis, and arthritis/arthralgia and accompanying skin findings. Its prevalence varies from society to society and changes in the range of 1/200-1/1000 on average. The gene responsible for FMF is the MEFV (Mediterranean Fever) gene on chromosome 16, which encodes the pyrin protein. The problem in FMF is the change in pyrin protein due to the MEFV gene mutation. Mutation in pyrin reduces the activation threshold of the inflammasome, which excessively increases IL-1 secretion and initiates the inflammatory process. Mutations of M694V, V726A, M680I, and M694I are observed most frequently worldwide, and these are known as pathological mutations. The most feared complication is secondary AA-type amyloidosis. With the use of colchicine in the treatment, attacks are prevented, subclinical inflammation between attacks is taken under control, and the risk of amyloidosis is eliminated. Alternative treatments should be considered in the presence of partial remission with colchicine therapy, in cases of unresponsiveness to colchicine, or in cases of colchicine intolerance. TNF-a inhibitors, IL-1 inhibitors (anakinra, rilonacept, and canakinumab), and Janus kinase inhibitors are among alternative treatments.

It has been recently revealed that changes in DNA cannot be explained only by genetics, and the role of epigenetic mechanisms is also quite significant. In epigenetics, the DNA sequence does not change; however, since the promoter region of the gene changes, quantitative and qualitative changes emerge in gene transcription. As a result of transcriptional changes, the transcription of the relevant gene can be silenced or activated. These quantitative and qualitative changes are not permanent and can be regulated when needed. Furthermore, these alterations in gene transcription can be transferred to the following generations. When epigenetic mechanisms are mentioned, DNA methylation, histone acetylation, histone methylation, histone ubiquitination, histone phosphorylation, histone citrullination, histone ribosylation, non-coding RNA, and chromatin re-modeling come to mind.

Epigenetics tries to explain different phenotypes of FMF patients with the same genotype (patients with the same mutation and individuals from the same family), the absence of the clinical presentation of a patient with the mutation or the FMF clinical presentation of patients without the mutation, drug response or drug resistance. Histone

* Corresponding Author's E-mail: ekinbb_83@hotmail.com.

In: Epigenetics: Beyond the Genetics and Medicine
Editors: Sevgi Durna Daştan and Nazan Yurtcu
ISBN: 979-8-88697-228-3

modification, DNA methylation, and microRNA (miRNA) represent the epigenetic mechanisms that are accused the most of the correlation between FMF and epigenetics.

Keywords: Familial Mediterranean Fever, epigenetic, DNA methylation, histone modification

Introduction

Autoinflammatory diseases represent a group of diseases presenting with recurrent episodes of fever, increased activity of innate immune cells, and organ- or system-specific non-infectious inflammation. Innate immune cells that originate from the myeloid lineage (neutrophils, eosinophils) cause an overproduction of cytokines, e.g., IL-18 and IL-1B, and lead to uncontrolled inflammation. Pathological autoinflammatory phenotypes emerge as the result of errors in various signaling pathways that control innate immunity. Familial Mediterranean fever (FMF), which occurs as a result of the MEFV gene mutation, is one of these phenotypes.

FMF represents an autosomal recessive hereditary disease, which may have recurrent episodes of fever, serositis, and arthritis/arthralgia and accompanying skin findings. Patients are completely normal except for attacks. It is the most common monogenic disease in people who live in the Eastern Mediterranean. Its prevalence varies from society to society and changes in the range of 1/200-1/1000 on average. The gene responsible for FMF is the MEFV (Mediterranean Fever) gene on chromosome 16, which encodes the pyrin protein. Pyrin is produced from neutrophils, monocytes, fibroblasts, and dendritic cells. Pyrin is responsible for the activation of procaspase-1, a part of the inflammasome complex. Accordingly, IL-1b activation is regulated, and apoptosis and the activation of NF-kB are inhibited (Jesus et al., 2015). The problem in FMF is the change in the pyrin protein due to the MEFV gene mutation. Mutation in pyrin reduces the activation threshold of the inflammasome, which excessively increases IL-1 secretion and initiates the inflammatory process. Moreover, leukocyte apoptosis is inhibited as a result of mutation (Manukyan et al., 2016).

Mutations of M694V, V726A, M680I, and M694I are observed most frequently worldwide, and these are known as pathological mutations. It has been found that the frequency of M694V, especially, is 15-60% in the Mediterranean population. The M694V variant is the most severe phenotype associated with amyloidosis, arthritis, frequent attacks, and erysipelas-like skin rash. The M694V mutation is detected most frequently in Turkey, followed by the M608I mutation. The E148Q variant is an insignificant variant observed in 25% of the eastern Mediterranean population. There is an association between the presence of the E148Q mutation and low disease activity. It has also been stated that this variant can also be found in the normal population, and its presence should not always be interpreted in favor of FMF (Roper et al., 2019).

FMF attacks start suddenly. It is impossible to predict the frequency of attacks, and it has been indicated that factors, including stress, cold, fatigue, trauma, surgery, dietary changes, contraceptive use, heavy exercise, infections, vitamin D deficiency, and menstruation, can trigger an attack. Some patients also describe prodromal findings. In general, attacks are self-limiting and end spontaneously within 72 hours. Fever, shivering, stabbing unilateral chest pain that increases with breathing and coughing, abdominal pain, erysipelas-like rash, erythro-arthritis in the form of monoarthritis in the lower extremities, arthralgia, and GIS complaints such as nausea/vomiting may be observed in the clinical picture. Secondary AA-type amyloidosis is the most feared complication. With the use of colchicine in the treatment, attacks are prevented, subclinical inflammation between attacks is taken under control, and the risk of amyloidosis is eliminated. Alternative treatments should be considered in the presence of partial remission with colchicine therapy, in cases of unresponsiveness to colchicine, or in cases of colchicine intolerance. Colchicine treatment should be continued when considering these treatments. TNF-a inhibitors, IL-1 inhibitors (rilonacept, anakinra, and canakinumab), IL-6 blockers (Yılmaz et al., 2015), and Janus kinase inhibitors (Gök et al., 2017) are among alternative treatments.

Recent studies have revealed that non-MEFV genetic loci, epigenetic mechanisms, and environmental factors may affect pyrin protein and lead to FMF clinical diversity. Patients without FMF mutation but with the clinical picture of FMF have been found to have a milder course, the disease begins at an older age, and a family history of FMF is observed at a lower rate. Different gene mutations or epigenetic mechanisms are suspected in these patients (Alvarez-Errico et al., 2017). Therefore, the absence of mutations does not exclude the diagnosis of FMF. Sometimes, the patient with a mutation may not show clinical signs. This again indicates the importance of epigenetic and environmental factors.

The change in disease activity in people who live in countries in the eastern Mediterranean and have migrated to other regions also suggests the presence of epigenetic and environmental factors (Özen et al., 2017).

The fact that monozygotic twins with the same genotype appear to have completely different phenotypic characteristics due to the difference in environmental factors to which they are exposed can also be explained by epigenetic mechanisms (Martin, 2005).

The fact that viruses can change human epigenetics through DNA methylation is on the agenda (Tao & Robertson, 2003).

Epigenetic Mechanisms

Deletions, mutations, and insertions that affect genes are inherited during transcription and cause permanent changes.

It has been recently revealed that changes in DNA cannot be explained only by genetics, and the role of epigenetic mechanisms is quite significant. Epigenetic mechanisms are known as mechanisms that do not alter the nucleotide sequence, but rather change chromatin. In other words, the DNA sequence does not change; however, since the gene's promoter region changes, quantitative and qualitative changes in gene transcription emerge. The transcription of the relevant gene can be silenced or activated as a result of transcriptional changes. These quantitative and qualitative changes are not permanent and can be regulated when needed. Moreover, these alterations in gene transcription can be transferred to the next generations (Morgan et al., 1999).

When epigenetic mechanisms are mentioned, DNA methylation, histone acetylation, histone methylation, histone ubiquitination, histone phosphorylation, histone citrullination, histone ribosylation, non-coding RNAs, and chromatin re-modeling come to mind.

Cytosine methylation is known to be the best among epigenetic mechanisms. When cytosine is methylated, it becomes thymine. Thymine pairs with adenine at the next replication, which results in a point mutation. Due to this mutation, transcription is silenced, and this change is passed on to the next generations by mitosis. Again, one of the X chromosomes in females is inactivated by DNA methylation.

The impacts of environmental factors on epigenetic mechanisms have also been on the agenda recently. Epigenetic changes emerge as a result of hypermethylation in individuals who consume a diet rich in S-adenosine methionine (SAM) or who consume SAM as a supplement (Jiang et al., 2004).

DNA forms a helix around the histone complex (H2a, H2b, H3, and H4), and the nucleosome structure occurs. Owing to histone methylation, histone phosphorylation, histone acetylation, histone ubiquitination, histone citrullination, and histone ribosylation, the DNA-histone relationship is influenced, and chromatin structure is changed. When histones are acetylated, DNA is released, and transcription starts. When the acetyl groups in histone are removed, cytosine is methylated, and transcription stops. The histone acetyl transferase enzyme is responsible for the binding of the acetyl group, whereas the histone deacetyl transferase enzyme is responsible for its removal.

Histone methylation also activates or silences transcription, depending on the location of the methyl group. Histone methylation occurs when 1, 2, or 3 methyl groups are added to amino acids (lysine, arginine, serine, and threonine) in histone proteins by histone methyl transferase enzymes. H3K4me3 modification activates transcription, while H3K9me3 is associated with gene silencing.

Non-coding RNAs (nc-RNA) appear to be the active molecules of RNA. These molecules are involved in many biological events. Non-coding RNA actually represents an umbrella term. Subgroups involve piwi-interacting RNA, small nucleolar RNAs, small interfering RNAs, microRNAs, antisense RNAs, circular RNAs, and long intergenic non-coding RNA. However, studies have included especially microRNA and long intergenic non-coding RNA (Pea et al., 2021).

It is possible to classify non-coding RNAs as long or small in accordance with the nucleotide number they carry. microRNAs (miRNAs) constitute a known subgroup of short, non-coding RNAs with an essential role in the regulation of host gene expression at the post-transcriptional level. Hence, they are considered to involve in phenotypic heterogeneity. They are usually 20 to 25 nucleotides long, do not code proteins but ensure regulating gene expression. Approximately 2656 mature miRNAs have been found in humans, and they are considered to provide regulating 60% of gene expression (Kumar et al., 2010). A single miRNA is capable of regulating the expression of a large number of genes as a result of inhibiting protein translation or cleaving mRNA (Garzon et al., 2010). The miRNA expression pattern of each cell type contributes to the formation of tissue-specific features and functions. miRNAs are capable of changing gene expression in their genes and function as intercellular communication molecules. Research conducted recently has demonstrated that miRNAs are packaged and released into surrounding tissues or circulation. Based on all this information, miRNAs are thought to be a significant clinical marker in the diagnosis and follow-up of treatment (Adams et al., 2017).

Epigenetics and FMF

Different phenotypes of FMF patients with the same genotype (patients with the same mutation and individuals from the same family), the absence of the clinical presentation of patients with mutation or the FMF clinical picture of patients without mutations, drug response or drug resistance have recently been tried to explain by epigenetic and environmental factors, the presence of a new mutation not checked in routine genetic analyzes, dysfunction in other genes regulating gene expression, and dysfunction associated with protein transport and the polygenic and multigenic nature of the disease, in addition to genetics (Batu et al., 2016).

Environmental factors have been researched for many years. When patients with FMF of the same lineage in Germany and Turkey were screened for FMF severity, environmental factors contributed by 12% to the variation in FMF severity (Ben-Zvi et al., 2012). Moreover, a relatively low incidence of amyloidosis in the Armenians living in the USA has been attributed to environmental factors. A milder course of the disease has been observed in subjects with FMF who migrated to Europe. It is considered that climatic factors, dietary habits, etc. determine the clinical picture of FMF and the risk of amyloidosis through genetic effects (Özen, 2009).

Phenotypic differences in patients with the same genotype suggest the fact that some genes are silenced, or some genes are activated. These concepts have necessitated understanding epigenetic mechanisms.

Histone modification, DNA methylation, and microRNA (miRNA) represent the epigenetic mechanisms that are accused the most of the relationship between FMF and epigenetics (Randa et al., 2021).

DNA methylation usually occurs in a region rich in cytosine and guanine bases, called the CpG island, by binding the methyl group to the 5th carbon of the cytosine base. S-adenosyl methionine (SAM) is a methyl donor, and the enzyme DNA methyltransferase catalyzes the reaction. As a result of this reaction, transcription is suppressed through the inhibition of RNA polymerase 2 transcription. Nevertheless, studies on this issue yield contradictory results. Some studies detected that MEFV mRNA expression decreased as a result of methylation in patients with MEFV mutations, while other studies revealed that MEFV mRNA expression increased (Notarnicola et al., 2002). A study carried out in Turkey detected an increase in MEFV gene methylation and a decrease in MEFV expression in peripheral leukocytes in subjects with FMF (Kireçtepe et al., 2011).

The pyrin protein is encoded by the MEFV gene, and higher DNA methylation on the second exon has been determined in subjects with FMF than in healthy controls. This shows the correlation between FMF and methylation (Erdem et al., 2017).

Acetylation of lysine residues, phosphorylation, methylation, ubiquitination, and ribosylation of arginine residues, and phosphorylation of threonine and serine residues are among posttranslational histone modifications. Histone-histone or histone-DNA interactions emerge due to histone modifications. In this way, gene expression is regulated by turning the relevant gene on or off. The H3K4me3 modification has frequently been identified at the promoter and transcription start site, where the CpG island is located. This indicates that histone modification and DNA methylation are not completely independent entities. An article published by Fidan B et al. in 2015 suggests that the H3K4me3 modification may be associated with DNA methylation and inflammation in patients with FMF (Fidan et al., 2015).

Recent studies have revealed that miRNAs are involved in regulating inflammatory pathways. It is thought that miRNAs have a role in the formation and differentiation of B and T cells, the proliferation of neutrophils and monocytes, the activation of antibodies, and the release of inflammatory regulators (Wang et al., 2016).

Many miRNAs, e.g., miR-155 and miR-146a, have been accused in the etiology of different diseases, including multiple sclerosis (MS), rheumatoid arthritis (RA), systemic lupus erythematosus (SLE), and bacterial infections (Perez-Hernandez et al., 2015).

miR-21 is considered to take a crucial part in the pathogenesis of autoimmune diseases (psoriasis, type I diabetes, MS, Sjögren's syndrome (SS), SLE) and in the regulation of autoimmune responses (Wu et al., 2015).

Wada et al. detected that circulating miRNA levels altered in the course of FMF attacks in subjects from different subgroups of FMF (Wada et al., 2017).

Latsoudis et al. revealed considerably increased miR-4520a expression in human pre-monocytic cells, after the silencing of the MEFV gene (Latsoudis et al., 2017).

In the research by Amarilyo et al., the blood analysis taken from 10 subjects with FMF having the M694V homozygous mutation showed that the expression of miR-144-3p, miR-21-5p, miR-4454, and miR-451a was elevated in subjects with FMF compared to healthy controls, while the expression of miR-107, let 7d-5p, and miR-148b-3p was reduced (Amarilyo et al., 2018).

The expression of miR-204-3p was identified to decrease in the serum of subjects with FMF. The release of inflammatory cytokines is thought to be inhibited by miR-204-3p via the phosphoinositide 3-kinase gamma pathway, and miR-204-3p may be used as a good biomarker (Tomohiro et al., 2018).

Another study performed on FMF patients examined miR-197-3p, a subtype of miRNA with anti-inflammatory properties, and detected that this subtype decreased in FMF patients (Akkaya et al., 2021). Furthermore, miR-197-3p has also been identified in non-small cell lung cancer, p53-dependent lung cancer, and hepatocellular carcinoma (Ni et al., 2018).

Conclusion

FMF represents an autosomal recessive hereditary disease that may have recurrent episodes of fever, serositis, and arthritis/arthralgia and accompanying skin findings. Amyloid accumulation in the kidneys is the most feared complication. Different phenotypes of FMF patients with the same genotype are tried to be explained by environmental factors and epigenetics in addition to genetics. Epigenetics is a collection of mechanisms that do not alter the DNA base sequence but cause changes in chromatin. Quantitative and qualitative changes in gene transcription emerge as a result of changes in chromatin. Thus, the transcription of the relevant gene is silenced or activated. The mentioned quantitative and qualitative changes are not permanent and are regulated when needed. Moreover, these alterations in gene transcription can be transferred to the following generations. Histone modification, DNA methylation, and microRNA (miRNA) are among the epigenetic mechanisms, especially those accused in FMF.

References

Adams, B. D., Parsons, C., Walker, L., Zhang, W. C. & Slack, F. J (2017). Targeting noncoding RNAs in disease. *J. Clin. Invest.* 127, 761-771.

Álvarez-Errico, D., Vento-Tormo, R. & Ballestar, E. (2017). Genetic and epigenetic Determinants in Autoinflammatory Diseases. *Frontiers in Immunology*, 8:318. http://doi: 10.3389/fimmu.2017.00318.

Amarilyo, G., Pillar, N., Ben-Zvi, I., Weissglas-Volkov, D. & Zalcman, J. (2018). Analysis of microRNAs in familial Mediterranean fever. *PLoS ONE* 13(5), e0197829.

Batu, E. D., Kara Eroğlu, F., Tsoukas, P., Hausmann, J. S., Bilginer, Y. & Kenna, M. A. (2016). Periodic fever, aphthosis, pharyngitis, and adenitis syndrome: Analysis of patients from two geographic areas. *Arthritis Care Res.* (Hoboken), 68:1859-65.

Ben-Zvi, I., Brandt, B., Berkun, Y., Lidar, M. & Livneh, A. (2012). The relative contribution of environmental and genetic factors to phenotypic variation in familial Mediterranean fever (FMF). *Gene,* 491:260-3. doi:10.1016/j. gene.2011.10.005 38.

Dogan, E., Gursoy, S., Bozkaya, G., Camlar, S., Kilicarslan, O. & Soylu, A. (2019). The effects of epigenetic regulation on phenotypic expressivity in Turkish patients with familial Mediterranean fever. *Indian Journal of Rheumatology,* 14(4):297-303. doi:10.4103/injr.injr_24_19.

Erdem, G. C., Erdemir, S., Abaci, I., Kirectepe, A. K., Everest, E., & Turanli, E. T. (2017). Alternatively spliced MEFV transcript lacking exon 2 and its protein isoform pyrin-2d implies an epigenetic regulation of the gene in inflammatory cell culture models. *Genetics and Molecular Biology,* 40, 3, 688-697.

Fidan, B., Karacan, I., Ozdogan, Ugurlu, S., Seyahi, E., Turanli, T. E. (2015). Analysis of Histone Modification in Familial Mediterranean Fever Patients. *The European Human Genetics Conference 2015*, 6-9 June, Glasgow, Scotland, UK.

Garzon, R., Marcucci, G. & Croce, C. M (2010). Targeting microRNAs in cancer: Rationale, strategies and challenges. *Nat. Rev. Drug Discov.* 9(10), 775-789.

Gök, K., Cengiz, G., Erol, K. & Ozgecmen, S. (2017). Tofacitinib suppresses disease activity and febrile attacks in a patient with coexisting rheumatoid arthritis and familial medşterranean fever. *Acta Rheumatol. Port.,* 42(1):88-90. PMID:28371574.

Javier Perez-Hernandez, Maria J. Forner, Carolina Pinto, Felipe J. Chaves, Raquel Cortes & Josep Redon (2015). Increased urinary exosomal microRNAs in patients with systemic lupus erythematosus. *PLoS ONE* 10, e0138618.

Jesus, A. A., Canna, S. W., Liu, Y. & Goldbach-Mansky, R. (2015). Molecular mechanisms in geneticallly defined autoinflammatory diseass: disorders of amplified danger signaling. *Annu. Rev. Immunol.,* 33:823-74.

Jiang, Y. H., Bressler, J. & Beaudet, A. L. (2004). Epigenetics and human disease. *Annu. Rev. Genomics Hum. Genet.,* 5:479-510.

Jun-Sheng Ni, Hao Zheng, Zhi-Ping Huang, Yong-Gang Hong, Yang-Liu Ou, Yuan-Ping Tao, Meng-Chao Wang, Zhen-Guang Wang, Yuan Yang & Wei-Ping Zhou (2018). microRNA-197-3p acts as a prognostic marker and inhibits cell invasion in hepatocellular carcinoma. *Oncol. Lett.* 17(2), 2317-2327.

Kirectepe, A. K., Kasapcopur, O., Arisoy, N., Celikyapi Erdem, G., Hatemi, G. & Ozdogan, H. (2011). Analysis of MEFV exon methylation and expression patterns in familial Mediterranean fever. *BMC Med. Genet.* 12:105. doi:10.1186/1471-2350-12-105.

Koga, T., Migita, K., Sato, T., Sato, S., Umeda, M., Nonaka, F., Fukui, S., Kawashiri, S., Iwamoto, N., Ichinose, K., Tamai, M., Nakamura, H., Origuchi, T., Ueki, Y., Masumoto, J., Agematsu, K., Yachie, A., Yoshiura, K., Eguchi, K., & Kawakami, A. (2018). MicroRNA-204-3p inhibits lipopolysaccharide-induced cytokines in familial Mediterranean fever via the phosphoinositide 3-kinase γ pathway. *Rheumatology* (Oxford) 57(4), 718-726.

Kumar, M., Nath, S., Prasad, H. K., Sharma, G. & Li, Y (2012). MicroRNAs: A new ray of hope for diabetes mellitus. *Protein Cell.* 3(10), 726-738.

Latsoudis, H., Mashreghi, M. F. & Grün, J. R (2017). Differential expression of miR-4520a associated with pyrin mutations in familial Mediterranean fever (FMF). *J. Cell. Physiol.* 232(6), 1326-1336.

Manukyan, G., & Amninov, R. (2016). Update on pyrin functions and mechanisms of familial Mediterranean fever. *Frontiers in Microbiology*, 7:456.

Martin, G. M. (2005). Epigenetic drift in aging identical twins. *Proc. Natl. Acad. Sci. USA*, 102:10413-4.

Morgan, H. D., Sutherland, H. G. E. & Martin, D. L. K. (1999). Epigenetic inheritance at the agouti locus in the mouse. *Nat. Genet.,* 23:314-8.

Notarnicola, C., Didelot, M. N., Koné-Paut, I., Seguret, F., Demaille, J. & Touitou, I. (2002). Reduced MEFV messenger RNA expression in patients with familial Mediterranean fever. *Arthritis Rheum.,* 46:2785-93.

Özen, S. (2009). Changing concepts in familial Mediterranean fever: Is it possible to have an autosomal-recessive disease with only one mutation? *Arthritis & Rheumatism,* 60(6):1575-7. doi:10.1002/art.2456.

Özen, S., Batu, E. D. & Demir, S. (2017). Familial Mediterranean fever: recent developments in pathogenesis and new recommendations for management. *Front. Rheumatol.,* 8:253.

Pea, A., Jamieson, N. B. & Braconi, C. (2021). Biology and clinical application of regulatory RNAs in hepatocellular carcinoma. *Hepatology.* 73(S1):38-48. doi:10.1002/hep.31225.

Randa, S., Lotfy, Ola S. M. Ali, Waheba A. Zarouk, Hala T. El-Bassyouni &Ghada M. Shehata (2021). Epigenetics and Familial Mediterranean fever, *Azhar. Int. J. Pharm. Med. Sci.*, Vol 1 (1):1-12.

Tao, Q. & Robertson, K. D. (2003). Stealth technology: how Epstein-Barr virus utilizes DNA methylation to cloak itself from immune detection. *Clin. Immunol.,* 10:53-63.

Wada, T., Toma, T. & Matsuda, Y (2017). Microarray analysis of circulating microRNAs in familial Mediterranean fever. *Mod. Rheumatol.* 6, 1-18.

Wang, S., Wan, X. & Ruan, Q (2016). Te MicroRNA-21 in autoimmune diseases. *Int. J. Mol. Sci.* 17(6), 864.

Westwell-Roper, C., Niemietz, I., Tucker, L. B. & Brown, K. L. (2019). Periodic fever syndromes: beyond the single gene paradigm. *Pediatric Rheumatology,* 17:22. https://doi.org/10.1186/s12969-019-0324-7.

Wu, M., Barnard, J., Kundu, S. & McCrae, K. R (2015). A novel pathway of cellular activation mediated by antiphospholipid antibodyiNduced extracellular vesicles. *J. Tromb. Haemost.* 13, 1928-1940.

Yeliz Z. Akkaya-Ulum, Tayfun Hilmi Akbaba, Zeynep Tavukcuoglu, Jae Jin Chae, Engin Yilmaz, Seza Ozen & Banu Balci-Peynircioglu (2021). Familial Mediterranean fever-related miR-197-3p targets IL1R1 gene and modulates inflammation in monocytes and synovial fibroblasts. *Scientifc Reports | (2021)* 11:685 | https://doi.org/10.1038/s41598-020-80097-4.

Yılmaz, S., Cinar, M., Simsek, I., Erdem, H. & Pay, S. (2015). Tocilizumab in the treatment of patients with AA amiloidosis secondary to familial Mediterranean fever. *Rhematology,* 54(3):564-5. PMID:25504961.

Chapter 13

Epigenetics in Neurobiological and Neurobehavioral Diseases

Aslihan Sanri*, **MD**
Department of Pediatric Genetics,
Samsun Education and Research Hospital, Samsun, Turkey

Abstract

Genetic and environmental interactions have a significant role in the evolution, development, and functioning of the central nervous system. Epigenetic mechanisms including, DNA methylation, non-coding RNAs, and histone modifications are important to clarify how genetic and environmental interactions alter neurobiology and behavior. Alterations in epigenetic mechanisms induce remarkable changes in cognitive and behavioral phenotypes. It is becoming apparent that the epigenetic machinery is involved in the pathogenesis of neurobehavioral and neurobiological disorders. A better understanding of the altered epigenetics mechanism underlying these disorders is important to inventing new therapies for neurobiological disorders.

Keywords: epigenetics, DNA methylation, histone modification, non-coding RNA, neurobiological disorder, neurobehavioral disorder

Introduction

Epigenetics is defined as heritable changes that alter gene expression without changes in the DNA sequence. Epigenetics is implicated in numerous biological pathways such as embryogenesis, neural cell, and other cell types differentiation. Therefore, epigenetics may be the most fundamental mechanism for understanding the pathogenesis of a variety of neurobehavioral and neurobiological disorders (Kubota et al., 2012).

The main epigenetic mechanisms are DNA methylation, histone protein modifications, and non-coding RNA (ncRNA) (Qureshi & Mehler, 2013). DNA methylation is the addition of methyl groups (-CH3) to cytosine residues. DNA methylation is catalyzed by the enzymes DNA methyltransferases (DNMTs). DNA methylation mainly concerns the CpG islands (CGIs) which are located on the gene promoters (Kocerha & Aggarwal, 2018). When cytosines are methylated, they bind repressor proteins, such as histone deacetylases (HDACs) and the

* Corresponding Author's E-mail: aslihanaltunoglu@gmail.com.

In: Epigenetics: Beyond the Genetics and Medicine
Editors: Sevgi Durna Daştan and Nazan Yurtcu
ISBN: 979-8-88697-228-3

methyl-binding domain (MBP) protein. DNA methylation leads to higher affinity between DNA and histone core. The higher affinity interaction between DNA and histone proteins finally blocks the transcription and gene expression (Roth, 2012).

Histone modification is a well-understood epigenetic mechanism. Histone modification is related to a variety of neurological disorders. Histones are elementary proteins that have a role in the packaging of DNA and the formation of nucleosomes (Rosales-Reynoso et al., 2016). Histone posttranslational modifications (PTM), including acetylation, methylation, and phosphorylation, direct the interactions between histones and DNA and alter gene transcription (Roth, 2012). Enzymes involved in PTMs are HDACs, histone methyltransferases, histone acetyltransferases (HATs), and histone demethylases (Qureshi & Mehler, 2013). Histone acetylation decreases the affinity between histones and DNA. A lower affinity interaction between DNA and histone core causes activation of the transcriptional machinery. Therefore, histone acetylation is usually related to active gene expression (Roth, 2012).

Non-coding RNAs (ncRNAs) are a cluster of RNAs, which do not encode functional proteins, but instead have a role in the regulation of gene expression at the posttranscriptional level (Rosales-Reynoso et al., 2016). ncRNAs can be divided into regulatory ncRNAs and housekeeping ncRNAs. Regulatory ncRNAs are divided into two groups according to size: short-chain ncRNAs including siRNAs, piRNAs, and miRNAs, and long ncRNAs (lncRNAs). Growing evidence suggests that ncRNAs have a significant role in epigenetic modification and regulation of gene expression (Wei et al., 2017). In recent years, they have been frequently mentioned in the etiology of neurobiological diseases.

In this brief review, we try to summarize the description of neurobehavioral and neurobiological disorders caused by epigenetic alterations.

Epigenetic Mechanisms in Autism and Related Disorders

Autism is one of the most common neurobiological disorders, affecting nearly 100 (range 34 to 264) per 10000 children all over the world. Autism is characterized by problems in social interaction, impaired communication, and repetitive behaviors (Grafodatskaya et al., 2010, Kubota et al., 2012). The molecular etiology of most cases of autism spectrum disorders (ASD) is not fully understood (Grafodatskaya et al., 2010). Both environmental and genetic factors have been implicated. Environmental factors, such as malnutrition, maternal care, mental stress, drugs, and neuronal stimulation, may alter the epigenetic machinery; thus, they have the potential to affect brain functions. The main link connecting genetic and environmental factors contributing to brain dysfunction seems to be epigenetics (Kubota et al., 2012).

Recent genetic reports have demonstrated mutations in at least 20 genes in a group of autistic children. Many of these mentioned genes encode proteins that are related to synaptic function, such as synaptic scaffolding proteins, transporters, receptors, and neuronal cell adhesion molecules. Therefore, autism may be a disorder of synapses (Kubota et al., 2012).

Any disruptions in the functions of genes that regulate epigenetic mechanisms lead to epigenetic syndromes comorbid with ASD including Rett Syndrome (RTT), Fragile-X Syndrome, Angelman Syndrome, and Prader-Willi Syndrome can be divided into two groups. The first group involves genes regulating epigenetic marks including, enzymes such as DNMT, MBD proteins, and enzymes that affect histone modification. The second group consists of genes that are regulated by epigenetic mechanisms, like imprinted genes (Grafodatskaya et al., 2010).

Rett syndrome is a neurodevelopmental disorder characterized by early normal development followed by arrest between 6 and 18 months of age, then regression of acquired skills, speech loss, acquired microcephaly, stereotypes (especially in hands), seizures, ataxia, and severe intellectual disability. RTT is caused by a mutation in the methyl-CpG-binding protein 2 (MECP2) gene which is located on X-chromosome. Recent research suggests that MECP2 has multiple roles in transcription regulation, assisting histone modifications, chromatin looping, inhibition of transcription factor binding, and alternative RNA splicing. MECP2 is expressed abundantly in mature neurons, which is evidence of the critical role of MECP2 in the maturation of hippocampal neurons (Grafodatskaya et al., 2010). Mutations in the MECP2 gene result in a dysfunctional protein which leads to disruption of gene expression in the central nervous system (CNS) leading to manifestations of RTT such as autism. Recent studies have revealed that MECP2 controls some neuronal gene expressions, such as brain-derived neurotrophic factor (BDNF), insulin-like growth factor binding protein 3 (IFGBP3), distal-less homeobox-5 (DLX5), and protocadherin-beta 1 (PCDHB1) and protocadherin 7 (PCDH7). These findings suggest that MECP2 is also possibly associated with autism by epigenetic dysregulation of genes that encode synaptic molecules (Kubota et al., 2012).

Epigenetic Mechanisms in Neurodegenerative Disorders

Neurodegenerative diseases such as Alzheimer's disease (AD), and Huntington's disease (HD) are quite common worldwide. Although several genes have been implicated in the etiology of these diseases, none of the genes alone causes directly the manifestations of the disorders (Gapp et al., 2014). They appear to be related to altered epigenetic mechanisms (Rosales-Reynoso et al., 2016).

Alzheimer's disease is one of the most common neurodegenerative diseases associated with dementia. AD affects approximately 6% of people over 65 years of age worldwide (Gapp et al., 2014). AD is associated with the aggregation of extracellular plaques of amyloid peptides produced by mishandling of the amyloid precursor protein (APP), and neurofibrillary tangles in different areas of the brain (Rosales-Reynoso et al., 2016). Neurofibrillary tangles consist of hyperphosphorylated tau proteins. Several genes have been associated with AD including amyloid-beta a4 precursor protein (APP), apolipoprotein E (APOE), beta-site AAP cleaving enzyme 1 (BACE1), and presenilins 1 and 2 (PSEN1, PSEN2) K6 M. Recent opinion revealed that aberrant histone modification especially acetylation and DNA methylation contribute to the etiology of AD (Roth, 2012). DNA hypomethylation is the most frequently reported epigenetic mechanism in AD. In cell culture studies, PSEN1 promoter hypomethylation leads to increased presenilin expression, and as a result amyloid plaque formation (Rosales-Reynoso et al., 2016). Histone acetylation is overall increased, and histone PTMs are also dysregulated in AD. It was thought to be due to the interaction between the APP C-terminal peptide (AICD), a product of APP cleavage, and HAT TIP60 which leads to increased acetylation. Lastly, environmental factors such as heavy metal exposure, trauma-induced brain injury, and early stressful life events have been proposed to predispose to AD. All these environmental factors can induce a variety of epigenetic alterations in the genome and contribute to the development of AD (Gapp et al., 2014).

Huntington's disease is a rare devastating neurodegenerative disorder characterized by psychiatric, motor, and cognitive dysfunction. Cognitive impairment, memory loss, personality changes, and uncoordinated movement including chorea, rigidity, and dystonia are typical features of HD (Walker, 2007). Impulsivity, psychotic symptoms, and depression are related to personality changes. The progressive deterioration of inhibitory GABAergic neurons in the caudate nucleus and putamen which have a role in the motor system underlies the pathophysiology of AD. (Gapp et al., 2014). HD results from mutations in the huntingtin gene (HTT) encoding the huntingtin protein. Huntingtin is a nuclear protein expressed in many tissues and regulates transcription by binding to several transcription factors (Rosales-Reynoso et al., 2016). In HD, the trinucleotide CAG repeats expansion in the HTT are responsible for pathophysiology. Increased CAG repeats revealed the production of widespread huntingtin that aggregates and as a result forms inclusions in the cells (Walker, 2007). In several studies, histone methylation and acetylation have been shown to change in HD (Gapp et al., 2014; Rosales-Reynoso et al., 2016). Supporting this data, animal models have found reduced histones H3 and H4 acetylation and increased methylation. In cell cultures, polyglutamine binding to HAT proteins reduces HAT activity and the level of acetylation of histones H3 and H4 has been observed (Gapp et al., 2014; Rosales-Reynoso et al., 2016).

Epigenetic Mechanisms in Psychotic Disorders

Schizophrenia (SZ) is a relatively common mental illness. SZ is characterized by positive and negative psychotic symptoms. Positive symptoms are disordered thoughts, hallucinations, illusions, and delirium. Negative symptoms include apathy, social isolation, and motivation loss (Rosales-Reynoso et al., 2016). For the diagnosis of SZ according to the Diagnostic and Statistical Manual of Mental Disorder fourth edition (DSM-IV), at least two of symptoms the mentioned are needed for a period of more than 1 month: hallucinations, apathy, disorganized speech, delusions, disorganized or catatonic behavior, alogia, and lack or decline in motivation (Smith & Huang, 2012).

The etiology of SZ is not fully understood. Both genetic and environmental factors during prenatal and postnatal development may lead to SZ. Current knowledge suggests that epigenetics especially histones and DNA methylation is involved in SZ (Kocerha & Aggarwal, 2018). Significantly reduced mRNA levels of reelin have been shown in the brain tissue of SZ patients. Reelin is an extracellular matrix protein encoded by the reelin gene (RELN) and involved in neuronal cell migration. This finding supports that, DNA hypermethylation in the promoter of the RELN may take a part in SZ pathophysiology (Rosales-Reynoso et al., 2016). It was speculated that altered DNA methylation of the RELN and glutamate decarboxylase 1 (GAD1) genes may cause GABAergic neurondysfunctions and altered GABAergic neural activity appears to be responsible for some phenotypes of SZ (Grayson et al., 2009; Roth, 2012). In another study, hypermethylation of genes takes part in dopamine metabolism including RELN, and membrane-bound catechol-O-methyl transferase (MB-COMT) was found in SZ (Guidotti, 2000; Smith & Huang, 2012).

Not only DNA methylation and histone modifications, but also ncRNAs are implicated in the SZ. There is growing evidence indicating miRNAs' role in SZ (Kocerha et al., 2015). miR-137 is one of the well-established ncRNAs in the etiology of SZ. The target genes of miR-137 are known as schizophrenia risk genes including calcium channel, voltage-dependent, L type, alpha-1c subunit (CACNA1C), transcription factor 4 (TCF4), zinc finger protein 804a (ZNF804A), erb-b2 receptor tyrosine kinase 4 (ERBB4), glutamate receptor, ionotropic, n-methyl-d-aspartate, subunit 2a (GRIN2A), gamma-aminobutyric acid receptor, alpha-1 (GABRA1), glutamate receptor, metabotropic 5 (GRM5), glycogen synthase kinase 3-beta (GSK3B), neuregulin 2 (NRG2) and 5-hydroxytryptamine 2c (HTR2C) (Kim et al., 2012, Kwon et al., 2013). miR-137 is considered a risk allele for SZ patients and is associated with severe symptoms, lower white matter integrity, significantly disrupted functional connectivity, smaller hippocampus, and enlarged lateral ventricles. Another ncRNA, miR-219, has an important role in the methyl D- aspartate receptor (NMDA-R) signaling pathway (Kocerha & Aggarwal, 2018). NMDA-R signaling is one of the most emphasized pathways in SZ. NMDA-R signaling is firmly controlled by miR-219. miR-219 is the most abundant miRNA in the human synapses (Kocerha et al., 2015). Disruption of the mature miR-219 transcript leads to molecular and behavioral changes (Kocerha et al., 2009). In two different studies that miR-219 dysregulation was reported in the cortical tissue of SZ patients. Post-mortem miRNA expression profiling has identified a global increase in miRNA expression in the prefrontal cortex of SZ when compared to controls (Kocerha et al., 2015). SZ susceptibility loci are also controlled epigenetically by several known lncRNAs (Kocerha & Aggarwal, 2018). One of the disrupted schizophrenia 1 (DISC1) gene polymorphisms is associated with negative and positive symptoms (Chubb et al., 2008, Wei, 2017). A lncRNA termed Gomafu mediates some specific variants of the DISC1 splice site in SZ. Gomafu is related to neural development, and Gomafu expression is suppressed in the cortical tissue of patients with SZ (Kocerha & Aggarwal, 2018).

Epigenetic Mechanisms in Mood Based Disorders

Major depressive disorders (MDD) are defined by the fifth edition of DSM (DSM-V) as a heterogeneous syndrome characterized by sleep disruption, anhedonia, reduced appetite, deficient energy, depressive mood, distractibility, and suicidal ideation. Alterations in epigenetic mechanisms, in response to stressful experiences and environmental factors, may have a significant role in MDD (Saavedra et al., 2016). Altered patterns of DNA methylation, histone modification, and ncRNA expression have been detected in both human and animal models of MDD (Kocerha & Aggarwal, 2018). There are several studies on the DNA methylation pattern in MDD. In the study by Córdova-Palomera et al., DNA methylation differences in MDD were evaluated by monozygotic twins (Cordova-Palomera et al., 2015). They identified differentially methylated regions in wd repeat-containing protein 26 (WDR26), CACNA1C, mitogen-activated protein kinase 11 (MAPK11), and insulin-like growth factor II (IGF2) genes (Wray et al., 2012; Cordova-Palomera et al., 2015). Sabunciyan et al., conducted a genome-wide DNA methylation scan in MDD and identified over 200 candidate regions having significant DNA methylation differences in regions harboring genes crucial for neuronal development and differentiation (Sabunciyan et al., 2012). The most significant DNA methylation difference was observed in the proline-rich membrane anchor 1 (PRIMA1) gene. A 12% to 15% increase in DNA methylation in PRIMA1 was observed in the MDD group than in controls (Sabunciyan et al., 2012; Saavedra et al., 2016). Stenz et al., described a correlation between the methylation of the BDNF gene promoter in blood samples and post-mortem brain tissue from MDD patients (Stenz et al., 2015).

Few studies have investigated the role of histone modification in conducted by MDD. HDACs dysfunction may influence the pathophysiology of mood disorders (Saavedra et al., 2016). Hobara et al., investigated gene expression of HDAC2 and HDAC5 in patients with MDD during depressive and remissive episodes (Hobara et al., 2010). They revealed a significant increase in HDAC2 and HDAC5 expression in the depressive episode in MDD patients compared to controls, whereas the expression of HDAC2 and HDAC5 was comparable to control in remissive episodes suggesting a state-dependent alteration in HDAC expression (Hobara et al., 2010; Saavedra et al., 2016).

The role of ncRNAs in MDD has drawn attention. A shred of growing evidence suggests significant roles for miRNA in MDD and other mood disorders. Global downregulation of miRNAs in MDD was identified (Kocerha et al., 2015). Smalheiser et al., revealed a significant downregulation of 21 miRNAs in the prefrontal cortex of patients who died by suicide in the MDD group than in the control group (Smalheiser et al., 2012). Defective miRNA biogenesis, such as the Digeorge syndrome critical region 8 (DGCR8) protein, is linked with a suicidal tendency (Kocerha & Aggarwal, 2018). Polymorphisms in miRNA-processing genes such as DGCR8, argonaute RISC component 1 (AGO1) and gem nuclear organelle-associated protein 4 (GEMIN4) genes may influence the risk and treatment of depression (He et al., 2012). The polymorphisms in these genes are also associated with a higher risk of suicidal incidence risk and determine the response to antidepressant medications (Kocerha et al., 2015). The miRNAs associated with MDD may function independently or cooperate with other ncRNAs. A link was identified between neural lncRNAs and the onset of the symptoms in patients diagnosed with MDD (Kocerha & Aggarwal, 2018).

Bipolar disorder (BD) is a severe psychiatric disturbance, characterized by recurrent depressive, manic, mixed, or hypomanic episodes. BD is often associated with functional impairment (Kocerha & Aggarwal, 2018). The definitive pathophysiology and etiology of BD have not been fully identified. Numerous genetic, neurochemical, and environmental factors are speculated to be responsible for BD. The role of epigenetics may be a link between these suggested factors. DNA methylation has been implicated in BD (Scaini et al., 2020). Family with sequence similarity 63, member b (FAM63B) gene hypomethylation was found in patients with BD and SZ, thus FAM63B is accepted as a risk factor for both SZ and BD (Starnawska et al., 2016). BD patients have some clinical signs that propose premature aging. A higher rate of aging-related findings, rapid cognitive decline, and shortened telomere length was observed in patients with BD compared to controls. More recently, the term "epigenetic age" or in other words "DNA methylation age" has been used to investigate the role of premature aging in BD, and advanced epigenetic aging was detected in patients with BD compared to controls (Scaini et al., 2020). The oxidative damage of DNA in patients with BD contributes to making disease progression worse. Besides DNA methylation, several alterations in miRNAs and lncRNAs have been detected in BD as epigenetic alterations (Kocerha & Aggarwal, 2018; Scaini et al., 2020).

Epigenetic Mechanisms in Addiction

Addiction disorders are characterized by rewarded behaviors for abused substances despite all the negative physical and psychological effects. Addiction can develop against illicit addictive substances such as cocaine and marijuana, alcohol, nicotine, gambling, and certain foods. The addiction cycle is composed of booze, withdrawal, and longing behaviors. With the first exposure to abused substances, the absence of addiction in everyone is associated with each substance having different addictive potentials, as well as personal genetic characteristics. The mesocorticolimbic system and associated brain structures are involved in addiction disorders. Apart from the dopaminergic mesocorticolimbic pathway, the GABAergic and glutamatergic pathways are also effective in the development of addictive behaviors. Epigenetics is another important mechanism in addiction. Cocaine and alcohol alter the gene expression in the glutamatergic and dopaminergic pathways by epigenetic modifications. Histone PTMs are everlastingly concerned with addiction pathophysiology (Kocerha & Aggarwal, 2018). For example, hyperacetylation or hypoacetylation of histones H3 and H4 induced by cocaine was observed in the nucleus accumbens of mice. Similarly, alcohol-induced hyperacetylation of histones H3 and H4 was detected in the frontal cortex and nucleus accumbens of rats (Kubota et al., 2012).

In addition to histone modification, alterations in ncRNAs mediated processes also lie behind addictive behaviors. Post-mortem analyses identified cocaine-associated lncRNAs dopamine neurons located in the midbrain (Kocerha & Aggarwal, 2018). In a study by Kumar et al., cocaine administration induced a rapid increase in histone acetylation of c-fos and fos genes were observed (Kumar et al., 2005). The C-fos and fos genes are known to have a critical role in cocaine-induced behaviors. Epigenetics alterations developed after exposure to cocaine seemed to last a certain time. For example, hyperacetylation of gene promoters following cocaine intake has been found to remain for a few days to weeks (Freeman et al., 2008). More recent work has analyzed the role of DNA methyltransferase 3A (DNMT3A) (K5) in the morphological and behavioral outcomes that may underlie cocaine addiction (Roth, 2012).

Alcoholism is a relevant topic in addiction because of its widespread cultural usage. The main epigenetic mechanism in alcohol addiction is histone modifications. Acute consumption of alcohol causes an anxiolytic response, resulting in chromatin relaxation. During the withdrawal phase, HDAC activity increases, histone acetylation decreases, and chromatin condensed. Condensed chromatin causes reduced gene expression, decreased the density of dendritic spine, and also anxiety, a prevalent adverse effect of alcohol addiction (Kocerha & Aggarwal, 2018). An important question is whether epigenetic modifications related to addiction are heritable or not. In response to this question, children of mothers with maternal exposure to alcohol during embryogenesis were shown to reveal the combination of a decrease in chromatin acetylation and dendritic branching, and an increase in anxiety resulting from alcohol-related behavior arising from excessive exposure to alcohol, especially during adolescence (Kocerha & Aggarwal, 2018).

Epigenetic Mechanisms in Anxiety, Stress, and Fear Disorders

Anxiety disorders (ADs) are a group of mental disorders characterized by uncontrollable feelings of anxiety and fear. Generalized anxiety disorder, panic disorder (PD), phobias, and post-traumatic stress disorders (PTSD) are some examples of ADs. Both genetic and environmental factors have a role in ADs. Stress, circadian rhythm, substance abuse, and the microbiota have been shown to have an impact on ADs. Epigenetic mechanisms have been implicated in ADs, including, histone modification, DNA methylation, and especially ncRNAs (Bartlett et al., 2017). A number of the ncRNAs are implicated in stress-related disorders

(Kocerha & Aggarwal, 2018). Studies have shown that miR-34 transcripts have a neurobehavioral impact. Overexpression of miR-34c in the central amygdala revealed an anxiolytic-like reaction in mice as a response to acute constriction. The target of miR-34c is the corticotropin-releasing hormone receptor 1 (CRHR1) gene, which is the key mediator of the stress response (Haramati et al., 2011). In the mice model, miR-34a was reported to mediate fear-related responses through the Notch signaling pathway (Dias et al., 2014). So, it can be elucidated that the miR-34 family is a cornerstone in stress, anxiety, and fear-associated behaviors (Kocerha & Aggarwal, 2018). Another ncRNA, miR-124 mediates anxiety and stress-related behaviors through corticosteroid signaling cascades (Mannironi et al., 2013). The enzymatic processing of ncRNA biogenesis can also cause anxiety-related behaviors. Dicer is one of the enzymes participating in miRNA biogenesis. Mice with knockout Dicer in the central amygdala exhibit anxiety, as well as other behaviors including front and hind limb clasping and ataxia (Kocerha et al., 2015; Kocerha & Aggarwal, 2018).

Panic disorder is unexpected, recurrent attacks of fear with accompanying palpitations, trembling, sweating, heat sensations, feeling dizzy, and other physical symptoms. The etiology of PD is still uncertain. Genetic, environmental, neurobiological, and psychopathological factors are enounced. One of the most studied genetic factors is the COMT Val158Met polymorphism. It has been implicated in the risk of PD, especially in female patients (Shulman et al., 1978). In some studies, adenosine a2a receptor (ADORA2A), neuropeptide y (NPY), dopamine receptor 2 (DRD2), gamma-aminobutyric acid receptor, beta-3 (GABRB3) genes have been related to PD (Kim & Kim, 2018). A limited number of epigenetic studies have been conducted so far about PD. Monoamine oxidase A (MAOA) hypomethylation showed a relation with panic disorder (Domschke et al. 2012). GAD1 hypomethylation was also concerned with PD (Kim & Kim, 2018). More recent studies identified the role of CRHR1 hypomethylation in PD. The result showed hypomethylation of CRHR1 and increased expression of CRHR1 in patients with PD (Schartner et al., 2017). Histone H3 acetylation and DNA methylation of the BDNF in the hippocampus are well-known epigenetic mechanisms in fear-related behaviors (Kocerha & Aggarwal, 2018). Human studies also revealed ncRNAs, especially miRNAs have a role in panic or fear responses. PD-related miRNAs are miR-22, miR-148a, miR-128, miR-138-2, and miR-488 B. High levels of miR-128 expression are found in animal models conditioned with fear extinction memory (Muinos-Gimeno et al., 2011).

Post-traumatic stress disorder is one of the ADs, that requires facing or witnessing a life-threatening experience or trauma. PTSD has both genetic and epigenetic associations. As genes are sensitive to stress, epigenetics has been speculated as the main mechanism for the development of PTSD. Regulation of COMT, a critical enzyme in the dopamine degradation process, aggravates PTSD behaviors. The specific COMT genotype has been associated with altered DNA methylation and impaired fear inhibition in PTSD (Kocerha & Aggarwal, 2018). Several altered miRNAtranscripts including miR-19b and miR-223 have been identified in veterans who experienced symptoms of PTSD. miRNA-19b and miR-223 were also concerned in the blood samples and amygdala of the animal model with PTSD. The miRNAs altered in the military veterans with active symptoms of PTSD. MiRNA are firmly associated with immunological pathways, demonstrating their role in the pathogenesis of PTSD (Kocerha et al., 2015).

Epigenetic Mechanisms in Circadian Rhythm

The circadian cycle is defined as a genetically determined clock that directs the cellular harmony of protein synthesis and metabolism. The circadian cycle continues to work in the absence of an environmental stimulus (Kocerha & Aggarwal, 2018). The circadian clock interacts with an environmentally driven cycle called the diurnal cycle. The diurnal cycle also drives protein synthesis and metabolism during night and day, hot and cold, light and dark, sleep and wake, satiety and hunger, and daily and seasonal sessions (Powell & LaSalle, 2015). In most cases, the two cycles work in close relationships and simultaneously. However, in some instances, the two can become asynchronous as in jet lag, starvation, sleep deprivation, and stationary darkness. Recent reports have revealed that epigenetic mechanisms such as DNA methylation allow the circadian clock to work in harmony with the diurnal cycle (Powell & LaSalle, 2015). Along with physiological diurnal cycles, cyclic DNA methylation profiles have been explored. To support this finding, potent fluctuations in promoter DNA methylation are prominent in vertebrate models (Kocerha & Aggarwal, 2018).

A panel of epigenetic factors has been reported as regulators of circadian functions, including miRNAs. miR-132 and miR-219 modulate circadian functions via the NMDA-R signaling (Asarnow et al., 2013). Similar to miRNAs, lncRNAs may also control the circadian rhythm. Profiling studies that, some lncRNAs, including natural antisense transcripts (NATs), regulate the circadian system (Coon et al., 2012).

Disrupted circadian rhythm and sleep patterns are compulsory outcomes in a subset of neuropsychiatric disorders. Patients diagnosed with particular congenital neurodevelopmental disorders, such as RTT and Angelman syndrome, demonstrate altered circadian rhythm and a wide range of abnormal behaviors, including disrupted sleep patterns (Kocerha & Aggarwal, 2018).

Conclusion

Various environmental factors are likely to reorganize epigenetic codes. Since epigenetic code is reversible, it is potentially treatable and preventable, discovering all its unknowns is crucial to discovering new therapies for neurobehavioral and neurobiological disorders. Epigenetic mechanisms have a central role in the development and functions of the CNS, and therefore any changes may lead to neurological deterioration leading to numerous neurobiological and neurobehavioral disorders including depression, drug dependency, neurodegenerative disorders, and schizophrenia. It is looking forward to in the coming years, epigenetic mapping will allow us to identify the pathophysiology of neurobiological and neurobehavioral disorders. Future perspectives will aim to detect epigenetics modifications that will permit identifying new therapeutic targets. New molecular techniques allow screening of whole-genome DNA methylation and chromatin modifications and will facilitate the recognition of crucial epigenetic marks of neurobiological and neurobehavioral disorders.

References

Asarnow, L. D., Soehner, A. M., & Harvey, A. G. (2013). Circadian rhythms and psychiatric illness. *Curr Opin Psychiatry, 26*(6), 566-571.

Balakathiresan, N. S., Chandran, R., Bhomia, M., Jia, M., Li, H., & Maheshwari, R. K. (2014). Serum and amygdala microRNA signatures of posttraumatic stress: fear correlation and biomarker potential. *J Psychiatr Res, 57*, 65–73.

Bartlett, A. A., Singh, R., & Hunter, R., G. (2017). Anxiety and Epigenetics. Adv Exp Med Biol, 978, 145-166. doi: 10.1007/978-3-319-53889-1_8Barry, G., Briggs, J. A., Vanichkina, D. P., Poth, E. M., Beveridge, N. J., Ratnu, V. S., Nayler, S. P., Nones, K., Hu, J., Bredy, T. W., Nakagawa, S., Rigo, F., Taft, R. J., Cairns, M. J., Blackshaw, S., Wolvetong, E. J., & Mattick, J. S. (2014). The long non-coding RNA Gomafu is acutely regulated in response to neuronal activation and involved in schizophrenia-associated alternative splicing. *Mol Psychiatry, 19*(4), 486-494.

Chubb, J. E., Bradshaw, N. J., Soares, D. C., Porteous, D. J., & Millar, J. K. (2008). The DISC locus in psychiatric illness. *Mol Psychiatry, 13*(1), 36-64.

Coon, S. L., Munson, P. J., Cherukuri, P. F., Sugden, D., Rath, M. F., Moller, M., Clokie, S. J. H., Fu, C., Olanich, M. E., Rangel, Z., Werner, T., Mullikin, J. C., & Klein, D. C. (2012). Circadian changes in long noncoding RNAs in the pineal gland. *Proc Natl Acad, 109*(33), 13319-133124.

Coppedè, F. (2014). Epigenetics and cognitive disorders, in: J. Peedicayil, D. R. Grayson, D. Avramopoulos (Eds.), Epigenetics in Psychiatry, *Academic Press*, 343–367.

Cordova-Palomera, A., Fatjo-Vilas, M., Gasto, C., Navarro, V., Krebs, M. O., & Fananas, L. (2015). Genome-wide methylation study on depression: Differential methylation and variable methylation in monozygotic twins. *Transl. Psychiatry, 5*, 557.

Dias, B. G., Goodman, J. V., Ahluwalia, R., Easton, A. E., Andero, R., & Ressler, K. J. (2014). Amygdala-dependent fears memory consolidation via miR-34a and Notch signaling. *Neuron, 83,* 906–918.

Domschke, K., Tidow, N., Kuithan, H., Schwarte, K., Klauke, B., Ambree, O., Reif, A., Schmidt, H., Arolt, V., Kersting, A., Zwanzger, P., &, J. (2012). Monoamine oxidase A gene DNA hypomethylation—a risk factor for panic disorder? *Int J Neuropsychopharmacol, 15*, 1217.

Freeman, W. M., Patel, K. M., Brucklacher, R. M., Lull, M. E., Erwin, M., Morgan, D., Roberts, D. C. S., & Vrana, K. E. (2008). Persistent alterations in mesolimbic gene expression with abstinence from cocaine self-administration. *Neuropsychopharmacology, 33*(8), 1807–1817.

Gapp, K., Woldemichael, B., T., Bohacek, J., & Mansuy, I., M. (2014). Epigenetic regulation in neurodevelopment and neurodegenerative diseases. *Neuroscience, 4*(264), 99-111. doi: 10.1016/j.neuro science.2012.11.040.

Grafodatskaya, D., Chung, B., Szatmari, P., & Weksberg, R. (2010). Autism spectrum disorders and epigenetics. *J Am Acad Child Adolesc Psychiatry, 49*, 794–809. doi: 10.1016/j.jaac.2010.05.005.

Grayson, D., Chen, Y., Dong, E., Kundakovic, M., & Guidotti, A. (2009). From trans-methylation to cytosine methylation: Evolution of the methylation hypothesis of schizophrenia. *Epigenetics, 4*(3), 144–149.

Guidotti, A., Auta, J., Davis, J. M., Di-Giorgi-Gerevini, V., Dwivedi, Y., Grayson, D. R., Impagnatiello, F., Pandey, G., Pesold, C., Sharma, R., Uzunov, D., & Costa, E. (2000). Decrease in reelin and glutamic acid decarboxylase67 (GAD67) expression in schizophrenia and bipolar disorder: a postmortem study. *Arch Gen Psychiatry, 57,* 1061-1069.

Haramati, S., Navon, I., Issler, O., Ezra-Nevo, G., Gil, S., Zwang, R., Hornstein, E., & Chen, A. (2011). MicroRNA as repressors of stress-induced anxiety: the case of amygdalar miR-34. *J Neurosci, 31*(40), 14191-14203.

He, Y., Zhou, Y., Xu, Q., Cui, H., Luo, T., Song, H., Nie, X., Wang, L., Ying, B. (2012). Genetic variations in microRNA processing genes are associated with susceptibility to depression. *DNA Cell Biol, 31*, 1499–1506.

Hobara, T., Uchida, S., Otsuki, K., Matsubara, T., Funato, H., Matsuo, K., Suetsugi, M., & Watanabe, Y. (2010). Altered gene expression of histone deacetylases in mood disorder patients. *J. Psychiatr. Res,* 44, 263–270.

Kim, A. H., Parker, E. K., Williamson, V., McMichael, G. O., Fanous, A. H., & Vladimirov, V. I. (2012). Experimental validation of candidate schizophrenia gene ZNF804A as target for hsa-miR-137. *Schizophr Res, 141*, 60–64.

Kim, E. J., & Kim, Y. K. (2018). Panic disorders: The role of genetics and epigenetics. AIMS *Genetics, 5*(3), 177–190. https://doi.org/10.3934/genet.2018.3.177.

Kocerha, J., & Aggarwal, N. (2018). Chapter 8-Epigenetics in Neurobehavioral Disease. Tollefsbol, Trygve O. Epigenetics in Human Disease. San Diego, *Academic Press*: 251-267.

Kocerha, J., Dwivedi, Y., & Brennand, K. J. (2015). Noncoding RNAs and neurobehavioral mechanisms in psychiatric disease. *Mol Psychiatry, 20*(6), 677-684. doi: 10.1038/mp.2015.30.

Kocerha, J., Faghihi, M. A., Lopez-Toledano, M. A., Huang, J., Ramsey, A. J., Caron, M. G., Sales, N., Willoughby, D., Elmen, J., Hansen, H. F., Orum, H., Kauppinen, S., Kenny, P. J., & Wahlestedt, C. (2009). MicroRNA-219 modulates NMDA receptor-mediated neurobehavioral dysfunction. *Proc Natl Acad, 106*(9), 3507-3512.

Kubota, T., Miyake, K., & Hirasawa, T. (2013). Epigenetics in Neurodevelopmental and Mental Disorders. *Med Epigenet, 1*, 52–59. doi: 10.1159/000354718.

Kubota, T., Miyake, K., Hirasawa, T., Onaka, T., & Yamasue, H. (2012). Chapter 10- Epigenetic Modulation of Human Neurobiological Disorders. Tollefsbol, Trygve O. Epigenetics in Human Disease. San Diego, *Academic Press*: 193-203.

Kumar, A., Choi, K.-H., Renthal, W., Tsankova, N. M., Theobald, D. E. H., Truong, H. T., Russo, S. J., Laplant, Q., Sasaki, T. S., Whistler, K. N., Neve, R. L., Self, D. W., & Nestler, E. J. (2005). Chromatin remodeling is a key mechanism underlying cocaine-induced plasticity in the striatum. *Neuron, 48*(2), 303–314.

Kwon, E., Wang, W., & Tsai, L. H. (2013). Validation of schizophrenia-associated genes CSMD1, C10orf26, CACNA1C, and TCF4 as miR-137 targets. *Mol Psychiatry*, 18, 11–12.

Lahiri, D., Maloney, B., & Zawia, N. (2009). The LEARn model: an epigenetic explanation for idiopathic neurobiological diseases. *Mol Psychiatry, 14*, 992–1003 https://doi.org/10.1038/mp.2009.82.

LaPlant, Q., Vialou, V., Covington, H. E., Dumitriu, D., Feng, J., Warren, B. L., Maze, I., Dietz, D. M., Watts, E. L., Iniguez, S. D., Koo, J. W., Mouzon, E., Renthal, W., Hollis, F., Wang, H., Noonan, M. A., Ren, Y., Eisch, A. J., Bolanos, C. A., Kabbaj, M., Xiao, G., Neve, R. L., Hurd, Y. L., Oosting, R. S., Fan, G., Marrison, J. H., & Nestler, E. J. (2010). Dnmt3a regulates emotional behavior and spine plasticity in the nucleus accumbens. *Nature Neuroscience, 13*(9), 1137–1143.

Mannironi, C., Camon, J., De Vito, F., Biundo, A., De Stefano, M. E., Persiconi, I., Bozzoni, I., Fragapane, P., Mele, A., & Presutti, C. (2013). Acute stress alters amygdala microRNA miR-135a and miR-124 expression: inferences for corticosteroid dependent stress response. *PLoS One, 8,* 73385. doi: 10.1371/journal.pone.0073385.

Mastroeni, D., Grover, A., Delvaux, E., Whiteside, C., Coleman, P. D., & Rogers, J. (2011). Epigenetic mechanisms in Alzheimer's disease. *Neurobiol Aging, 32*(7), 1161-1180. doi: 10.1016/j.neurobiolaging.2010.08.017.

Muinos-Gimeno, M., Espinosa-Parrilla, Y., Guidi, M., Kagerbauer, B., Sipila, T., Maron, E., Pettai, K., Kananen, L., Navines, R., Martin-Santos, R., Gratacos, M., Metspalu, A., Hovatta, I., & Estivill, X. (2011). Human microRNAs miR-22, miR-138-2, miR-148a, and miR-488 are associated with panic disorder and regulate several anxiety candidate genes and related pathways. *Biol Psychiatry, 69,* 526–533.

Powell, W. T., & LaSalle, J. M. (2015). Epigenetic mechanisms in diurnal cycles of metabolism and neurodevelopment. *Human Molecular Genetics, 24,* R1–R9. https://doi.org/10.1093/hmg/ddv234.

Qureshi, I. A., & Mehler, M. F. (2013). Understanding neurological disease mechanisms in the era of epigenetics. *JAMA Neurology, 70*(6), 703–710.

Rosales-Reynoso, M. A., Ochoa-Hernández, A. B., Juárez-Vázquez, C. I., & Barros-Núñez, P. (2016. Epigenetic mechanisms in the development of memory and their involvement in certain neurological diseases. *Neurologia, 31*(9), 628-638. doi: 10.1016/j.nrl.2014.02.004.

Roth, T. L. (2012). Epigenetics of neurobiology and behavior during development and adulthood. *Dev Psychobiol, 54*(6), 590-597. doi: 10.1002/dev.20550.

Saavedra, K., Molina-Márquez, A., Saavedra, N., Zambrano, T., & Salazar, L. (2016). Epigenetic Modifications of Major Depressive Disorder. *International Journal of Molecular Sciences, 17*(8), 1279. https://doi.org/10.3390/ijms17081279.

Sabunciyan, S., Aryee, M. J., Irizarry, R. A., Rongione, M., Webster, M. J., Kaufman, W. E., Murakami, P., Lessard, A., Yolken, R. H., Feinberg, A. P., & Potash, J. B. (2012). Genome-wide DNA methylation scan in major depressive disorder. *PLoS One, 7,* 34451.

Scaini, G., Valvassori, S., S., Diaz, A., P., Lima, C., N., Benevenuto, D., Fries, G., R., & Quevedo, J. (2020). Neurobiology of bipolar disorders: a review of genetic components, signaling pathways, biochemical changes, and neuroimaging findings. *Braz J Psychiatry, 42*(5), 536-551. doi: 10.1590/1516-4446-2019-0732.

Schartner, C., Ziegler, C., Schiele, M. A., Kollert, L., Weber, H., Zwanger, P., Arolt, V., Pauli, P., Deckert, J., Reif, A., Domschke, K. (2017). CRHR1 promoter hypomethylation: An epigenetic readout of panic disorder? *Eur Neuropsychopharmacol, 27*, 360–371.

Shulman, R., Griffiths, J., & Diewold, P. (1978). Catechol-O-methyl transferase activity in patients with depressive illness and anxiety states. *Br J Psychiatry, 132,* 133–138.

Smalheiser, N. R., Lugli, G., Rizavi, H. S., Torvik, V. I., Turecki, G., & Dwivedi, Y. (2012). MicroRNA expression is down-regulated and reorganized in the prefrontal cortex of depressed suicide subjects. *PloS One, 7,* 33201.

Smith, C. L., & Huang, K. (2012). *Epigenomics in Neurobehavioral Diseases*. doi:10.1016/B978-0-388415-2.00007-X.

Starnawska, A., Demontis, D., McQuillin, A., O'Brien, N. L., Staunstrup, N. H., Mors, O., Nielsen, A. L., Børglum, A. D., & Nyegaard, M. (2016). Hypomethylation of FAM63B in bipolar disorder patients. *Clin Epigenetics, 8,* 52. https://doi.org/10.1186/s13148-016-0221-6.

Stenz, L., Zewdie, S., Laforge-Escarra, T., Prados, J., La Harpe, R., Dayer, A., Paoloni-Giacobino, A., Perroud, N., & Aubry, J. M. (2015). Bdnf promoter I methylation correlates between post-mortem human peripheral and brain tissues. *Neurosci. Res, 91,* 1–7.

Walker, F. O. (2007). Huntington's disease. *Lancet,* 369, 218-228.

Wei, J. W., Huang, K., Yang, C., & Kang, C. S. (2017). Non-coding RNAs as regulators in epigenetics (Review). *Oncol Rep, 37*(1), 3-9. doi: 10.3892/or.2016.5236.

Wray, N. R., Pergadia, M. L., Blackwood, D. H., Penninx, B. W., Gordon, S. D., Nyholt, D. R., Ripke, S., MacIntyre, D. J., McGhee, K. A., Maclean, A. W., Smith, J. H., Hottenga, J. J., Willemsen, G., Guide, E. J. C., Lewis, C. M., McGuffin, P., Hickie, B., Van den Oord, E. J. C. G., Lui, J. Z., Macgregor, S., McEvory, B. P., Byrne, E. M., Medland, S. E., Statham, D, J., Henders, A. K., Heath, A. C., Montgomery, G. W., Martin, N. G., Boomsma, D. I., Madden, P. A. F., & Sullivan, P. F. (2012). Genome-wide association study of major depressive disorder: New results, meta-analysis, and lessons learned. *Mol. Psychiatry, 17*, 36–48.

Chapter 14

The Role of Epigenetics in Fetal Brain Development

Fatih Kılıcbay[1,*], MD and Huseyin Erdal[2], PhD
[1]Division of Neonatology, Department of Pediatrics,
Sivas Cumhuriyet University Faculty of Medicine, Sivas, Turkey
[2]Department of Medical Genetics, Faculty of Medicine,
Aksaray University, Aksaray, Turkey

Abstract

The physiological and behavioral development of an individual is a dynamic event that includes the interaction between genes and the environment. The brain and nerve development period of the baby in the womb is between the 4th and 10th weeks of pregnancy. Although the early stages of the brain development are affected by genetic factors, the decision of where and how genes are utilized is determined by environmental factors. This situation solely depends on the pregnancy period of the mother, meaning it is tightly related to the level of food intake and stress exposure which affects the early phases of brain architecture. Environmental factors and experience leave traces on certain parts of genes, and these epigenetic changes can change the activity or expression of the genes.

Keywords: newborn, epigenetics, fetal brain, DNA methylation

Introduction

The physiological and behavioral development of an individual is a dynamic event involving the interaction between the individual's genes and experiences or the environment. Human brain development is regulated by the genes that interact with early experiences. There are certain delicate terms in the advancement of specific abilities. These are very important periods during the development of the brain while certain areas are the most sensitive to specific experiences. The perinatal period, early childhood, and puberty are periods when the brain is particularly susceptible to reconstruction by the environmental factors (Yurdakök & Çelik, 2019).

During prenatal and postnatal early childhood, rapid changes occur in the brain that result in the formation, proliferation, and development of neuronal pathways. Experiences after preterm birth play a major role in revealing the functional capacity of the nervous system responsible for emotional, physiological, and social situations. The normal development of the

* Corresponding Author's E-mail: fatihkilicbay@cumhuriyet.edu.tr.

In: Epigenetics: Beyond the Genetics and Medicine
Editors: Sevgi Durna Daştan and Nazan Yurtcu
ISBN: 979-8-88697-228-3

nervous systems is provided by the acquisition of the necessary experiences at the appropriate time. Having bad experiences such as neglect, abuse or encountering other stressors in the early stages of life can cause harmful consequences such as stress-related cardiovascular and metabolic diseases, perceptual, mental and behavioral disorders in adulthood. This concept is called "early life programming." There are many strong data supporting that exposure to stress in early life period leads to long-term changes in gene functions with permanent changes in individuals (Maccari et al., 2014).

Billions of cells in multicellular organisms have the same DNA. However, these cells differentiate to possess various different structures and functions as a result of epigenetics-mediated changes in gene expression pattern during pre- and post-natal development along with the rest of the life (Murgatroyd & Spengler, 2011). In this way, the adaptation of the organism to the changing environment takes place. Epigenetic changes caused by experiences in the early stages of life, such as intrauterine, neonatal, and early infancy; enable these experiences to be embedded in the genome and programming of hormonal and observable responses in adulthood. Among the mechanisms that lead to these epigenetic changes, the most well-known are the modification of histone proteins that allow DNA to be packaged into chromatin, and DNA methylation that occurs at the cytosine side chain. (Murgatroyd & Spengler, 2011). DNA methylation inhibits the active transcription of some genes and causes genes to remain silent (Yurdakök & Çelik, 2019).

Previous studies have shown that there is a causative connection between the stress that the mother is exposed to during pregnancy and the postnatal environment and DNA methylation (Maccari et al., 2014). In this review, we will highlight the effects of the role of epigenetics on fetal brain development.

Definition of Epigenome

The epigenome occurs not only on the chromatin level but also on DNA level with a covalent bound formation by methylation of cytosine nucleotide. (Szyf et al., 2007). It has an important role in the accessibility of transcription machinery. For this reason, genes that cannot be accessed are silenced, and those that can be accessed are expressed. Recent studies have reported the discovery of another new level of epigenetic regulation by microRNAs (miRNA).

DNA Methylation

In multicellular organisms, the insertion of methyl groups (CH_3) into DNA on the cytosine nucleotide at the 5th position results in the methylation of the cytosine-guanine (CpG) dinucleotide (5-methylcytosine) (Hesson & Pritchard, 2019). DNA methylation causes the genes to be silent by preventing the active transcription of some genes (Yurdakök & Çelik, 2019). Since DNA methylation is very stable compared to other epigenetic markers, its diagnostic potential is quite high. (Szyf et al., 2007). The establishment of the DNA methylation pattern occurs during development and is subsequently maintained by DNA methyl transferase throughout life. While most authors hold the notion that DNA methylation is irreversible, recent studies have shown that DNA methylation is potentially reversible even in post-mitotic tissues (Szyf et al., 2007). Recent studies have shown that the DNA methylation pattern in neurons is dynamic and has a vital role in memory and fear conditioning. In vertebrates, DNA methylation is related to formation of chromatin. While the chromatin structure that provides gene expression is hypo-methylated, the inactive chromatin structure is hyper-methylated (Szyf et al., 2007). The methylation of DNA is considered to have a significant role in the regulation of gene expression. Gene expression is silenced by DNA methylation through two main mechanisms. The first mechanism involves the direct interference of a methyl residue in a recognition element for a transcription factor with transcription factor binding those results in silencing of gene expression (Hesson & Pritchard, 2019). The second mechanism takes place indirectly. A specific concentration of DNA methylation found in a gene region allows binding of methylated-DNA-binding proteins such as MeCP2 that engages with other proteins and enzymes responsible for histone modification which eventually causes more compact chromatin structure and gene silencing.

Brain Development Based on Experience

The organization and regulation of brain development are affected by chemical agents, hormones, and growth factors. Acceleration of growth and functional differentiation during brain development make it more sensitive to the external factors, such as toxic chemicals, radiation, infection, and the emergence of sensitive situations. In addition to care and attention, the developmental process is affected by the interaction of both genetic and epigenetic factors (Yurdakök, 2014).

The highest proportion of the brain growth and development occurs after the postnatal period. An infant's brain between 2-4 weeks corresponds roughly 36% of an adult brain in size. By 1 year of age, the brain grows to approximately 70% of its adult size and to approximately 80% of its adult size at the end of 2nd year (Knickmeyer et al., 2008) Neuronal proliferation and migration occur in the prenatal period. In this period, there is a systemic neuronal proliferation that continues with extensive axonal migration and synapse formation starting from the 6th week of pregnancy.

Relation of Epigenetic Programming Mechanisms with Maternal Care

Studies on the development of the brain and the effects of its practices on it are limited due to the lack of appropriate methodological tools. However, the results obtained from studies with animal models for many years have revealed valuable findings in this regard. Laboratory studies, especially on rats, have shown that bad experiences during fetal or infancy cause changes in the structure and functions of the brain. A previous study investigating the effect of the social environment on the epigenetic programming is one of the best understood epigenetic regulations, which focuses on the effect of maternal care on the glucocorticoid gene expression in the hippocampus of the offspring (Szyf et al., 2007).

A few weeks after the beginning of the pregnancy, the human brain development begins. In this process, several cellular events occur e.g., differentiation, neuronal proliferation and migration, axonal growth, cell death, myelination, and synapse formation. Organization of the brain development process and its regulation are affected by chemical stimuli, hormones, neurotropins, growth factors, and neurotransmitters such as acetylcholine, norepinephrine, dopamine, etc.). The place and densities of target receptors change over time along with the brain development. The rapid growth and differentiation stages that occur in brain development lead to the emergence of critical periods regarding genetic and epigenetic factors, where sensitivity to love and attention is greater, as well as to environmental influences such as nutrients, hazardous agents including endocrine confounders, radiation, and infection (Yurdakök, 2014).

It has been shown that the predisposition and the sensitivity to epigenetic changes in humans extend to early childhood from the preconception period. The epigenome is reported to be sensitive to the disorganization during lifetime, but it is considered to be the most sensitive to the exogenous factors during embryogenesis due to the rapid cell division and prevalent epigenetic remodeling. After fertilization, the motifs of DNA methylation are broadly erased and reconfigured during the mammalian maturation by adapting a complicated pattern (Perera & Herbstman, 2011).

While maintaining the imprinted genes during the preimplantation term is vital to typical embryonic progress, the demethylation of other genes is required to switch the target genes on. So, a common demethylation takes place across the genome, except imprinted genes, in between fertilization-implantation period. Between day 5 and day 7 post-fertilization in humans, the required methylation patterns are reinstalled de novo in unimprinted gene regions by DNA methyltransferases (DNMT3a, DNMT3b) (Foley et al., 2009). The maintenance of DNA methylation motifs after DNA replication, i.e., full or hemi-methylation, is handled by DNMT1, which is required for healthy development. The prenatal period, including the first few hours after birth, is the most sensitive period in the neonatal period. Neuron augmentation and immigration to form several parts of the brain occur mostly in the prenatal period, starting from the 6th week of pregnancy.

In 1992, Barker et al. proposed the "fetal basis of adult disease" (FEBAD) hypothesis. According to this hypothesis, they stated that the main factor determining the physiological and metabolic adaptation of organs in the adult period is to be programmed in the antenatal period and environmental and nutritional factors that may disrupt this programming and increase the risk of diseases that may occur in the adult period (Law, Barker, Osmond, Fall, & Simmonds, 1992). They showed that abdominal obesity, a marker of enhanced risk of cardiovascular disease and diabetes apart from body mass, is related to delayed fetal growth, suggesting a persistent response to unfavorable circumstances during fetal life.

With the FEBAD hypothesis, it has been shown that especially fetal nutritional status, other intrauterine factors, and environmental factors can lead to nasty consequences in adult life, such as cardiovascular disease, type 2 diabetes mellitus, depression disorder, and an increase in some cancer diseases by reprogramming of operational capacity of organs (Perera & Herbstman, 2011).

There is persuasive evidence that epigenetic disorder is based on the relationships observed between adult disease and the negative environmental / nutritional conditions of development. For example, Heijmans et al. found a lower insulin-like growth factor II (IGF2) and less DNA methylation in fasted individuals. IGF2 has a critical role in infant growth and development. Exposure to lower IGF2 levels during the gestational period is believed to have an important role in the development of schizophrenia and coronary heart disease in adulthood (Heijmans et al., 2008).

Especially in recent published studies with animals, it has been shown that the baby is also affected by the stress experienced by the mother while in the womb (Weaver et al., 2005; Perera

& Herbstman, 2011). The main factor caused the stress condition in the baby was considered as the increase in the mother's glucocorticoid levels regulated by the hypothalamus-pituitary-adrenal (HPA) axis. HPA is an essential system associated with the expression of stress-related genes whose dysregulation can cause developmental disorders in the brain (Gudsnuk & Champagne, 2012).

Changes in gene expression due to epigenetic factors are associated with the severity of prenatal disorders. In addition, dysregulation in gene activity continues throughout adulthood. Studies on mice have shown that exposure to various degrees of stress during pregnancy causes neurobiological effects in the long-term. (Yurdakök & Çelik, 2019). Diethyl stilbesterol (DES), a pharmaceutical substance that causes reproductive dysfunction and cancer due to in-utero exposure to drugs in girls, has been shown to lead to epigenetic changes by causing methylation in mice (Perera & Herbstman, 2011). Environmental toxic substances can cause epigenetic changes which may result in the alteration of gene expression profiles. In particular, air pollution has been shown to be associated with intrauterine growth restriction.

Exposure to Environmental Pollutants before Birth and Its Impact on Health and Epigenetics Dysregulation

In the studies carried out by Baccarelli and Bollati, it has been shown that epigenetic changes can appear due to the exposure of concourse to the air bone pollutants, benzene, and permanent natural contaminants (Baccarelli & Bolatti 2009). It has been shown that as a result of prenatal exposure to toxic chemicals, air bone pollutants, and endocrine disruptors, epigenetic programming can deteriorate and cause several abnormalities affecting up to 3rd generations.

Neural Stem Cell Fate under Epigenetic Control Mechanisms

The underlying mechanisms which are responsible for neuronal stem cell-derived differentiation of several cell types are of pivotal importance in shaping the central nervous system (CNS). The previous and ongoing studies underline that the primary regulatory system among these mechanisms is epigenetics which controls cellular growth and differentiation (Noctor et al., 2001). The most prominent epigenetics control mechanisms are, but not limited to, a close relation of neuronal transcription factors with chromatin remodeling enzymes, a sustainable genome stability of neuronal cells, and the role of non-coding RNA (ncRNA) world in the decision of neuronal cell fate. In this context, inter-cellular signaling pathways partially play a role by interfering with the aforementioned various epigenetics activities (Hsieh & Gage, 2004).

Inhibitory Effect of Signaling Molecules on Glial Genes to Promote Non-Glial Cells

Several extracellularly acting molecules have been discovered so far which take part in neuronal stem cell differentiation, of which transmit their signals through transcription factors to regulate the expression of target genes. It is evident now that epigenetics mechanisms, which particularly modify the DNA methylation pattern and/or histone composition, coordinate the pathways of these signals (Hsieh & Gage, 2004). Since long time the scientists have focused on the differentiation process of mature neurons, which take place before astrocytes in the telencephalon, to find out the mechanism underlying selective inhibition of glia-specific genes e.g., astrocyte specific glial fibrillary acidic protein (GFAP). It was reported in a previously defined epigenetics system that GFAP activation was inhibited in neuroepithelial cells of early telencephalon though blockage of signal transducer and activator of transcription 3 (STAT3) binding due to CpG methylation in neurons after mitosis (Hsieh & Gage, 2004).

Activation of Neuronal and Glial Biogenesis

In recent years, the mechanisms in the differentiation of neuronal and glial cells have begun to be understood. One of the transcription factors involved in the regulation of the bHLH gene in precursor cells of the brain cortex is called neurogenin 1 (NEUROG1) (Sun et al., 2001). Intriguing results of a previous study by Sun et al. demonstrated that NEUROG1 upregulation notably favored neuronal differentiation over glial one even under the glial factors' stimuli such as LIF and ciliary neurotrophic factor (CNTF) (Sun et al., 2001). They introduced a model called "sequestration" to articulate the control mechanism to shift from neurogenesis to gliogenesis, in which NEUROG1 suppresses differentiation of gliocytes by isolating activator complexes from gliocyte-specific genes and by blocking STAT3 induction in case the neurogenic fate is executed in cortical progenitor cells. As components of the activator complex and the downstream molecules of the bone morphogenetic proteins (BMPs) pathway, CBP/p300 and SMAD1 can interact with STAT proteins to promote gene expression (Hsieh & Gage, 2004). During gestational development, astrogenesis predominantly progresses through the formation of an activator complex with STAT3, SMAD1, and p300. Moreover, histone methylation has also recently been claimed to be involved in the regulation of GFAP gene expression (Desai et al., 2019).

The Implication of ncRNAs during Early Neural Development

As a member of the epigenetics regulatory players, ncRNAs function to mediate several vital biological processes in various species such as X-inactivation, transcriptional gene silencing, and spatiotemporal expression of certain genes (Hsieh & Gage, 2004). Micro RNAs (miRNA), as a prominent member of ncRNAs, have been identified in various species e.g., yeasts, animals, plants, etc., and have been demonstrated to target specific mRNAs to interfere with translation. A previous study conducted with mouse bone marrow tissue revealed that miRNAs take part in the regulation of lineage dependent differentiation of hematopoietic stem cells during mammalian development (Hsieh & Gage, 2004). The accumulating evidence underline the fact that small ncRNAs together with other epigenetic players can be promising molecules in stem cell biology as well as in the regulation of developmental stages in mammals.

Infant Outcomes of Maternal Prenatal Stress

Exposure to early life stress causes alterations in the pathways pertaining to stress response, mainly affects the HPA stress response of the fetus in the prenatal period or the infant in the postnatal period, and leads to dysregulation. An external stressor in the HPA pathways leads to neuronal activation that triggers the secretion of two major hormones in the hypothalamus i.e., corticotropin-releasing factor (CRF) and arginine vasopressin (AVP). AVP and CRF trigger the release of adrenocorticotropic hormone (ACTH) from the pituitary gland. Thereafter, ACTH provides the release of glucocorticoids (GCs), e.g., cortisol in humans, corticosterone in rodents, by adrenal gland cortex. GCs induce physiological changes in numerous tissues and result in psycho-biological changes associated with the stress experience e.g., elevated heart rate, blood sugar, and blood pressure and aberrations in sleep-wake rhythms (Yurdakök &

Çelik, 2019). While the effects of GCs within short periods are mostly adaptive, they increase alertness to threat, but severe and/or extended exposure to fear/stress in the developing brain may lead to hyperactivation of the HPA axis and increase in GCs. Low and stable levels of GCs are required for normal development of the central nervous system early in the life. Prolonged, severe, or unexpected stress early in the life can cause long-term alterations in the cognitive, stress, and emotion-regulating areas of the brain (Maccari et al., 2014; Yurdakök & Çelik, 2019).

The mechanism of the effects of prenatal psychosocial stress on the fetus has been understood mainly by studies with laboratory rodents. Since women frequently face social-based stresses such as bullying, work pressure, heavy workload, close friend or spouse abuse, physical or mental violence, or social disadvantage during pregnancy, those with a social component were examined from these animal models (Mahenge et al., 2013). In these studies, pregnant rats/mice were exposed to various stressors throughout pregnancy and fetal development, neurobiology, and behavior were evaluated.

When hamsters are left to face the social stress of a dominant group early in pregnancy, both female and male offspring have been shown to be born with significantly smaller sizes and low birth weight. A significant decrease in the number of male offspring was also observed as an indication of selective resorption or spontaneous abortion in the womb (Pratt & Lisk, 1991). The epigenetic consequences of prenatal chronic variable stress have been investigated in mice for several target genes, such as CRF and GR. The amount of DNA methylation was measured in the promoter sequence of these genes, which is the critical DNA region in gene regulation. It was determined that there was a decrease in DNA methylation of the CRF gene promoter region and an increase in the methylation of the GR promoter region in the hypothalamic tissue in adult male fetuses exposed to prenatal stress (Yurdakök & Çelik, 2019). Exposure to prenatal social stress has been shown to have sex-based effects on insulin, glucose, and lipid homeostases in adult rats. Prenatal stress caused stress-related hyperglycemia in males and hyperinsulinemia response to glucose loading in females. Thus, it was thought that prenatal social stress may be correlated with an increased risk of insulin resistance and metabolic dysfunction in adulthood (Mahenge et al., 2013).

Epigenetic Changes due to Hypoxic Ischemic Damage

The intra uterine environment is the development of the fetus in a hypoxic niche compared to normal ambient conditions. This hypoxic condition is required for the normal brain development of the fetus because exposure to a high amount of oxygen may be harmful to the developing brain of the fetus. However, it may cause serious damage to the fact that the amount of oxygen falls below the tolerable level. This may cause hypoxic brain damage to preterm and term newborns, causing retardation of permanent neuromotor development and mortality (Cristancho & Marsh, 2020). Prenatal and perinatal hypoxic injuries can result in several neurodevelopmental disorders (NDDs) such as mental and developmental disabilities, epilepsy, autism, and cerebral palsy.

Despite ranging between a broad spectrum, injuries caused by hypoxia can be classified into two main groups which are acute and chronic hypoxic injuries. Irrelevant from the type of the injury, acute and chronic hypoxia-induced NDDs manifest the whole pattern of NDDs however, which may appear at various stages in each individual. For example, chronic in utero hypoxia can be highly dependent on the external factors e.g., altitude, placental insufficiency due to maternal obesity, smoking, drug use, etc., and fetal anomalies such as congenital heart failures (Cristancho & Marsh, 2020).

Epigenic mechanisms also have a critical role in response to in utero hypoxia, of which the canonical response promotes the upregulation of a transcriptional regulatory protein called hypoxia inducible factor 1 alpha (HIF1α) that is a critical protein for sustaining cellular functions under decreased oxygen levels and whose expression is corroborated by hypoxia (Semenza, 2014). The response triggered by HIF1α varies, including induction of hematopoiesis and angiogenesis, regulation of metabolic events, and gain of nutrient intake for cell survival.

It is a well-known issue from previous studies that epigenetics mechanisms are involved in the regulation of HIF1α action against the response to the hypoxic attacks in several cell types. Especially, HIF1α promoter is presumed to be implicated in the adjustment of intracellular HIF1α levels owing to its CG/CH methylation-oriented modifications. Furthermore, the binding affinity of HIF1α can also be dramatically altered by the methylation status of its target response element, i.e., 5′-RCGTG-3′, which comprises a CpG dinucleotide. HIF1α also takes part in the upregulation of some chromatin remodeling enzymes called Jumonji chromatin demethylases. Since the methylation patterns of HIF1α target sites in the developing brain are still unknown, the engagement of HIF1α to its binding regions in various developmental periods of the brain as well as in different cell types can provide an adaptable response of the brain against the hypoxic damages especially by controlling Jumonji C-domain proteins. Children with NDDs, caused by genetic factors, have been claimed to possess similar epigenetics alterations which have been shown to be involved in the hypoxia-induced brain injuries (Cristancho & Marsh, 2020).

Postnatal Epigenetic Effects

As in prenatal life, postnatal life is critical in terms of epigenetic changes. It is suggested that the quality and/or quantity of mother-infant interactions lead to individual differences in physiological and behavioral development that can be stimulated by the environment (Yurdakök & Çelik, 2019).

The newborn brain seeks out various types of stimuli to facilitate the development of its neuronal circuits. Scent, auditory, visual, and tactile (tactile) stimuli from the environment have an important role in brain development and have effects that can be seen in future generations on the neuroendocrine systems that regulate social and emotional behaviors (Yurdakök, 2014).

Environmental stimuli create various synaptic formations with neuronal connections in the developing brain. These synapses can modify and adapt by the time in response to experience and the intensity of stimuli (synaptic plasticity). Neurons that are not used in synapses undergo selective apoptosis in the postnatal period and die. This can result in the loss of up to 50% of neurons in the brain cortex. Newborn infants should be exposed to the required positive stimuli and expected experiences throughout this critical period in terms of brain organization (Yurdakök & Çelik, 2019).

The bound between mother and infant is a special type of emotional attachment and is a unique event in providing the appropriate stimuli for normal brain improvement in newborn infants. A safe mother-infant attachment is thought to depend on physical contact between mother and infant. The primary objective of this attachment is to preserve the connection between the infant and the caregiver, ensuring the infant's survival and proper growth and development. The attachment between mother and infant is bi-directional and encompasses the neurobehavioral and chemical-sensory systems of both mother and infant. The first sign of the baby's attachment to the mother is that a full-term baby recognizes his mother's smell and voice at birth with the effect of the amniotic fluid in the mother's womb and the stimulus from the intrauterine environment and turns toward the mother. Amniotic fluid and breast milk originate from the mother's circulatory system and carry a chemically similar “aromatic signature” for the fetus and the newborn. The milk, sweat, and saliva of a mother contain the similar odors with amniotic fluid. If the newborn baby is slowly placed on the mother's stomach immediately after birth, it will crawl toward the scent of the mother's breast and the nipple of the nipple to suckle with a crawling motion. The first hours after birth are a sensitive period for the development of the sense of smell. The exposure to amniotic fluid and breast milk in this sensitive period affects mother-infant relations and breastfeeding later on.

Breastfeeding increases oxytocin in the brains of both mother and baby. Breastfeeding stimulates nerve endings in the nipple and areola, stimulating the release of oxytocin from the pituitary gland in the mother's brain. Maternal oxytocin levels are associated with attachment to the baby and affectionate mothering behavior (Feldman et al., 2007). Oxytocin has opposite effects to cortisol. Mother-infant attachment significantly affects the baby's sociability in later life. The central oxytocin pathways of the infant have a critical role in the development of social relations. A decrease in social relations, an increase in aggression and impulsive, and repetitive behaviors were observed in monkeys who were separated from their mothers shortly after birth and raised in standard care conditions. Oxytocin levels in the cerebrospinal fluid of these monkeys were determined to be significantly reduced compared to those of monkeys raised by their mothers.

The effect of tactile stimulus in infancy is also discovered using the stimulation of a paint brush to ensure the licking effect of puppy rats on the epigenetic pathways. In artificially reared offspring (e.g., cubs bred in the absence of mother), in which minimal level of tactile warning is sufficient for survival and increasing the frequency of this warning in the newborn period, it has been shown to be able to significantly correct (Gonzalez et al., 2001).

Conclusion

The fact that the healthy individuals should have appropriate social and emotional functions should be provided with a stress-free environment starting from the mother's stomach to the early periods of life for a healthy neural system. In order to prevent maltreatments including the neglect and the abuse against pregnancies and infants, to provide adequately psychological support to mothers in pregnancy and postpartum, it is vital importance for mothers to support the contact with their babies to able to improve the behavior of infants and the bonds with them.

Especially in the hospitalized newborn babies, the painful and unexpected attempts need to be avoided as much as possible. Besides the babies should be treated and handled sufficiently for pain relief and/or relaxing practices. The fact that the brain of the baby is shaped by environmental factors in the early life can be the ground for physical and mental problems that they will face in their next life. Last but not least, the epigenetic effects in the critical times of neural development can make the individuals encounter less physical and spiritual problems in the future.

References

Baccarelli, A., & Bollati, V. (2009). Epigenetics and environmental chemicals. *Current Opinion in Pediatrics, 21*(2), 243–251. https://doi.org/10.1097/mop.0b013e32832925cc.

Cristancho, A. G., & Marsh, E. D. (2020). Epigenetics modifiers: potential hub for understanding and treating neurodevelopmental disorders from hypoxic injury. *Journal of Neurodevelopmental Disorders, 12*(1), 37. https://doi.org/10.1186/s11689-020-09344-z.

Desai, M., Han, G., Li, T., & Ross, M. G. (2019). Programmed Epigenetic DNA Methylation-Mediated Reduced Neuroprogenitor Cell Proliferation and Differentiation in Small-for-Gestational-Age Offspring. *Neuroscience, 412*, 60–71. https://doi.org/10.1016/j.neuroscience.2019.05.044.

Feldman, R., Weller, A., Zagoory-Sharon, O., & Levine, A. (2007). Evidence for a neuroendocrinological foundation of human affiliation: plasma oxytocin levels across pregnancy and the postpartum period predict mother-infant bonding. *Psychological Science, 18*(11), 965–970. https://doi.org/10.1111/j.1467-9280.2007.02010.x.

Foley, D. L., Craig, J. M., Morley, R., Olsson, C. A., Dwyer, T., Smith, K., & Saffery, R. (2009). Prospects for epigenetic epidemiology. *American Journal of Epidemiology, 169*(4), 389–400. https://doi.org/10.1093/aje/kwn380.

Gonzalez, A., Lovic, V., Ward, G. R., Wainwright, P. E., & Fleming, A. S. (2001). Intergenerational effects of complete maternal deprivation and replacement stimulation on maternal behavior and emotionality in female rats. *Developmental Psychobiology, 38*(1), 11–32. https://doi.org/10.1002/1098-2302(2001)38:1<11::aid-dev2>3.0.co;2-b.

Gudsnuk, K., & Champagne, F. A. (2012). Epigenetic influence of stress and the social environment. *ILAR Journal, 53*(3-4), 279–288. https://doi.org/10.1093/ilar.53.3-4.279.

Heijmans, B. T., Tobi, E. W., Stein, A. D., Putter, H., Blauw, G. J., Susser, E. S., Slagboom, P. E., & Lumey, L. H. (2008). Persistent epigenetic differences associated with prenatal exposure to famine in humans. *Proceedings of the National Academy of Sciences of the United States of America, 105*(44), 17046–17049. https://doi.org/10.1073/pnas.0806560105.

Hesson, L. B., & Pritchard, A. L. (Eds.). (2019). *Clinical Epigenetics*. Springer Nature. https://doi.org/10.1007/978-981-13-8958-0.

Hsieh, J., & Gage, F. H. (2004). Epigenetic control of neural stem cell fate. *Current Opinion in Genetics & Development, 14*(5), 461–469. https://doi.org/10.1016/j.gde.2004.07.006.

Knickmeyer, R. C., Gouttard, S., Kang, C., Evans, D., Wilber, K., Smith, J. K., Hamer, R. M., Lin, W., Gerig, G., & Gilmore, J. H. (2008). A structural MRI study of human brain development from birth to 2 years. *The Journal of Neuroscience: The Official Journal of the Society for Neuroscience, 28*(47), 12176–12182. https://doi.org/10.1523/JNEUROSCI.3479-08.2008.

Law, C. M., Barker, D. J., Osmond, C., Fall, C. H., & Simmonds, S. J. (1992). Early growth and abdominal fatness in adult life. *Journal of Epidemiology and Community Health, 46*(3), 184–186. https://doi.org/10.1136/jech.46.3.184.

Maccari, S., Krugers, H. J., Morley-Fletcher, S., Szyf, M., & Brunton, P. J. (2014). The consequences of early-life adversity: neurobiological, behavioural and epigenetic adaptations. *Journal of Neuroendocrinology, 26*(10), 707–723. https://doi.org/10.1111/jne.12175.

Mahenge, B., Likindikoki, S., Stöckl, H., & Mbwambo, J. (2013). Intimate partner violence during pregnancy and associated mental health symptoms among pregnant women in Tanzania: a cross-sectional study. *BJOG: An International Journal of Obstetrics and Gynaecology, 120*(8), 940–946. https://doi.org/10.1111/1471-0528.12185.

Murgatroyd, C., & Spengler, D. (2011). Epigenetics of early child development. *Frontiers in Psychiatry, 2*, 16. https://doi.org/10.3389/fpsyt.2011.00016.

Noctor, S. C., Flint, A. C., Weissman, T. A., Dammerman, R. S., & Kriegstein, A. R. (2001). Neurons derived from radial glial cells establish radial units in neocortex. *Nature, 409*(6821), 714–720. https://doi.org/10.1038/35055553.

Perera, F., & Herbstman, J. (2011). Prenatal environmental exposures, epigenetics, and disease. *Reproductive Toxicology (Elmsford, N.Y.), 31*(3), 363–373. https://doi.org/10.1016/j.reprotox.2010.12.055.

Pratt, N. C., & Lisk, R. D. (1991). Role of progesterone in mediating stress-related litter deficits in the golden hamster (Mesocricetus auratus). *Journal of Reproduction and Fertility, 92*(1), 139–146. https://doi.org/10.1530/jrf.0.0920139.

Semenza G. L. (2014). Oxygen sensing, hypoxia-inducible factors, and disease pathophysiology. *Annual Review of Pathology, 9*, 47–71. https://doi.org/10.1146/annurev-pathol-012513-104720.

Sun, Y., Nadal-Vicens, M., Misono, S., Lin, M. Z., Zubiaga, A., Hua, X., Fan, G., & Greenberg, M. E. (2001). Neurogenin promotes neurogenesis and inhibits glial differentiation by independent mechanisms. *Cell, 104*(3), 365–376. https://doi.org/10.1016/s0092-8674(01)00224-0.

Szyf, M., Weaver, I., & Meaney, M. (2007). Maternal care, the epigenome and phenotypic differences in behavior. *Reproductive Toxicology (Elmsford, N.Y.), 24*(1), 9–19. https://doi.org/10.1016/j.reprotox.2007.05.001.

Weaver, I. C., Champagne, F. A., Brown, S. E., Dymov, S., Sharma, S., Meaney, M. J., & Szyf, M. (2005). Reversal of maternal programming of stress responses in adult offspring through methyl supplementation: altering epigenetic marking later in life. *The Journal of neuroscience: the official journal of the Society for Neuroscience, 25*(47), 11045–11054. https://doi.org/10.1523/JNEUROSCI.3652-05.2005.

Yurdakök, K. (2014). Neonatal maltreatment and brain development. *Journal of Pediatric and Neonatal Individualized Medicine (JPNIM), 3*(2), e030228-e030228.

Yurdakök, K., & Çelik, M. (2019). Epigenetic effects of child abuse and neglect. *Çocuk Sağlığı ve Hastalıkları Dergisi (Journal of Pediatric Health and Disease) 62*: 17-30.

Chapter 15

Epilepsy and Epigenetics

Arzuhan Cetindag Ciltas*, **PhD**
Sivas Cumhuriyet University Vocational School of Health Services,
Department of Therapy and Rehabilitation, Turkey

Abstract

Epilepsy is a common neurological disorder manifested by recurrent seizures, and its underlying causes could be significantly associated with genetic. Epigenetic hereditary changes in gene expression that are not caused by changes in the DNA sequence.

DNA methylation, post-transcriptional changes of histones, and the action of non-coding RNA molecules are currently the most well-researched epigenetic mechanisms. These processes control gene expression, and interruption of these molecular pathways can lead to disease development. Investigating the epigenetic processes involved in epilepsy is a potential avenue of search that will lead to a better understanding of the etiology and treatments of epilepsy.

Keywords: epilepsy, epileptogenesis, epigenetics, epigenetics mechanism

Introduction

Epilepsy is a serious neurological condition manifesting itself by recurrent and spontaneous seizures starting in the hippocampus or cerebral cortex of the brain (Avanzini and Franceschetti, 2003; Pitkänen and Sutula, 2002). Despite the effectiveness of current anti-epileptic drugs (AEDs), almost 25% of the patients with epilepsy are resistant to medical treatment (Rana and Musto, 2018). However, many AEDs are unable to control seizures in nearly 25% of patients diagnosed with epilepsy, and none of the current treatment options can alter the pathophysiology of the disease, only reducing or alleviating symptoms (Kwan and Brodie, 2000). Therefore, there is a significant need for new treatment approaches.

Epileptogenesis refers to the pathological condition which can lead to spontaneous seizures as a result of direct or indirect damage to the brain and pathophysiological events and its progressive course (Pitkänen and Sutula, 2002; Vezzani and Rüegg, 2017). These damages can be genetic, congenital, or acquired. Traumas, infections, cerebrovascular accidents, or febrile convulsions may trigger epileptogenesis (Terrone et al., 2016). The pathophysiology of

* Corresponding Author's E-mail: acetindag@cumhuriyet.edu.tr.

In: Epigenetics: Beyond the Genetics and Medicine
Editors: Sevgi Durna Daştan and Nazan Yurtcu
ISBN: 979-8-88697-228-3

epilepsy remains as a mystery. Although there are studies conducted on animal models where certain neuronal networks contribute to seizure formation and creep, the datum obtained from the patients with epilepsy are insufficient (Khoshkhoo et al., 2017). This may be evidenced by the complexity of the neuronal networks involved in the epilepsy process (Pfisterer et al., 2020).

Recently, epilepsy and cognitive functions have been amalgamated with epigenetic mechanisms. A great deal of research on identifying epigenetic processes has focused on temporal lobe epilepsy (TLE). Current research has indicated that several epigenetic mechanisms, such as chemical modifications in DNA, the activity of several non-coding RNA molecules, and post-translational changes in DNA wrapping proteins have a remarkable impact on these gene networks in the experiments with the patients with epilepsy (Hauseret al., 2018).

Epigenetic control of gene transcription has become a focal point of research for the potential capability of the permanent and dynamic modulation of gene expression in the brain. It has been shown that the epigenetic mechanisms which were thought to be non-divisible and static in extremely differentiated cells tend to be dynamic and active in the adult brain and are vital for the care of basic neuronal functions. The identical epigenetic mechanisms regulating normal brain function are marked as dysregulated systems in various neuronal diseases besides epilepsy. These biochemical markers could be significant biomarkers in the epileptogenesis process or work as new and promising therapeutic approaches for the management or alleviation of epileptic symptoms (Hauser et al., 2018).

Major Epigenetic Mechanisms

Epigenetics is a sub-field of genetics exploring the changes in the physical structure promoting genes and is derived from the Greek word "epi" meaning upon or above (Gräff et al., 2011). Epigenetics, which was first used in 1940 to identify hereditary changes independent of shifts in DNA code, is now widely used to identify chromatine sequencing and structure (Henshall and Kobow, 2015). In other words, epigenetics refers to those changes that occur in phenotype without a genotypic change. In recent years, thanks to advances in technology, many studies have been carried out in the area of epigenetics. The significant effects of epigenetic mechanisms, especially on humans, have drawn attention to their association with diseases. Many diseases arise from malfunctions in epigenetic mechanisms. The interaction and regulation of epigenetic mechanisms in accordance with each other is a very important process for the organism to have a normal embryonic development (Guler and Peynircioglu, 2016). Epigenetic modifications can enable a gene to function and be silenced, as well as determine the location, time, and manner of the gene expression, and which proteins are then transcribed (Portela and Esteller, 2010). The purpose of epigenetic mechanisms is to regulate gene expression by creating reversible modifications on DNA and/or histones (Li, 2002). Epigenetic mechanisms include DNA methylations, chromatine changes (histonic modifications) and RNA-based mechanisms [MicroRNAs (MiRNA), non-codingRNA] (Al Aboud et al., 2018). The epigenetic mechanisms may be affected by the factors in environmental and lifestyle (Chen et al., 2017).

DNA Methylation

One of the recently popular epigenetic mechanisms is DNA methylation. In mammals, transcription begins in the promoter regions, which are rich in CG sequence. These sequences, where guanine is arranged after cytosine and these two bases are linked by phosphate, thus called as the CpG region. These regions in DNA, which are rich in CpG, are called CpG islands (Teperek and Miyamoto, 2013). DNA methylation takes place when a methyl (-CH3) group is bound to DNA bases via covalent bonding. Although methylation reactions are rarely seen on other bases, they occur by binding to the 5th carbon (5-mC) of cytosine, and DNA methylation actually refers to 5-mC. These methylation reactions occur on CpG islands in the density-reşated promoter region of the gene, thereby being inhibited (Gibney and Nolan, 2010). This chemical event is catalyzed by DNA methyl transferases (DNMT). There are 5 different DNA Methyltransferases (DMNT) enzymes identified in mammals: These enzymes are called DNMT1, DNMT2, DNMT3A, DNMT3B, and DNMT3L. Of these, DNMT1, DNMT2, and DNMT3L, are involved in the methylation pattern during embryo and gamete formation as well as tissue development. The other enzymes, which include DNMT3A and DNMT3B), are required for new DNA methylation (Subramaniam et al., 2014).

Histonic Modifications

Histones are positively charged proteins that wrap around DNA and allow it to have a three-dimensional structure. In this way, the DNA wrapped by different types of histone proteins create the nucleosome, which is the most fundamental component of chromatine (Luger et al., 1997). The control of gene expression is provided by changes in the structure of chromatine (Orcan and University, 2006). The chromatine is divided into two basic structures: The heterochromatine is denser, compact, and transcriptionally silent, while euchromatine is less dense and transcriptionally active (Kanwal and Gupta, 2012).

Histones are structures that wrap around DNA and form chromatine. The histones with DNA wrapped around them are called nucleosomes or histone octamers. The N-terminus of the outer surface of nucleosomes contains positively charged amino acids. This structure, consisting of 15-38 amino acids, is called the histone tail. In a nucleosome, each consisting of two molecules, H2A, H2B, H3, and H4 histone proteins wrap around a 147 base DNA molecule (Mariño-Ramírez et al., 2014). The tails of histones at the N-terminus are involved in post-translational gene regulation with a range of different modifications such as methylation, acetylation, phosphorylation, ubiquitination, sumoylation, and deimination (Chen et al., 2010; Mottamal et al., 2015). These modifications may tend to alter DNA-histone interactions. Histonic modifications are reversible (Virani et al., 2012). Histonic acetylation and histonic methylation are the most widely studied histonic modifications. The histonic acetylation is involved in many physiological events. Generally, hyperacetylation occurs in the eukramatine region of the chromosomes, and transcription is active. However, in the heterochromatin region, hypoacetylation (a decrease in the acetylation level of histones) occurs in silent genomic regions.

While histonic acetylation is initiated by histone acetyl transferase (HAT), histonic deacetylation is initiated by histone deacetylase (HDAC) (Brait and Sidransky, 2011). Histonic modifications have a very important role in the development of chromatine structures and coding of epigenetic changes such as mitosis, DNA replication, recombination, gene transcription, and X chromosome inactivation (Chen et al., 2010; Virani et al., 2012).

RNA Based Mechanisms (Non-Coding RNA)

The rapid development of sequencing techniques has resulted in substantial findings with human genome sequencing. Only 2% of the genome of eukaryotic organism synthesizes protein-coding messenger RNAs (mRNAs). The remaining 98% are not converted into protein and expressed as non-coding RNA (ncRNA). The end product RNA molecules (non-coding RNA: ncRNA) that are not converted into protein and called as non-coding RNA (ncRNA), are synthesized (Akkaya and Dinçer, 2013; Ricciuti et al., 2014). Some of these ncRNAs have been reported to be involved in epigenetic processes (Hatipoğlu et al., 2017). It is stated that some ncRNAs can suppress gene expression by breaking mRNAs in the cytoplasm or by blocking translation while some ncRNAs inhibit the transcription step in the nucleus (Bodur and Demirpençe, 2010; Güzelgül and Aksoy, 2009). ncRNAs are also thought to be propulsive for the initiation of histonic modifications and DNA methylation, thus contributing to the formation of the heterochromatine region and keeping the DNA silent (Akkaya and Dinçer 2013; Hatipoğlu et al., 2017). ncRNAs are involved in many biological processes such as cellular defense, transcriptional gene silencing, and chromosome remodeling. This mechanism is impaired in many diseases, including cancer. ncRNAs are examined in two categories according to their sizes (Gurel et al., 2016). Those shorter than 50 nucleotides are called short ncRNAs, while ncRNAs longer than 200 nucleotides are called long ncRNAs (Li et al., 2014). Short ncRNAs are molecules with a length of 18-28 nucleotides. The main short, non-coding RNAs that have an important role in gene silencing include micro RNA (miRNA), small interfering (siRNA), and piwi RNA (piRNA) (Huang et al., 2013). miRNAs are single-stranded RNAs with a length of 18-26 nucleotides that cannot be converted into proteins. miRNAs initially suppress protein expression by degradation of the target mRNA or inhibition of translation. Genes can be targeted by many miRNAs, and each miRNA can directly or indirectly affect hundreds of mRNAs (Rönnau et al., 2014). Long, non-coding RNAs (lncRNAs) are located in the nuclear or cytosolic areas. It is known that IncRNAs are involved in many physiological processes including responding to stress, physical development, embryonic stem cell potential, chromatine re-modification, cell cycle, migration, and metabolism (Zhang et al., 2013).

Epilepsy and Epigenetic Mechanisms

The underlying causes of many epileptic disorders have not been entirely clarified. The interfering mechanism here may develop mostly as a result of a mutation in the ion channel or a stimulatory /suppressive neurotransmission element (Thomas and Berkoviç, 2014). Other types of epileptic disorders include focal epilepsy, which is associated with neuronal loss called hippocampal sclerosis and gliosis, and temporal lobe epilepsy (TLE) caused by trauma and infection, often characterized by seizures stemming from the hippocampus (Blümcke et al., 2013). Most patients with temporal lobe epilepsy are pharmacologically resistant to AEDs and surgical resection is recommended for the treatment of the disease (Wiebe et al., 2001). The molecular causes of such diseases are not entirely identified, and effective treatments are too slow to be used. In recent years, it has been emphasized that there may be a relationship between epigenetic mechanisms and epilepsy. Many studies have been conducted on temporal lobe epilepsy in order to identify the epigenetic processes involved in epilepsy. Nevertheless, it is thought that epigenetics may also have an important role in other epileptic diseases (Hauser et al., 2018).

Through neuro- and gliogenesis, as well as activity-dependent synaptic plasticity, changes found in the developmental phases of epigenetic processes support the structural and functional functions of the brain. Besides misregulations during neuronal development, epigenetic perturbations can result in a various of pathological conditions which include changes in neurogenesis, abnormal neuronal formation, and structural changes in individual cells even large networks; these factors might all have a role in the development of hyperexcitable cycles and epileptic seizures. (Kobow and Blümcke, 2014).

Epigenetic Mechanisms Affected in Epilepsy

DNA Methylation in Epilepsy

Recent research has provided valuable evidence indicating the possible contribution of abnormal changes in DNA methylation to epileptogenesis. One of the major epigenetic modifications is known to be DNA methylation. It happens mainly in parts of DNA with CpG regions, identified as cytosine residues near those of guanine in the underlying DNA sequence. DNMTs having different and specific activities attach methyl groups to DNA bases. While DNMT3a and DNMT3b are mainly responsible for the addition of new methylation markers, DNMT1 is primarily associated with DNA methylation maintenance. (Okano et al., 1999). Typically, when a DNA region is methylated, transcription of the corresponding gene is typically suppressed. Gene suppression occurs through DNA methylation by either providing binding sites for transcription regulating proteins or by preventing transcription factor binding. The mentioned factors will enable the compression or unwinding of the DNA and will make the corresponding sequence accessible for transcription by the RNA polymerase to some extent. It is possible to find DNA methylation all over the genome, but due to the regulatory potential for significant alterations in the linked transcription of the gene, the presence of methylation in promoter regions is especially notable. DNA methylation, which was previously assumed to be a stable structure, is now known to be a very dynamic process. (Ma et al., 2009).

TLE has been associated with changes in DNA methylation. Several genome-wide investigations have reported that the progression of epilepsy is followed by dramatic changes in the methylome. In human tissue in TLE, genome-wide methylation alterations support dynamic protein production of DNA-modifying enzymes. For example, DNMT3a and DNMT1 enzymesare upregulated in TLE hippocampal tissue and are abundant in neuronal cells, indicating the involvement of novo DNA methylation in TLE (Zhu et al., 2012).

Since DNA methylation and hydroxymethylation have an essential role in regulating the genome by permitting or preventing regulatory protein binding, methyl-binding proteins are thought to manage the course of epilepsy besides basal methylation changes (Ni et al., 2015).

The methyl binding proteins attach to methylated DNA regions and could interfere with transcriptional suppression or bound sequence activation. In another recent study, 321 genes in total demonstrated changes in DNA methylation after exposure to epilepticus status or seizures. 90% of these genes contained reduced levels of DNA methylation (i.e., hypomethylation) (Miller-Delaney et al., 2012).

In a pilocarpine-induced rat model, hypermethylation was found to be prominent and interrelated with specific diminished expression of genes (Kobow et al., 2013). Furtherresearch revealed that abnormal DNA methylation in epilepsy most likely arises from the disruption in TLE levels of the DNA-modifying enzyme upregulated primarily in neuronal cells (DNMT1 and DNMT3a) (Zhu et al., 2012). William–Karnesky et al., indicated that in different seizure models, inhibition of DNA methylation would modulate epileptogenesis. Moreover, supplementary adenosine was specifically used to reverse DNA hypermethylation, which was found to inhibit mossy fiber spreading in the hippocampal tissue and prevent epilepsy progression for approximately three months. By reversing the progression of the disease, the role of altered DNA methylation was highlighted in the epileptogenic process (Williams-Karnesky et al., 2013).

On the other hand, Tailiani et al., (2009) state that it is possible to manipulate DNA methylation by the oxidation of 5mC to 5-hydroxymethylcytosine (5hmC), which is conducted by 10-11 translocation enzymes (TETs) and is very prominent in the brain. Hence, as a major factor in the regulation of the neuronal activity, it has become a focus of research (Kriaucionis and Heintz, 2009; Münzel et al., 2010; Seritrakul and Gross, 2017). It has been reported by genome-wide studies that 5hmC is present at transcriptional repression and activation sites, however, predominantly linked to escalated gene expression (Xu et al., 2011). However, the precise role of 5hmC in epilepsy has not yet been determined. Reduced levels of 5hmC were reported in the CA3 region of the hippocampus following kainic acid-induced seizures connected with decreased TET1 levels (Parrish et al., 2013).

Histonic Modifications in Epilepsy

Histonic modifications connected with epilepsy and its progressive course include several different events such as histonic phosphorylation, methylation, and acetylation. Histone modifications have a well-known important role in epilepsy and in the process of epilepsy, and recent studies indicate their increasing importance. (Kobow and Blumcke, 2018; Citraro et al., 2017; Younus and Reddy, 2017). Histones can be exposed to change at their N-terminus, usually by lysine or arginine residues (Hauser et al., 2018).

Altered histonic acetylation, which is catalyzed by histone deacetylases (HDACs), promotes changes in gene expression connected with epilepsy and the development of epilepsy. It has been reported that following the induction of status epilepticus (SE), the glutamate receptor encoding the GluR2 gene is epigenetically controlled through an H4 reduced histonic acetylation and decreases total mRNA expression. Therefore, therapeutic inhibition of histone deacetylases through specific inhibitors (HDACs) is considered an effective treatment to enhance neuronal protection and interfere with epileptogenesis. In contrast, Huang et al., (2002) reported that following SE in the pilocarpine rat model, this process increased histonic acetylation at the brain-induced neurotrophic factor (BDNF) promoter, indicating increased activation of c-fos and c-jun during the development of epilepsy, and the obtained data suggest that acetylation mediates a number of epileptic factors (Sng et al., 2006).

It is notable that AEDs targeting histonic modifications are utilized to mitigate epilepsy. It is known that Valproic acid, one of the leading drugs used for treating epilepsy, have lysine deacetylase (KDAC) inhibitory properties, and in certain genes in the hippocampus, it affects DNA methylation. (Milutinovic et al., 2007; Aizawa and Yamamuro, 2015; Detich et al., 2003). Furthermore, behavioral phenotypes, including nutrition, stress, and enhanced physical activity, can trigger changes in histonic acetylation (Weaver et al., 2004). More significantly, administering an HDAC inhibitor could reserve some of these phenotypes (Weaver et al., 2006).

Many studies have revealed that histonic methylation has important functions in neuronal functions and regulates cognitive processes such as learning and memory (Gupta-Agarwal et al., 2012; Gupta et al., 2010). The rrole these dynamic changes might be vital in the development of epilepsy, since histonic modifications are very important in the regulation of chromatine structure and gene expression as well. As environmental factors change, histones can be rapidly manipulated to adapt the cell better to a new environment (Hauser et al., 2018). Histonic modifications are potentially promising in the regulation of chromatine structure and gene expression for the treatment of epilepsy. However, farther studies are necessary to develop advanced treatment methods.

Non-Coding RNAs in Epilepsy

MicroRNAs (miRNAs) are a family of small non-coding RNAs regulating gene expression by reducing mRNA stability and translation. There may be regulatory mechanisms and therapeutic targets in the epileptogenesis (Henshall et al., 2016). In humans, there are approximately 1,600 miRNAs regulating more than half of the protein-coding genes. Each miRNA has the ability to regulate more than one protein. Functional research has identified strong seizure-regulatory effects of at least a dozen different miRNAs so far (Jimenez-Mateos and Henshall, 2013). Neuronal miR-124 levels were reported to decrease following kainic acid-induced in rats. Neuron-restrictive silencing factor, a transcriptional repressor that coordinately represses diverse genes along the development of epilepsy, is the main target of miR-124 (Brennan et al., 2016). In their study, Wang et al., found that pre-treatment with miR-124 decreased severity in seizures induced by pilocarpine and pentylenetetrazole in rats (Wang et al., 2016).

Unlike miRNAs, non-coding RNAs (lncRNAs) received little attention in the field of epilepsy, and the studies are limited. IncRNAs are about 200 nucleotides in length. IncRNAs have a role in the regulation of many neuronal mechanisms such as cognition and memory (Hauser et al., 2018). A genome-wide study has shown that lncRNAs have irregular adjacent protein-coding genes of lncRNAs in pilocarpine and kainate models. Therefore, neuron differentiation and morphogenesis are important functions related to lncRNA (Lee et al., 2015).

Conclusion

It is thought that epilepsy occurs mainly as a result of the imbalance in glutamate and GABA levels, but the exact etiology of epilepsy remains unclear. Genetic research has identified a single point mutation in genes occurring in voltage-gated sodium, potassium and calcium channels, and acetylcholine receptors (Meldrum and Rogawski, 2007). Based on this information, the pharmaceutical industry has developed and approved DNMT and HDAC inhibitor drugs by focusing on studies on DNA methylation and histonic acetylation for the care of diseases such as epilepsy and stroke. Similarly, drugs targeting ncRNA may be effective for the treatment of epilepsy by affecting several paths (Hauser et al., 2018). In addition to these treatments, environmental factors, epigenetic regulations, and approaches that include genome expression are among the issues that need to be focused on (Chen et al., 2017). Today, the majority of epilepsy patients are resistant to antiepileptic drugs. Therefore, the development of new drugs is of great importance for the treatment modalities. Especially, recent intensive studies on epigenetics are considered as strong potential targets both for epilepsy and for the prevention of other diseases. However, more studies are needed to make epigenetic mechanisms effective in the treatment of epilepsy and for the improving of novel treatment options.

References

Aizawa, S. and Yamamuro, Y. (2015). Valproate administration to mice increases hippocampal p21 expression by altering genomic DNA methylation. *Neuroreport*, *26*(15), 915-920.

Akkaya, Z. and Dinçer, P. (2013). The new era in therapeutic approaches: Non-coding RNAs and diseases. *Marmara Medical Journal*, *26*(1), 5-10.

Avanzini, G. and Franceschetti, S. (2003). Cellular biology of epileptogenesis. *The Lancet Neurology*, *2*(1), 33-42.

Blümcke, I. Thom, M. Aronica, E. Armstrong, D. D. Bartolomei, F. Bernasconi and Spreafico, R. (2013). International consensus classification of hippocampal sclerosis in temporal lobe epilepsy: a Task Force report from the ILAE Commission on Diagnostic Methods. *Epilepsia*, *54*(7), 1315-1329.

Bodur, E. and Demirpençe, E. (2010). Non-coding RNAs and gene silencing. *Hacettepe Tıp Dergisi*, *41*(8), 82-89.

Brait, M. and Sidransky, D. (2011). Cancer epigenetics: above and beyond. *Toxicology Mechanisms and Methods*, *21*(4), 275-288.

Brennan, G. P. Dey, D. Chen, Y. Patterson, K. P. Magnetta, E. J. Hall, A. M. and Baram, T. Z. (2016). Dual and opposing roles of microRNA-124 in epilepsy are mediated through inflammatory and NRSF-dependent gene networks. *Cell Reports*, *14*(10), 2402-2412.

Chen, T. Giri, M. Xia, Z. Subedi, Y. N. and Li, Y. (2017). Genetic and epigenetic mechanisms of epilepsy: a review. *Neuropsychiatric Disease and Treatment*, *13*, 1841.

Chen, Z. Wang, L. Wang, Q. and Li, W. (2010). Histone modifications and chromatin organization in prostate cancer. *Epigenomics*, *2*(4), 551-560.

Citraro, R. Leo, A. Santoro, M. D'agostino, G. Constanti, A. and Russo, E. (2017). Role of histone deacetylases (HDACs) in epilepsy and epileptogenesis. *Current Pharmaceutical Design*, *23*(37), 5546-5562.

Detich, N. Bovenzi, V, and Szyf, M. (2003). Valproate induces replication-independent active DNA demethylation. *Journal of Biological Chemistry*, *278*(30), 27586-27592.

Gibney, E. R. and Nolan, C. M. (2010). Epigenetics and gene expression. *Heredity*, *105*(1), 4-13.

Gräff, J. Kim, D. Dobbin, M. M. and Tsai, L. H. (2011). Epigenetic regulation of gene expression in physiological and pathological brain processes. *Physiological Reviews*, *91*(2), 603-649.

Gupta, S. Kim, S. Y. Artis, S. Molfese, D. L. Schumacher, A. Sweatt, J. D. and Lubin, F. D. (2010). Histone methylation regulates memory formation. *Journal of Neuroscience*, *30*(10), 3589-3599.

Gupta-Agarwal, S. Franklin, A. V. DeRamus, T. Wheelock, M. Davis, R. L. McMahon, L. L. and Lubin, F. D. (2012). G9a/GLP histone lysine dimethyltransferase complex activity in the hippocampus and the entorhinal cortex is required for gene activation and silencing during memory consolidation. *Journal of Neuroscience*, *32*(16), 5440-5453.

Güler, C. and Peynircioğlu, B. B. (2016). DNA Methylatıon and Its Relatıon wıth Dıseases. *Acıbadem Üniversitesi Sağlık Bilimleri Dergisi*, (2), 61-68.

Gürel, Ç. Nursal, A. F. and Yiğit, S. (2016). Epigenetics and Cancer. *Turkiye Klinikleri J Radiat Oncol-Special Topics*, *2*(1), 45-51.

Güzelgül, F. and Aksoy, K. (2009). Kodlanmayan RNA'ların İşlevi ve Tıpda Kullanım Alanları [*Function of Non-Coding RNAs and Their Use in Medicine*]. *Arşiv Kaynak Tarama Dergisi*, *18*(3), 141-155.

Hatipoğlu, Ö. F. Ertuğrul, K. A. Y. A. Yaykaşlı, E. and Yaykaşlı, K. O. (2012). Epigenetic Mechanisms and Cancer. *Duzce Medical Journal*, *14*(3), 58-68.

Hauser, R. M. Henshall, D. C. and Lubin, F. D. (2018). The epigenetics of epilepsy and its progression. *The Neuroscientist*, *24*(2), 186-200.

Henshall, D. C. and Kobow, K. (2015). Epigenetics and epilepsy. *Cold Spring Harbor Perspectives in Medicine*, *5*(12), a022731.

Henshall, D. C., Hamer, H. M. Pasterkamp, R. J. Goldstein, D. B. Kjems, J. Prehn, J. H. and Rosenow, F. (2016). MicroRNAs in epilepsy: pathophysiology and clinical utility. *The Lancet Neurology*, *15*(13), 1368-1376.

Huang, T. Alvarez, A. Hu, B. and Cheng, S. Y. (2013). Noncoding RNAs in cancer and cancer stem cells. *Chinese Journal of Cancer*, *32*(11), 582.

Huang, Y. Doherty, J. J. and Dingledine, R. (2002). Altered histone acetylation at glutamate receptor 2 and brain-derived neurotrophic factor genes is an early event triggered by status epilepticus. *Journal of Neuroscience*, *22*(19), 8422-8428.

Jimenez-Mateos, E. M. and Henshall, D. C. (2013). Epilepsy and microRNA. *Neuroscience*, *238*, 218-229.

Kanwal, R. and Gupta, S. (2012). Epigenetic modifications in cancer. *Clinical Genetics*, *81*(4), 303-311.

Khoshkhoo, S. Vogt, D. and Sohal, V. S. (2017). Dynamic, cell-type-specific roles for GABAergic interneurons in a mouse model of optogenetically inducible seizures. *Neuron*, *93*(2), 291-298.

Kobow, K. and Blümcke, I. (2014). Epigenetic mechanisms in epilepsy. *Progress in Brain Research*, *213*, 279-316.

Kobow, K. and Blümcke, I. (2018). Epigenetics in epilepsy. *Neuroscience Letters*, *667*, 40-46.

Kobow, K. Kaspi, A. Harikrishnan, K. N. Kiese, K. Ziemann, M. Khurana, I. and Blümcke, I. (2013). Deep sequencing reveals increased DNA methylation in chronic rat epilepsy. *Acta Neuropathologica*, *126*(5), 741-756.

Kriaucionis, S. and Heintz, N. (2009). The nuclear DNA base 5-hydroxymethylcytosine is present in Purkinje neurons and the brain. *Science*, *324*(5929), 929-930.

Kwan, P. and Brodie, M. J. (2000). Early identification of refractory epilepsy. *New England Journal of Medicine*, *342*(5), 314-319.

Lee, D. Y. Moon, J. Lee, S. T. Jung, K. H. Park, D. K. Yoo, J. S. and Lee, S. K. (2015). Dysregulation of long non-coding RNAs in mouse models of localization-related epilepsy. *Biochemical and Biophysical Research Communications*, *462*(4), 433-440.

Li, E. (2002). Chromatin modification and epigenetic reprogramming in mammalian development. *Nature Reviews Genetics*, *3*(9), 662-673.

Li, P. F. Chen, S. C. Xia, T. Jiang, X. M. Shao, Y. F. Xiao, B. X. and Guo, J. M. (2014). Non-coding RNAs and gastric cancer. *World Journal of Gastroenterology: WJG*, *20*(18), 5411.

Luger, K. Mäder, A. W. Richmond, R. K. Sargent, D. F. and Richmond, T. J. (1997). Crystal structure of the nucleosome core particle at 2.8 Å resolution. *Nature*, *389*(6648), 251-260.

Ma, D. K. Jang, M. H. Guo, J. U. Kitabatake, Y. Chang, M. L. Pow-Anpongkul, N. and Song, H. (2009). Neuronal activity–induced Gadd45b promotes epigenetic DNA demethylation and adult neurogenesis. *Science*, *323*(5917), 1074-1077.

Mariño-Ramírez, L. Kann, M. G. Shoemaker, B. A. and Landsman, D. (2005). Histone structure and nucleosome stability. *Expert Review of Proteomics*, *2*(5), 719-729.

Meldrum, B. S. and Rogawski, M. A. (2007). Molecular targets for antiepileptic drug development. *Neurotherapeutics*, *4*(1), 18-61.

Miller-Delaney, S. F. Das, S. Sano, T. Jimenez-Mateos, E. M. Bryan, K. Buckley, P. G. and Henshall, D. C. (2012). Differential DNA methylation patterns define status epilepticus and epileptic tolerance. *Journal of Neuroscience*, *32*(5), 1577-1588.

Milutinovic, S. D'Alessio, A. C. Detich, N. & Szyf, M. (2007). Valproate induces widespread epigenetic reprogramming which involves demethylation of specific genes. *Carcinogenesis*, *28*(3), 560-571.

Mottamal, M. Zheng, S. Huang, T. L. and Wang, G. (2015). Histone deacetylase inhibitors in clinical studies as templates for new anticancer agents. *Molecules*, *20*(3), 3898-3941.

Münzel, M. Globisch, D. Brückl, T. Wagner, M. Welzmiller, V. Michalakis, S. and Carell, T. (2010). Quantification of the sixth DNA base hydroxymethylcytosine in the brain. *Angewandte Chemie International Edition*, *49*(31), 5375-5377.

Ni, G. Qin, J. Li, H. Chen, Z. Zhou, Y. Fang, Z. and Zhou, L. (2015). Effects of antiepileptic drug monotherapy on one-carbon metabolism and DNA methylation in patients with epilepsy. *PLoS One*, *10*(4), e0125656.

Okano, M. Bell, D. W. Haber, D. A. and Li, E. (1999). DNA methyltransferases Dnmt3a and Dnmt3b are essential for de novo methylation and mammalian development. *Cell*, *99*(3), 247-257.

Parrish, R. R. Albertson, A. J. Buckingham, S. C. Hablitz, J. J. Mascia, K. L. Haselden, W. D. and Lubin, F. D. (2013). Status epilepticus triggers early and late alterations in brain-derived neurotrophic factor and NMDA glutamate receptor Grin2b DNA methylation levels in the hippocampus. *Neuroscience*, *248*, 602-619.

Pfisterer, U. Petukhov, V. Demharter, S. Meichsner, J. Thompson, J. J. Batiuk, M. Y. and Khodosevich, K. (2020). Identification of epilepsy-associated neuronal subtypes and gene expression underlying epileptogenesis. *Nature Communications*, *11*(1), 1-19.

Pitkänen, A. and Sutula, T. P. (2002). Is epilepsy a progressive disorder? Prospects for new therapeutic approaches in temporal-lobe epilepsy. *The Lancet Neurology*, *1*(3), 173-181.

Portela, A. and Esteller, M. (2010). Epigenetic modifications and human disease. *Nature Biotechnology*, *28*(10), 1057-1068.

Rana, A. &and Musto, A. E. (2018). The role of inflammation in the development of epilepsy. *Journal of Neuroinflammation*, *15*(1), 1-12.

Ricciuti, B. Mecca, C. Crinò, L. Baglivo, S. Cenci, M. and Metro, G. (2014). Non-coding RNAs in lung cancer. *Oncoscience*, *1*(11), 674.

Rönnau, C. G. H. Verhaegh, G. W. Luna-Velez, M. V. and Schalken, J. (2014). Noncoding RNAs as novel biomarkers in prostate cancer. *BioMed Research International*, *2014*.

Seritrakul, P. and Gross, J. M. (2017). Tet-mediated DNA hydroxymethylation regulates retinal neurogenesis by modulating cell-extrinsic signaling pathways. *PLoS Genetics*, *13*(9), e1006987.

Sng, J. C. Taniura, H. and Yoneda, Y. (2006). Histone modifications in kainate-induced status epilepticus. *European Journal of Neuroscience*, *23*(5), 1269-1282.

Subramaniam, D. Thombre, R. Dhar, A. and Anant, S. (2014). DNA methyltransferases: a novel target for prevention and therapy. *Frontiers in Oncology*, *4*, 80.

Tahiliani, M. Koh, K. P. Shen, Y. Pastor, W. A. Bandukwala, H. Brudno, Y. and Rao, A. (2009). Conversion of 5-methylcytosine to 5-hydroxymethylcytosine in mammalian DNA by MLL partner TET1. *Science*, *324*(5929), 930-935.

Teperek, M. and Miyamoto, K. (2013). Nuclear reprogramming of sperm and somatic nuclei in eggs and oocytes. *Reproductive Medicine and Biology*, *12*(4), 133-149.

Terrone, G. Pauletti, A. Pascente, R. and Vezzani, A. (2016). Preventing epileptogenesis: a realistic goal? *Pharmacological Research*, *110*, 96-100.

Thomas, R. H. and Berkovic, S. F. (2014). The hidden genetics of epilepsy—a clinically important new paradigm. *Nature Reviews Neurology*, *10*(5), 283-292.

Vezzani, A. and Rüegg, S. (2017). Introduction to the 2nd meeting on Immunity and Inflammation in Epilepsy (IIE 2016). *Epilepsia*, *58*, 7-10.

Virani, S. Colacino, J. A. Kim, J. H. and Rozek, L. S. (2012). Cancer epigenetics: a brief review. *Ilar Journal*, *53*(3-4), 359-369.

Wang, W. Wang, X. Chen, L. Zhang, Y. Xu, Z. Liu, J. ... and Luo, J. (2016). The microRNA miR-124 suppresses seizure activity and regulates CREB1 activity. *Expert Reviews in Molecular Medicine*, *18*.

Weaver, I. C. Cervoni, N. Champagne, F. A. D'Alessio, A. C. Sharma, S. Seckl, J. R. and Meaney, M. J. (2004). Epigenetic programming by maternal behavior. *Nature Neuroscience*, *7*(8), 847-854.

Weaver, I. C. Meaney, M. J. and Szyf, M. (2006). Maternal care effects on the hippocampal transcriptome and anxiety-mediated behaviors in the offspring that are reversible in adulthood. *Proceedings of the National Academy of Sciences*, *103*(9), 3480-3485.

Wiebe, S. Blume, W. T. Girvin, J. P. and Eliasziw, M. (2001). A randomized, controlled trial of surgery for temporal-lobe epilepsy. *New England Journal of Medicine*, *345*(5), 311-318.

Williams-Karnesky, R. L. Sandau, U. S. Lusardi, T. A. Lytle, N. K. Farrell, J. M. Pritchard, E. M, and Boison, D. (2013). Epigenetic changes induced by adenosine augmentation therapy prevent epileptogenesis. *The Journal of Clinical Investigation*, *123*(8), 3552-3563.

Xu, Y. Wu, F. Tan, L. Kong, L. Xiong, L. Deng, J. and Shi, Y. G. (2011). Genome-wide regulation of 5hmC, 5mC, and gene expression by Tet1 hydroxylase in mouse embryonic stem cells. *Molecular Cell*, *42*(4), 451-464.

Younus, I. and Reddy, D. S. (2017). Epigenetic interventions for epileptogenesis: a new frontier for curing epilepsy. *Pharmacology & Therapeutics*, *177*, 108-122.

Zhang, H. Chen, Z. Wang, X. Huang, Z. He, Z. and Chen, Y. (2013). Long non-coding RNA: a new player in cancer. *Journal of Hematology & Oncology*, *6*(1), 1-7.

Zhu, Q. Wang, L. Zhang, Y. Zhao, F. H. Luo, J. Xiao, Z. ... and Wang, X. F. (2012). Increased expression of DNA methyltransferase 1 and 3a in human temporal lobe epilepsy. *Journal of Molecular Neuroscience*, *46*(2), 420-426.

Chapter 16

Epigenetics and Cardiovascular Diseases

Yücel Karaca[*], MD and Çetin Mirzaoğlu, MD
Department of Cardiology, Elazığ Fethi Sekin City Hospital, Elazığ, Turkey

Abstract

Epigenetic mechanisms occurring in DNA methylation, histone modification, and RNA-based mechanisms may generate heritable phenotypic changes without a change in DNA sequence. The disruption of gene expression patterns governed by epigenetics may lead to various diseases such as cardiovascular diseases, autoimmune diseases, and cancers. Genetic studies guide for preventive measures, appropriate treatment selection, drug interactions, drug efficacy, and patient compliance. Cardiovascular diseases (CVDs) are the most common cause of mortality worldwide. The increase in risk factors is predictive of the fact that the frequency of CVDs will further increase. Thus, detailed genetic data screening will become important in the diagnosis and prevention of CVD in the near future.

Keywords: DNA methylation, epigenetics, histone, cardiovascular diseases, RNA

Introduction

While cardiovascular diseases (CVDs) are the most common cause of death worldwide, it is predicted that their incidence will increase, especially with the increase in risk factors (Benjamin et al., 2017). Therefore, it has become increasingly important to carry out detailed genetic data screening and determine risk factors in the diagnosis and prevention of CVDs (Katrancıoğlu et al., 2012).

Genetic factors have a significant role in all cardiovascular events. Therefore, studies aimed at determining the genetic variations that can be used in the diagnosis of disease have been accelerated (Katrancıoğlu et al., 2012; Altıparmak & Özer, 2017). Genetic defects are held responsible for the malformations of the heart and blood vessels, which make up the majority of congenital anomalies. There are studies indicating genetic predisposition for common complex phenotypes such as cardiomyopathies, long QT syndrome, atherosclerosis, and hypertension (Richard et al., 2003; Wang et al., 2003; Bhagavatula et al., 2004; Ozaki et al., 2004). Genetic studies will guide for preventive measures, appropriate treatment selection, drug

[*] Corresponding Author's E-mail: yucel_karaca@hotmail.com.

In: Epigenetics: Beyond the Genetics and Medicine
Editors: Sevgi Durna Daştan and Nazan Yurtcu
ISBN: 979-8-88697-228-3

treatment effectiveness, drug interactions, and ensuring patient compliance with treatment (Katrancıoğlu et al., 2012; Altıparmak & Özer, 2017).

In ancient Greek, the prefix "epi" means "above," "over," and "beyond." Nowadays, epigenetics is used in the meaning of "genetics over genes" (Gunes & Kulac, 2013). The word epigenetics was first used scientifically by Conrad Waddington in 1942. According to Waddington, epigenetics is the branch of science that investigates how the genotype creates the phenotype during development (Goldberg et al., 2007). Nowadays, the most commonly used and accepted definition of it is as follows: Epigenetics is the branch of science that investigates differences in gene expression not caused by genotypic changes (Holliday, 2006; Martin et al., 2007). The cell or organism is directly affected by these differences; however, no change occurs in the DNA (deoxyribonucleic acid) sequence (Bird, 2007). Despite the presence of the same DNA sequence in all somatic cells of an organism, the expression of the gene largely varies between different cell types. The mitotic and/or meiotic inherited changes in the gene function that cannot be explained by changes in DNA sequence constitute the definition of epigenetics (Felsenfeld, 2014). The gene activity can be affected by epigenetic mechanisms through transcriptional and post-transcriptional and/or translational and post-translational modifications (Beckers et al., 2018). Epigenetics has a complex molecular basis, which determines when and how certain genes are activated. In this process, events such as cell regeneration, gene expression, and X chromosome inactivation occur in adults (Bond & Finnegan, 2007; Meissner et al., 2008). On the other hand, disruption of the process leads to the emergence of problems such as cardiovascular, cancer, autoimmune, and neurological diseases (Herman & Baylin, 2003; Jones & Baylin, 2007; Portela & Esteller, 2010; Turgeon et al., 2014).

Both genetic and environmental factors may affect such epigenetic mechanisms, which potentially have a wide range of consequences. Epigenetic modifications that start from the embryonal period and continue at every stage of life are reversible and transferable to the next generations (Haluskova, 2010). The fact that some epigenetic markers are reversible has encouraged many researchers to focus on epigenetic therapy (Bali et al., 2011).

Epigenetic Mechanisms

Epigenetic modifications allow each cell type in a multicellular organism to express specific genes required for its existence and to transfer information to new cells. Epigenetic modifications frequently take place throughout an organism's lifetime, and furthermore, if they occur in germ cells, these modifications can be transferred to the next generations (Chandler, 2007). Paramutation, imprinting, gene silencing, carcinogenic processes, teratogenic effects, X chromosome inactivation, reprogramming, maternal characteristics, the regulation of histone modifications, and cloning are known to include epigenetic processes. Epigenetic control occurs mainly with DNA methylation, histone modifications, and microRNAs (Beckers et al., 2018).

DNA Methylation

The most well-known and most functional of the modifications at the DNA level is DNA methylation (Waterland & Michels, 2007). DNA methylation is a covalent modification and is characterized by the formation of 5-methyl cytosine (5m-C) structure by attaching a methyl group (-CH3) to the 5th carbon of the cytosine (C) base (Bird, 2002). DNA methyltransferases (DNMTs) catalyze this chemical reaction. These enzymes take the methyl group from the methyl group donor S-adenosyl-L-methionine and transfer it to the 5th carbon of cytosine. There are five known DNA methyltransferase enzymes in mammals: DNMT1, DNMT3A, DNMT3B, DNMT3L, and DNMT2. DNMT1, DNMT3A, and DNMT3B are the enzymes with the most important catalytic activities. DNMT1 is responsible for transferring the methylation patterns established in the DNA chain to new chains. DNMT3A and DNMT3B are called de novo methyltransferases and are responsible for the formation of the first methylation patterns established early in development (Denis et al., 2011).

DNA methylation occurs in the regions of the genome formed by the sequencing of cytosine (C) and guanine (G) pairs and where CpG sequences are concentrated. The human genome contains approximately 28 million CpG sequences. Less than 10% of these sequences are present in the regions larger than 500 base pairs, which are called CpG islands, with a GC content of more than 55%. CpG islands conserved in the evolutionary process are generally present in the promoter regions of genes (Takai & Jones, 2002; Smith & Meissner, 2013).

Until the present day, the great majority of studies on DNA methylation have focused on methylation in the promoter region. Actually, the association between promoter region methylation and gene silencing was described in the 1970s. The discovery of the methylation of CpG islands in the promoter region and its suppression of gene expression contributed to the shaping of the general perception of the function of DNA methylation (Jones, 2012).

Homocysteine (Hcy), a nonprotein-forming amino acid which is a possible causative factor in the pathogenesis of CVD, is one of the important amino acids in the methylation cycle (Wald, 2002). An increase in plasma Hcy, which is generally caused by dietary folate deficiency, contributes to the accumulation of S-adenosyl Hcy that inhibits transmethylation reactions and decreases methylation along the epigenome (Handy, 2011). Cancer with a poor prognosis (Hsiung et al., 2007; Li et al., 2014; Foy & Pickering, 2015) and autoimmune disorder (Wu et al., 2016) are among the known health problems of hypomethylation. However, their effect on cardiovascular physiology is controversial.

Gene studies testing associations between CVD risk and the methylation state of biologically genomic regions get evidence for DNA methylation in the pathogenesis of CVD. In the literature, the decreased methylation of genes in the inflammatory pathway is associated with incremented gene expression and reduced levels of circulating proinflammatory cytokines and is a marker of cardiovascular dysfunction. For instance, a study on the methylation of ANGPTL2, a gene encoding a proinflammatory protein, revealed that promoter methylation decreased in leukocytes taken from patients with acute coronary syndrome compared to healthy controls and there was a higher expression of ANGPTL2 (Nguyen et al., 2016). Another study on inflammatory protein (Yang et al., 2016), interleukin-6, demonstrated low levels of IL-6 methylation and high plasma IL-6 concentrations in patients with ischemic heart disease. Furthermore, it was found that hypermethylation of the ASC gene, which encodes a critical component of the inflammatory pathway, was associated with the improvement in heart failure (Butts et al., 2015). The mechanism of association between DNA methylation and CVD involves dyslipidemia, hypertension, and obesity, in addition to inflammation (Friso et al., 2008; Perkins et al., 2012; Deodati et al., 2013; Yoo et al., 2014; Guay et al., 2016).

Histone Modifications

Histone modifications are the factors that regulate the transcription step of the gene by interacting with chromatin-associated proteins. They change the expression of the gene by changing the structure and function of chromatin. Acetylation, methylation, phosphorylation, s-nitrosylation, ubiquitination, and sumoylation are the mechanisms included in the group of histone modifications. As a result of these mechanisms, they change the structure of chromatin as transcriptionally active (euchromatin) or inactive (heterochromatin) (Segre et al., 2011). Histone acetyltransferase, deacetylase, and histone methyltransferase contribute to various cardiovascular phenotypes by controlling the transcription. For example, both histone methylation and acetylation show different patterns according to plaque severity in human carotid arteries (Greissel et al., 2016). The relative ease of inhibiting histone modifications, when they are combined with the wide-ranging effects on cardiovascular physiology, makes them beneficial therapeutic targets.

RNA-Based Mechanisms

The role of microRNAs (miRNAs), which are small non-coding RNAs that stop translation or induce the deterioration of mRNA in the etiology of CVD, has been supported by studies. miRNAs that are significantly stabilized in human plasma have a dual potential as biomarkers of disease and as therapeutic targets (Mitchell et al., 2008). Some studies showed that miR-1 and miR-133 increased in patients with acute coronary syndrome and miR-499 was more sensitive than troponin T (Olivieri et al., 2013; Ahlin et al., 2016). Both miR-1 and miR-133 are miRNAs that designate cardiac development and demonstrate dysregulation in heart failure (Bostjancic et al., 2010).

The critical role of miRNA-based mechanisms in CVDs extends to regulating the risk phenotypes. In the literature, miR-148 has been demonstrated to change HDL and LDL cholesterol levels in animal models as a key player in lipid metabolism and by modulating LDLR and ABCA1 expression (Goedeke et al., 2015; Wagschal et al., 2015). miRNAs design the progression of atherosclerosis by their effects on endothelial function, plaque development and rupture, and blood vessel formation, besides their effects on cholesterol homeostasis (Madrigal-Matute et al., 2013). Based on the estimates suggesting that roughly 60%of all human genes (Zhang, 2008) are controlled by miRNAs, available evidence showing the association of miRNAs with CVD phenotypes constitutes the tip of the iceberg; however, it provides forced causes to maintain the development of miRNA-based treatments for CVDs.

Conclusion

The emergence of different functions of DNA methylation, which is a very critical mechanism in gene expression control, along with the fast-advancing technology, has contributed to the understanding of the pathogenesis of many diseases. Until the present day, the potential relationship between diseases and beyond promoter methylation has been greatly ignored. However, revealing the methylation states of different regions in the genome with high-scale technologies has been promising for understanding diseases whose mechanisms are not known exactly. The fact that the role of methylation in diseases with complex mechanisms such as inflammatory diseases is not exactly known will largely pave the way for new studies.

Considering the established importance of epigenetic regulation in the etiology of cancer, it is not surprising that progress in oncology has surpassed other fields. Nevertheless, CVD risk and disease phenotypes continue to be targets of epigenetic studies. Environmental and life-style factors that are well-known as the contributors to the CVD risk, such as diet and smoking, are also essential mediators of epigenetic processes such as DNA methylation. Furthermore, it is also acknowledged that the known biomarkers of CVD risk, such as Hcy, have an epigenetic role. Increasingly exciting developments in the field of epigenetics will make significant contributions to early diagnosis, drug development, and treatment opportunities for important diseases of our age, such as CVDs, as well as for understanding the pathogenesis of many diseases.

References

Ahlin, F., Arfvidsson, J., Vargas, K. G., Stojkovic, S., Huber, K., & Wojta, J. (2016). MicroRNAs as circulating biomarkers in acute coronary syndromes: A review. *Vascular Pharmacology*, *81*, 15–21. https://doi.org/10.1016/j.vph.2016.04.001

Altıparmak İ H, Özer A. Genetic Counseling in the Cardiovascular Diseases Prevention. *Turkiye Klinikleri J Cardiovasc. Surg- Special Topics,* 2017; 10(4):213-227.

Bali, P., Im, H. I., & Kenny, P. J. (2011). Methylation, memory and addiction. *Epigenetics*, *6*(6), 671–674. https://doi.org/10.4161/epi.6.6.15905.

Beckers, A., Petrossians, P., Hanson, J., & Daly, A. F. (2018). The causes and consequences of pituitary gigantism. *Nature reviews. Endocrinology*, *14*(12), 705–720. https://doi.org/10.1038/s41574-018-0114-1

Benjamin, E. J., Blaha, M. J., Chiuve, S. E., Cushman, M., Das, S. R., Deo, R., de Ferranti, S. D., Floyd, J., Fornage, M., Gillespie, C., Isasi, C. R., Jiménez, M. C., Jordan, L. C., Judd, S. E., Lackland, D., Lichtman, J. H., Lisabeth, L., Liu, S., Longenecker, C. T., Mackey, R. H., ... American Heart Association Statistics Committee and Stroke Statistics Subcommittee (2017). Heart Disease and Stroke Statistics-2017 Update: A Report From the American Heart Association. *Circulation*, *135*(10), e146–e603. https://doi.org/10.1161/CIR.0000000000000485.

Bhagavatula, M. R., Fan, C., Shen, G. Q., Cassano, J., Plow, E. F., Topol, E. J., & Wang, Q. (2004). Transcription factor MEF2A mutations in patients with coronary artery disease. *Human Molecular Genetics*, *13*(24), 3181–3188. https://doi.org/10.1093/hmg/ddh329.

Bird A. (2002). DNA methylation patterns and epigenetic memory. *Genes & Development*, *16*(1), 6–21. https://doi.org/10.1101/gad.947102.

Bird A. (2007). Perceptions of epigenetics. *Nature*, *447*(7143), 396–398. https://doi.org/10.1038/nature05913.

Bond, D. M., & Finnegan, E. J. (2007). Passing the message on: inheritance of epigenetic traits. *Trends in Plant Science*, *12*(5), 211–216. https://doi.org/10.1016/j.tplants.2007.03.010.

Bostjancic, E., Zidar, N., Stajner, D., & Glavac, D. (2010). MicroRNA miR-1 is up-regulated in remote myocardium in patients with myocardial infarction. *Folia Biologica*, *56*(1), 27–31.

Butts, B., Gary, R. A., Dunbar, S. B., & Butler, J. (2016). Methylation of Apoptosis-Associated Speck-Like Protein With a Caspase Recruitment Domain and Outcomes in Heart Failure. *Journal of Cardiac Failure*, *22*(5), 340–346. https://doi.org/10.1016/j.cardfail.2015.12.004.

Chandler V. L. (2007). Paramutation: from maize to mice. *Cell*, *128*(4), 641–645. https://doi.org/10.1016/j.cell.2007.02.007.

Denis, H., Ndlovu, M. N., & Fuks, F. (2011). Regulation of mammalian DNA methyltransferases: a route to new mechanisms. *EMBO Reports*, *12*(7), 647–656. https://doi.org/10.1038/embor.2011.110.

Deodati, A., Inzaghi, E., Liguori, A., Puglianiello, A., Germani, D., Brufani, C., Fintini, D., Cappa, M., Barbetti, F., & Cianfarani, S. (2013). IGF2 methylation is associated with lipid profile in obese children. *Hormone Research in Paediatrics*, *79*(6), 361–367. https://doi.org/10.1159/000351707.

Felsenfeld G. (2014). A brief history of epigenetics. *Cold Spring Harbor Perspectives in Biology*, *6*(1), a018200. https://doi.org/10.1101/cshperspect.a018200.

Foy, J. P., Pickering, C. R., Papadimitrakopoulou, V. A., Jelinek, J., Lin, S. H., William, W. N., Jr, Frederick, M. J., Wang, J., Lang, W., Feng, L., Zhang, L., Kim, E. S., Fan, Y. H., Hong, W. K., El-Naggar, A. K., Lee, J. J., Myers, J. N., Issa, J. P., Lippman, S. M., Mao, L., ... Saintigny, P. (2015). New DNA methylation markers and global DNA hypomethylation are associated with oral cancer development. *Cancer Prevention Research (Philadelphia, Pa.)*, *8*(11), 1027–1035. https://doi.org/10.1158/1940-6207.CAPR-14-0179.

Friso, S., Pizzolo, F., Choi, S. W., Guarini, P., Castagna, A., Ravagnani, V., Carletto, A., Pattini, P., Corrocher, R., & Olivieri, O. (2008). Epigenetic control of 11 beta-hydroxysteroid dehydrogenase 2 gene promoter is related to human hypertension. *Atherosclerosis*, *199*(2), 323–327. https://doi.org/10.1016/j.atherosclerosis.2007.11.029.

Goedeke, L., Rotllan, N., Canfrán-Duque, A., Aranda, J. F., Ramírez, C. M., Araldi, E., Lin, C. S., Anderson, N. N., Wagschal, A., de Cabo, R., Horton, J. D., Lasunción, M. A., Näär, A. M., Suárez, Y., & Fernández-Hernando, C. (2015). MicroRNA-148a regulates LDL receptor and ABCA1 expression to control circulating lipoprotein levels. *Nature Medicine*, *21*(11), 1280–1289. https://doi.org/10.1038/nm.3949.

Goldberg, A. D., Allis, C. D., & Bernstein, E. (2007). Epigenetics: a landscape takes shape. *Cell*, *128*(4), 635–638. https://doi.org/10.1016/j.cell.2007.02.006.

Greißel, A., Culmes, M., Burgkart, R., Zimmermann, A., Eckstein, H. H., Zernecke, A., & Pelisek, J. (2016). Histone acetylation and methylation significantly change with severity of atherosclerosis in human carotid plaques. *Cardiovascular Pathology: The Official Journal of the Society for Cardiovascular Pathology*, *25*(2), 79–86. https://doi.org/10.1016/j.carpath.2015.11.001.

Guay, S. P., Légaré, C., Brisson, D., Mathieu, P., Bossé, Y., Gaudet, D., & Bouchard, L. (2016). Epigenetic and genetic variations at the TNNT1 gene locus are associated with HDL-C levels and coronary artery disease. *Epigenomics*, *8*(3), 359–371. https://doi.org/10.2217/epi.15.120.

Güneş, S., & Kulaç, T. (2013). The role of epigenetics in spermatogenesis. *Turkish Journal of Urology*, *39*(3), 181–187. https://doi.org/10.5152/tud.2013.037.

Halusková J. (2010). Epigenetic studies in human diseases. *Folia biologica*, *56*(3), 83–96.

Handy, D. E., Castro, R., & Loscalzo, J. (2011). Epigenetic modifications: basic mechanisms and role in cardiovascular disease. *Circulation*, *123*(19), 2145–2156. https://doi.org/10.1161/CIRCULATIONAHA.110.956839.

Herman, J. G., & Baylin, S. B. (2003). Gene silencing in cancer in association with promoter hypermethylation. *The New England Journal of Medicine*, *349*(21), 2042–2054. https://doi.org/10.1056/ NEJMra023075.

Holliday R. (2006). Epigenetics: a historical overview. *Epigenetics*, *1*(2), 76–80. https://doi.org/10.4161/epi.1.2.2762.

Hsiung, D. T., Marsit, C. J., Houseman, E. A., Eddy, K., Furniss, C. S., McClean, M. D., & Kelsey, K. T. (2007). Global DNA methylation level in whole blood as a biomarker in head and neck squamous cell carcinoma. *Cancer Epidemiology, Biomarkers & Prevention: A Publication of the American Association for Cancer Research, Cosponsored by the American Society of Preventive Oncology*, *16*(1), 108–114. https://doi.org/10.1158/1055-9965.EPI-06-0636.

Jones P. A. (2012). Functions of DNA methylation: islands, start sites, gene bodies and beyond. *Nature Reviews. Genetics*, *13*(7), 484–492. https://doi.org/10.1038/nrg3230.

Jones, P. A., & Baylin, S. B. (2007). The epigenomics of cancer. *Cell*, *128*(4), 683–692. https://doi.org/10.1016/j.cell.2007.01.029.

Katrancıoğlu N, Özerdem G, Arslan S, Akgül A, Berkan Ö. Cardiovascular Disorders and Genetic. *Turkiye Klinikleri. J. Cardiovasc. Surg- Special Topics*, 2012;4(3),138-142.

Li, J., Huang, Q., Zeng, F., Li, W., He, Z., Chen, W., Zhu, W., & Zhang, B. (2014). The prognostic value of global DNA hypomethylation in cancer: a meta-analysis. *PloS One*, *9*(9), e106290. https://doi.org/10.1371/journal.pone.0106290.

Madrigal-Matute, J., Rotllan, N., Aranda, J. F., & Fernández-Hernando, C. (2013). MicroRNAs and atherosclerosis. *Current Atherosclerosis Reports*, *15*(5), 322. https://doi.org/10.1007/s11883-013-0322-z.

Martin, C., & Zhang, Y. (2007). Mechanisms of epigenetic inheritance. *Current Opinion in Cell Biology*, *19*(3), 266–272. https://doi.org/10.1016/j.ceb.2007.04.002.

Meissner, A., Mikkelsen, T. S., Gu, H., Wernig, M., Hanna, J., Sivachenko, A., Zhang, X., Bernstein, B. E., Nusbaum, C., Jaffe, D. B., Gnirke, A., Jaenisch, R., & Lander, E. S. (2008). Genome-scale DNA methylation maps of pluripotent and differentiated cells. *Nature*, *454*(7205), 766–770. https://doi.org/10.1038/nature07107.

Mitchell, P. S., Parkin, R. K., Kroh, E. M., Fritz, B. R., Wyman, S. K., Pogosova-Agadjanyan, E. L., Peterson, A., Noteboom, J., O'Briant, K. C., Allen, A., Lin, D. W., Urban, N., Drescher, C. W., Knudsen, B. S., Stirewalt, D. L., Gentleman, R., Vessella, R. L., Nelson, P. S., Martin, D. B., & Tewari, M. (2008). Circulating microRNAs as stable blood-based markers for cancer detection. *Proceedings of the National Academy of Sciences of the United States of America*, *105*(30), 10513–10518. https://doi.org/10.1073/pnas.0804549105.

Nguyen, A., Mamarbachi, M., Turcot, V., Lessard, S., Yu, C., Luo, X., Lalongé, J., Hayami, D., Gayda, M., Juneau, M., Thorin-Trescases, N., Lettre, G., Nigam, A., & Thorin, E. (2016). Lower Methylation of the ANGPTL2 Gene in Leukocytes from Post-Acute Coronary Syndrome Patients. *PloS One*, *11*(4), e0153920. https://doi.org/10.1371/journal.pone.0153920.

Olivieri, F., Antonicelli, R., Lorenzi, M., D'Alessandra, Y., Lazzarini, R., Santini, G., Spazzafumo, L., Lisa, R., La Sala, L., Galeazzi, R., Recchioni, R., Testa, R., Pompilio, G., Capogrossi, M. C., & Procopio, A. D. (2013). Diagnostic potential of circulating miR-499-5p in elderly patients with acute non ST-elevation myocardial infarction. *International Journal of Cardiology*, *167*(2), 531–536. https://doi.org/10.1016/j.ijcard.2012.01.075.

Ozaki, K., Inoue, K., Sato, H., Iida, A., Ohnishi, Y., Sekine, A., Sato, H., Odashiro, K., Nobuyoshi, M., Hori, M., Nakamura, Y., & Tanaka, T. (2004). Functional variation in LGALS2 confers risk of myocardial infarction and regulates lymphotoxin-alpha secretion in vitro. *Nature*, *429*(6987), 72–75. https://doi.org/10.1038/nature02502.

Perkins, E., Murphy, S. K., Murtha, A. P., Schildkraut, J., Jirtle, R. L., Demark-Wahnefried, W., Forman, M. R., Kurtzberg, J., Overcash, F., Huang, Z., & Hoyo, C. (2012). Insulin-like growth factor 2/H19 methylation at birth and risk of overweight and obesity in children. *The Journal of Pediatrics*, *161*(1), 31–39. https://doi.org/10.1016/j.jpeds.2012.01.015.

Portela, A., & Esteller, M. (2010). Epigenetic modifications and human disease. *Nature Biotechnology*, *28*(10), 1057–1068. https://doi.org/10.1038/nbt.1685.

Richard, P., Charron, P., Carrier, L., Ledeuil, C., Cheav, T., Pichereau, C., Benaiche, A., Isnard, R., Dubourg, O., Burban, M., Gueffet, J. P., Millaire, A., Desnos, M., Schwartz, K., Hainque, B., Komajda, M., & EUROGENE Heart Failure Project (2003). Hypertrophic cardiomyopathy: distribution of disease genes, spectrum of mutations, and implications for a molecular diagnosis strategy. *Circulation*, *107*(17), 2227–2232. https://doi.org/10.1161/01.CIR.0000066323.15244.54.

Segré, C. V., & Chiocca, S. (2011). Regulating the regulators: the post-translational code of class I HDAC1 and HDAC2. *Journal of Biomedicine & Biotechnology*, *2011*, 690848. https://doi.org/10.1155/2011/690848.

Smith, Z. D., & Meissner, A. (2013). DNA methylation: roles in mammalian development. *Nature reviews. Genetics*, *14*(3), 204–220. https://doi.org/10.1038/nrg3354.

Takai, D., & Jones, P. A. (2002). Comprehensive analysis of CpG islands in human chromosomes 21 and 22. *Proceedings of the National Academy of Sciences of the United States of America*, *99*(6), 3740–3745. https://doi.org/10.1073/pnas.052410099.

Turgeon, P. J., Sukumar, A. N., & Marsden, P. A. (2014). Epigenetics of Cardiovascular Disease - A New "Beat" in Coronary Artery Disease. *Medical Epigenetics*, *2*(1), 37–52. https://doi.org/10.1159/000360766.

Wagschal, A., Najafi-Shoushtari, S. H., Wang, L., Goedeke, L., Sinha, S., deLemos, A. S., Black, J. C., Ramírez, C. M., Li, Y., Tewhey, R., Hatoum, I., Shah, N., Lu, Y., Kristo, F., Psychogios, N., Vrbanac, V., Lu, Y. C., Hla, T., de Cabo, R., Tsang, J. S., … Näär, A. M. (2015). Genome-wide identification of microRNAs regulating cholesterol and triglyceride homeostasis. *Nature Medicine*, *21*(11), 1290–1297. https://doi.org/10.1038/nm.3980.

Wald, D. S., Law, M., & Morris, J. K. (2002). Homocysteine and cardiovascular disease: evidence on causality from a meta-analysis. *BMJ (Clinical Research Ed.)*, *325*(7374), 1202. https://doi.org/10.1136/bmj.325.7374.1202.

Wang, L., Fan, C., Topol, S. E., Topol, E. J., & Wang, Q. (2003). Mutation of MEF2A in an inherited disorder with features of coronary artery disease. *Science (New York, N.Y.)*, *302*(5650), 1578–1581. https://doi.org/10.1126/science.1088477.

Waterland, R. A., & Michels, K. B. (2007). Epigenetic epidemiology of the developmental origins hypothesis. *Annual Review of Nutrition*, *27*, 363–388. https://doi.org/10.1146/annurev.nutr.27.061 406.093705.

Wu, H., Zhao, M., Tan, L., & Lu, Q. (2016). The key culprit in the pathogenesis of systemic lupus erythematosus: Aberrant DNA methylation. *Autoimmunity Reviews*, *15*(7), 684–689. https://doi.org/10.1016/j.autrev.2016.03.002.

Yang, Q., Zhao, Y., Zhang, Z., & Chen, J. (2016). Association of interleukin-6 methylation in leukocyte DNA with serum level and the risk of ischemic heart disease. *Scandinavian Journal of Clinical and Laboratory Investigation*, *76*(4), 291–295. https://doi.org/10.3109/00365513.2016.1149616.

Yoo, J. Y., Lee, S., Lee, H. A., Park, H., Park, Y. J., Ha, E. H., & Kim, Y. J. (2014). Can proopiomelanocortin methylation be used as an early predictor of metabolic syndrome? *Diabetes Care*, *37*(3), 734–739. https://doi.org/10.2337/dc13-1012.

Zhang C. (2008). MicroRNomics: a newly emerging approach for disease biology. *Physiological Genomics*, *33*(2), 139–147. https://doi.org/10.1152/physiolgenomics.00034.2008.

Chapter 17

Epigenetics and Obesity

Handan Sarac*, PhD
Department of Plant and Animal Production,
Sivas Cumhuriyet University, Sivas, Turkey

Abstract

Obesity is an important health problem that has reached the level of pandemic today, has important effects on high prevalence diseases such as cardiovascular, diabetes, and cancer, and even leads to deaths. Obesity occurs from multifactorial effects, primarily genetic and environmental factors. Studies have identified a large number of genes that cause obesity, but the rapid increase in obesity in a short time cannot be explained only by genetic factors alone. Epigenetic changes that occur through environmental factors such as nutrition and physical activity also have an important role in the current increase in the incidence of obesity. Gene-environment interaction causes different phenotypic variations to occur in organisms. These different phenotypes, which occur without any changes in the DNA sequence, are explained by epigenetics. Therefore, the view that interindividual differences in susceptibility to obesity are due to epigenetic factors has recently gained considerable importance. Many studies have shown that epigenetic mechanisms such as DNA methylation, histone modifications, and non-coding RNAs are closely related to obesity.

The aim of this review is to present the relationship between epigenetics and obesity and the effects of epigenetic mechanisms on obesity.

Keywords: epigenetics, obesity, DNA methylation, histone modifications, non-coding RNAs

Introduction

The Concept of Epigenetics

DNA, which constitutes our genetic code, ensures that the characteristics it carries and that emerge as a result of gene expression are hereditarily transferred to new generations (Sırıken et al., 2018). Gregor Mendel, in his crossover studies with peas in the field of genetics, explained the rules for the transition of genes from parent to offspring, which he specified as inheritance factors (Liebers et al., 2014; Şahin et al., 2018). However, scientists have realized that not every phenotypic trait seen can be explained by Mendelian Genetics; for example, Mendelian Genetics is inadequate to explain the inheritance of quantitative traits. In the

* Corresponding Author's E-mail: handansarac@cumhuriyet.edu.tr.

In: Epigenetics: Beyond the Genetics and Medicine
Editors: Sevgi Durna Daştan and Nazan Yurtcu
ISBN: 979-8-88697-228-3

emergence of quantitative traits and phenotype, the environment is an important factor. Therefore, a significant amount of gene-environment interaction has a role in the emergence of such phenotypes (Şahin et al., 2018). Environmental factors can cause changes in gene expressions from embryo to the end of life (İnan, 2021). For this reason, in later years, some biologists emphasized that genetics and developmental biology should be handled together rather than separately and stated that these two fields could be related to each other and can be studied as a common discipline. Thus, the concept of epigenetics emerged (Şahin et al., 2018).

Epigenetics are heritable changes in gene expression that occur independently of the DNA sequence (He et al., 2019; Yavari and Borujeni, 2021). The origin of the word epigenetics is ancient Greek, the prefix "epi" means above and beyond, and when considered as a whole, it means above or beyond genetics (Şahin et al., 2018; İnan, 2021). It was first defined by Conrad Waddington in the 1940s as "a branch of science that examines how the genotype creates the phenotype during development." Today, the term is defined as "changes in gene function that can be inherited by mitosis and/or meiosis division, which cannot be explained by DNA sequence" (Koban et al., 2017; Sırıken et al., 2018; Izquierdo and Crujeiras, 2019; Ouni and Schürmann, 2020). The genetic code is the same in all cells of an organism, but the functions and characteristics of the cells differ depending on active and passive genes. The external causes that cause genes to be active or passive are explained by epigenetics (Izquierdo and Crujeiras, 2019; İnan, 2021).

Epigenetic Effects of Nutrition

Nutrition has a very important place in human health, as it is one of the most important factors affecting the risk of possible disease (Milagro et al., 2013; Geyik and Unaltuna, 2014; Özgür et al., 2020). As a result of human malnutrition habits, some mutations and modifications due to chemical or metabolic reasons may occur and gene expression may change. For example, types of over-fat, low-protein, low-calorie diet or high-calorie diet trigger changes in gene expression (Sırıken et al., 2018). Because epigenetics is one of the mechanisms by which the metabolic properties of nutrients and bioactive food components are affected (Milagro et al., 2013; Geyik and Unaltuna, 2014) and can influence epigenetic events by directly inhibiting enzymes that catalyze DNA methylation and histone modification and by changing the available substrates required for all enzymatic reactions (Sırıken et al., 2018). As a matter of fact, studies have revealed the existence of a relationship between people's eating habits and gene expression changes that cause epigenetic changes. There is a lot of evidence that the mother's nutritional status and father's eating habits, especially during pregnancy, have a role in the emergence of non-communicable diseases (such as diabetes mellitus, cardiovascular diseases (CVD), obesity and cancer) in the children to be born (van Dijk et al., 2015; Arslan and Yıldıran, 2021). In addition, maternal malnutrition in terms of methyl-supplying foods during pregnancy can cause methylation disorders during fetal development (Geyik and Unaltuna, 2014; Samblas et al., 2019). Low-birth-weight individuals have been shown to have fewer DNA methylation plastys (Hjort et al., 2017). The effect of prenatal nutrition on diseases that develop later in the offspring was observed in the winter famine in the Netherlands in 1944-1945, known as the "Dutch Hunger Winter." In this case, there was no effect on the birth weight of the children born when pregnant mothers were exposed to starvation in the first trimester of pregnancy, while an increased risk of obesity, hypercholesterolemia, and CVD was observed compared to those who were not exposed to starvation in adulthood (Sırıken et al., 2018; Samblas et al., 2019). On the other hand, epigenetic changes occur in response to environmental exposures such as overfeeding (Ouni and Schürmann, 2020). Malnutrition, especially in obese or diabetic patients, can change the epigenetic profile and take effect by transferring to offspring for generations (Sırıken et al., 2018). Furthermore, studies show that epigenetics is the reason behind the inability of obesity patients to lose weight (İnan, 2021).

Definition and Etiology of Obesity

Obesity is a chronic disease caused by excess energy taken into the body through nutrients and characterized by an increase in body fat mass compared to lean body mass (Izquierdo and Crujeiras, 2019). It is thought that the situation where the amount of energy taken is more than the amount of energy spent occurs due to the consequences of modern life such as sedentary life, lack of physical activity, and unhealthy nutrition (Kayar and Utku, 2013; Obri et al., 2020). Apart from these, obesity can also develop as a result of a genetic or epigenetic predisposition (Ouni and Schürmann, 2020). For this reason, obesity is a complex and important disease that can occur at any age and threatens human health, especially if genetic and environmental factors have a major role, depending on many factors (Chooi et al., 2019). The World Health Organization (WHO) describes obesity as excessive or abnormal fat accumulation in the adipose tissue that impairs the health of the organism (Chooi et al., 2019; Kurt el al., 2019).

WHO defines overweight, obese, and extremely obese based on body mass index (BMI = Weight [kg]/Height [m^2]). According to this; Overweight: BMI = 25.0-29.9 kg/m^2, Obese: BMI $\geq$ 30 kg/m^2 and Extremely obese: BMI $\geq$ 40 kg/m^2 (Herrera and Lindgren, 2010; Dönder and Önalan, 2018).

Worldwide, there has been a doubling in the incidence of obesity, especially since 1980, and almost a third of the world's population has been found to be overweight or obese (Dönder and Önalan, 2018; Chooi et al., 2019; Nettore et al., 2021). In this case, it can be said that the obesity epidemic has become a pandemic and has placed a serious burden on the world health system (Obri et al., 2020). In addition, according to estimates, by 2030 58% of the world's population will suffer from obesity (Geyik and Unaltuna, 2014). Today, smoking is the first cause of preventable death and obesity is the second. Therefore, the WHO has reported it as the most important health problem of the 21st century (Dönder and Önalan, 2018). In addition, obesity is known to be a risk factor for many diseases such as type 2 diabetes (T2D), CVD, cerebral vascular diseases, musculoskeletal disorders, and cancer (Herrera and Lindgren, 2010; He et al., 2019; Izquierdo and Crujeiras, 2019; Obri et al., 2020). WHO reports that at least 2.8 million people die each year due to diseases caused by overweight and obesity (WHO, 2021). For this reason, it is very important to determine the factors causing obesity, which is one of the biggest health problems of our time, and to develop treatment possibilities (Kayar and Utku, 2013).

Many factors such as genetic, environmental, hormonal, metabolic, neurological, physiological, biochemical, cultural and psychological factors have an interrelated role in the etiology of obesity (Kayar and Utku, 2013; Geyik and Unaltuna, 2014; Kurt et al., 2019). Differences occur between individuals in obesity, especially due to genetic predisposition (Geyik and Unaltuna, 2014). Studies have identified more than 20 genes that lead to obesity predisposition (Herrera and Lindgren, 2010; Ouni and Schürmann, 2020). However, genetics alone cannot explain the obesity pandemic (Obri et al., 2020). With extensive epigenome-wide association studies (EWAS), the identified risk variants explain only a small part of the heritability of obesity (de Mello et al., 2014; Samblas et al., 2019). Obesity is caused by the complex interaction of susceptibility genes with various environmental factors (e.g., stress, drug use, physical activity, nutrition) (Obri et al., 2020) and therefore more factors must be considered to understand the multifactorial pathology of obesity (Samblas et al., 2019). As a matter of fact, recent studies have determined that different mechanisms involved in the epigenetic regulation of gene expressions can cause both obesity and differences in obesity among individuals (Geyik and Unaltuna, 2014). The fact that obesity does not develop in all individuals exposed to the same environmental risk factors supports the hypothesis of the presence of epigenetic elements (Samblas et al., 2019). Thus, it has been understood that the main reason for individual differences in obesity is not only genetic characteristics, but also epigenetic mechanisms activated by environmental factors have an important role in the pathogenesis (Koban et al., 2017).

Table 1. Some obesity-related genes affected by epigenetic mechanisms

Gene Name	Symbol	Metabolic Function	Epigenetic Mechanism Affected	References
Leptin	LEP	Appetite control	DNA Methylation	(Samblas et al., 2019; Obri et al., 2020)
Melanocortin 4 receptor	MC4R	Appetite control	DNA Methylation	(Herrera and Lindgren, 2010; Obri et al., 2020)
Proopiomelanocortin	POMC	Appetite control	DNA and Histone Methylation	(Geyik and Unaltuna, 2014; Obri et al., 2020)
Tumor necrosis factor alpha	TNF	Insulin resistance	DNA Methylation	(Geyik ve Unaltuna, 2014)
Fatt mass and obesity	FTO	Appetite control	DNA Methylation	(Herrera and Lindgren, 2010)
Adrenoceptor beta 3	ADRB3	Regulation of lipolysis and thermogenesis	DNA Methylation	(Samblas et al., 2019)
Hypoxia inducible factor 3 alpha	HIF3A	Regulation of hypoxia	DNA Methylation	(Wang et al., 2015; Sayols-Baixeras et al., 2017)
Cut like homeobox 1	CUX1	Regulation of gene expression, morphogenesis, and differentiation	DNA Methylation	(Sayols-Baixeras et al., 2017)
Insulin-like growth factor 2	IGF2	Glucose homeostasis	DNA and Histone Methylation, Histone Acetylation	(de Mello et al., 2014)

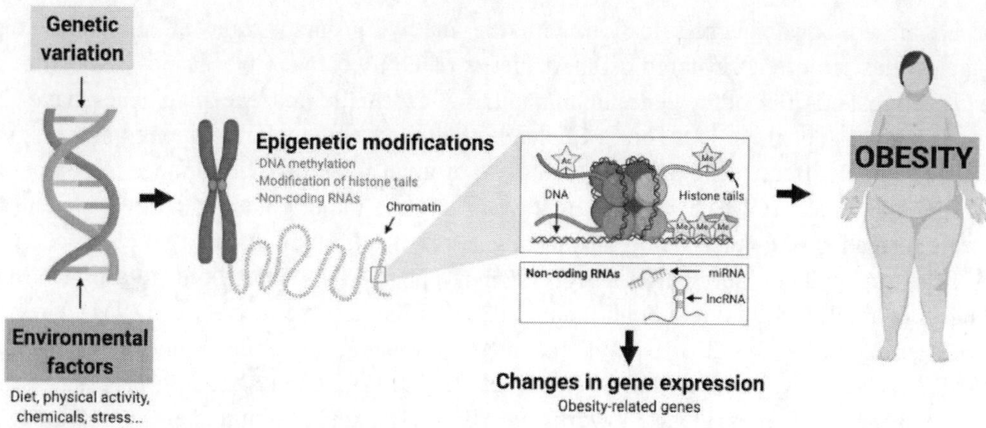

Figure 1. Contribution of the interaction between environmental factors and genetic variation to the development of obesity through epigenetic mechanisms (Obri et al., 2020).

Epigenetic Mechanisms Affecting Obesity

Among the factors leading to obesity are energy imbalances as well as epigenetic mechanisms (Geyik and Unaltuna, 2014). Epigenetic mechanisms control both gene activity and the development of the organism (Ling and Rönn, 2019). Therefore, they can contribute to environmentally induced phenotypic variations (Angers et al., 2010). For example, by influencing the expression of genes associated with obesity, they can have an important role in heredity and susceptibility to obesity (Herrera and Lindgren, 2010). Indeed, BMI is regulated by epigenetic mechanisms (He et al., 2019), and interindividual differences in susceptibility to obesity arise depending on epigenetic mechanisms (Geyik and Unaltuna, 2014; Ouni and Schürmann, 2020). Obese individuals show a different epigenetic pattern in DNA and histones compared to healthy normal weight individuals (Geyik and Unaltuna, 2014).

Today, researchers have focused on three main goals in epigenetic research on obesity. These include researching epigenetic biomarkers to predict future health problems or identifying the most at-risk individuals, understanding obesity-related environmental factors that can modulate gene expression by affecting epigenetic mechanisms, and working on new therapeutic strategies based on nutrition or pharmacological agents that affect epigenetic mechanisms (Milagro et al., 2013).

Epigenetic mechanisms affecting obesity; DNA methylation, histone modifications and non-coding RNAs (de Mello et al., 2014; Geyik and Unaltuna, 2014; Izquierdo and Crujeiras, 2019; Ling and Rönn, 2019; Ouni and Schürmann, 2020).

DNA Methylation

Among the epigenetic mechanisms, it is the most well-known and widespread modification in the organism (de Mello et al., 2014; Hjort et al., 2017; Izquierdo and Crujeiras, 2019; Arslan and Yıldıran, 2021). DNA methylation can be defined as the formation of 5-methyl cytosine (5 mC) by transfer of the methyl group (-CH3) in S-adenosyl methionine (SAM) to cytosine (C) located before guanine (G) (Yaykaşlı et al., 2012; Geyik and Unaltuna, 2014). Methylation of cytosine occurs specifically in cytosine-phosphate-guanine dinucleotides (CpG) (Ling and Rönn, 2019; Ouni and Schürmann, 2020). The cytosine base of the CpG dinucleotide is susceptible to covalent modification with the methyl group (Özgür et al., 2020). CpG dinucleotides are often clustered as short pieces of DNA called CpG islands (Koban et al., 2017). Almost 60-70% of the genes in human DNA, especially housekeeping genes, have CpG islands (Yaykaşlı et al., 2012). The CpG islands are linked to about half of the promoter regions of genes, which affects gene expression and are of great functional importance (Koban et al., 2017; Özgür et al., 2020). Therefore, methylation has a major role in the development and disease formation of eukaryotic organisms in general (Yaykaşlı et al., 2012).

DNA methylation is catalyzed by enzymes called DNA methyltransferase (DNMTs) (Angers et al., 2010; Ouni and Schürmann, 2020). So far, a large number of DNMT enzymes have been identified, but 3 of DNMT enzymes responsible for methylation in mammals are DNMT1, DNMT3A, and DNMT3B (Koban et al., 2017; Coco et al., 2019; Ling and Rönn, 2019). Of these enzymes, DNMT1 works mostly as a repair methyltransferase (Koban et al., 2017) and was responsible for copying methylation marks during DNA replication (Angers et al., 2010). Mutations in DNMT1 have been associated with neurodegenerative diseases such as hereditary sensory autonomic neuropathy and narcolepsy, which include dementia and hearing loss (Özgür et al., 2020). DNMT3A and DNMT3B enzymes are closely associated with increased leptin (LEP) promoter methylation when obesity is triggered by over-fat diet (Koban et al., 2017). These enzymes have a role both in regulating de novo methylation reactions during the development process and in the neural regulation of energy metabolism (Angers et al., 2010; Koban et al., 2017).

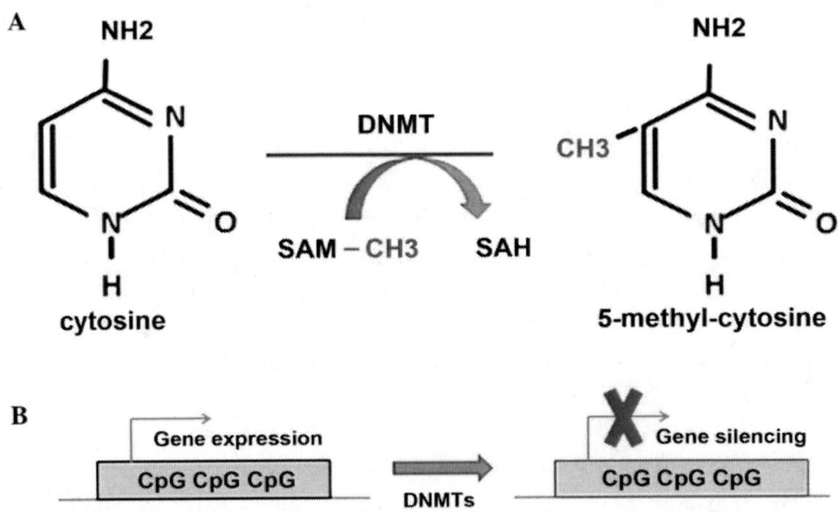

Figure 2. The mechanism of DNA methylation. (A) The methyl group (-CH3) from S-adenosyl methionine (SAM) is transferred to the 5′-position of cytosine by DNMTs and 5-methyl cytosine (5 mC) is formed. (B) Methylation of cytosine occurs specifically in CpG islands located in the promoter regions of genes and the gene is silenced (Cui et al., 2016).

DNA methylation provides regulation of gene expression by inhibiting the binding of the transcription factor(s) to DNA or by suppressing the gene (Moore et al., 2013; Gartstein and Skinner, 2018). Binding of methyl groups to gene regions prevents genes from expressing themselves, genes are closed or silenced, as a result, protein production cannot be achieved from this gene region (İnan, 2021). The level of DNA methylation in normal cells is well balanced, but epigenetic modifications in individual genomic regions are affected by genetic and environmental factors (Arslan and Yıldıran, 2021). Therefore, differences in methylation patterns were observed between obese and normal individuals (Geyik and Unaltuna, 2014). Current data support that changes resulting from DNA methylation play an important role in obesity. Methylation of some obesity-related genes affects body weight changes (de Mello et al., 2014; Sayols-Baixeras et al., 2017). In one of the experiments with agouti mice, the relationship between obesity and DNA methylation was demonstrated. In this experiment, a mutation in the Agouti locus, which controls the color of the fur in mice, causes the fur to turn yellow and binds to the melanocortin 4 receptor (MC4R) in the hypothalamus thereby impairing its antagonistic function, resulting in the expression of the agouti protein at an abnormal location, stimulating obesity. The Agouti gene is active when unmethylated, and produces yellow, obese, cancer-prone mice. But when pregnant mice are fed methyl-rich foods, the gene is methylated and silenced in most of the born mice, and the phenotypes of mice become brown and weak (Koban et al., 2017). In an EWAS, 37 CpG sites associated with BMI were identified (Nettore et al., 2021).

Histone Modifications

Histones are the essential proteins involved in the formation of eukaryotic chromatin and chromosome structure (Gartstein and Skinner, 2018; Şahin, et al., 2018). Thanks to the positively charged lysine and arginine amino acids they contain, they are positively charged and wrapped in negatively charged DNA (Şahin et al., 2018). There are 4 types of histone proteins in eukaryotic organisms. These are H2A, H2B, H3, H4. These histon proteins form the nucleosome structure by packaging and organizing DNA (Geyik and Unaltuna, 2014; Coco et al., 2019). Nucleosomes are the smallest functional unit of chromatin and are formed by 147 base pairs wrapping around two molecules each of the H2A, H2B, H3, and H4 proteins approximately twice (Yaykaşlı et al., 2012).

Histone modifications are a complex epigenetic mechanism that controls gene expression by changing chromatin structure, functions, and transcription activities in the cell (Koban et al., 2017; Arslan and Yıldıran, 2021). At least 8 different types of modification are known for histones. These are methylation, acetylation, phosphorylation, sumolization, ubiquitination, ADP-ribosylation, deamination, and proline isomerization (Gartstein and Skinner, 2018; Ling and Rönn, 2019). However, among these modifications, the most widely studied are histone acetylation and methylation (Coco et al., 2019; Özgür et al., 2020). There are many histone modifying enzymes (Ling and Rönn, 2019), these enzymes add or remove epigenetic marks on the N-terminal tails of histones. While histone acetyltransferases (HAT) or deacetylases (HDAC) are have a role in histone acetylation, histone methyltransferases (HMT) or demethylases (HDM) are have a role in histone methylation (Coco et al., 2019; Arslan and Yıldıran, 2021).

The acetylation of the lysine amino acid in the histone protein with HAT enzyme neutralizes the positive charge on the histone tail, allowing the chromatin structure to relax. This relaxed chromatin structure (eucromatin) allows transcription factors easier to reach the target gene. Thus, histone acetylation facilitates gene transcription. In contrast, HDACs remove acetyl groups from histones, and as a result of deacetylation, DNA becomes more tightly coiled and chromatin is condensed (heterochromatin). Thus, transcription becomes difficult and is prevented (Gartstein and Skinner, 2018; Coco et al., 2019).

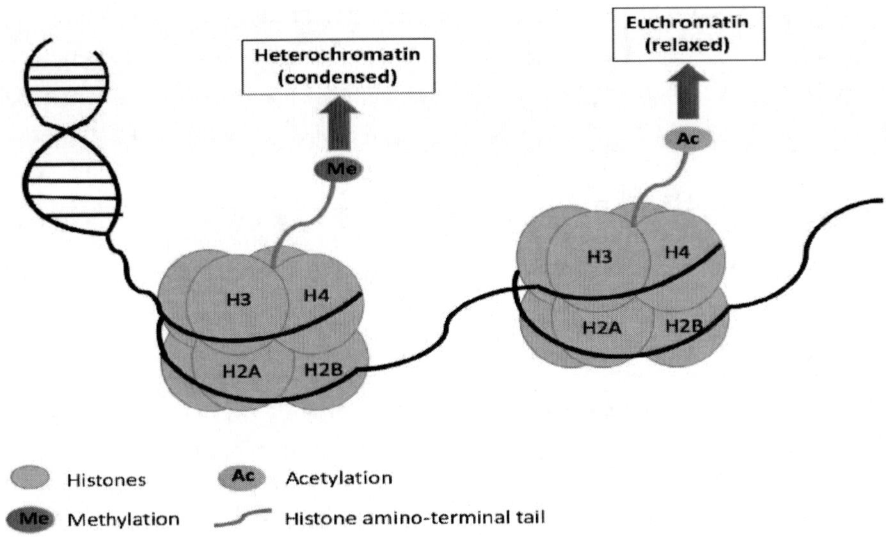

Figure 3. Histone methylation and acetylation. The addition of methyl groups to the N-terminal tails of histone proteins leads to histone methylation. This allows the chromatin structure to become more tightly packed and condense (heterochromatin). In heterochromatin states, chromatin structure silences transcriptional activities. On the other hand, acetylation of the lysine amino acid in the histone protein with the HAT enzyme provides relaxation of the chromatin structure (euchromatin). Euchromatin states facilitate transcription factors to reach target gene. Thus, transcriptional activation is ensured (Kim and Kaang, 2017).

Histone methylation leads to activation or suppression of gene expression, depending on the location and number of methyl groups (Gartstein and Skinner, 2018). For example, the gene is suppressed as a result of mono-methylation of the amino acid lysine of histones. On the other hand, in the case of di- or tri-methylation, gene transcription increases (Coco et al., 2019).

Transcriptional analyzes demonstrated the relationship between histone modifying enzymes and obesity. The expression of some histone deacetylases (HDACs) has been found to decrease some enzymes that regulate adipocyte differentiation and metabolism in the adipose tissue of obese women (Nettore et al., 2021).

Non-Coding RNAs

Transcripts that do not have protein-coding properties in the mammalian genome are called non-coding RNA (ncRNA) (Srijyothi et al., 2018). Although ncRNAs do not directly affect chromatin structure, they have important effects on transcriptional and post-transcriptional regulation of gene expression (Coco et al., 2019). They are passed on to the next generation by means of eggs from the mother and sperm from the father (Fitz-James and Cavalli, 2022).

ncRNAs include short microRNAs (miRNAs), Piwi interacting RNAs, and long non-coding RNAs (lncRNAs) that regulate genes (Gartstein and Skinner, 2018). Among these molecules, miRNAs are the most comprehensively studied and represent the main epigenetic regulators of gene expression (Coco et al., 2019).

miRNAs are small ncRNAs consisting of 21 to 25 nucleotides that function as post-transcriptional regulators of gene expression (Ouni and Schürmann, 2020). miRNAs bind to the cis-elements of the 3' untranslated region (3'UTR) of the target genes, inducing degradation and impairing stability, as well as acting as silencers by preventing translation (Herrera and Lindgren, 2010; Ouni and Schürmann, 2020).

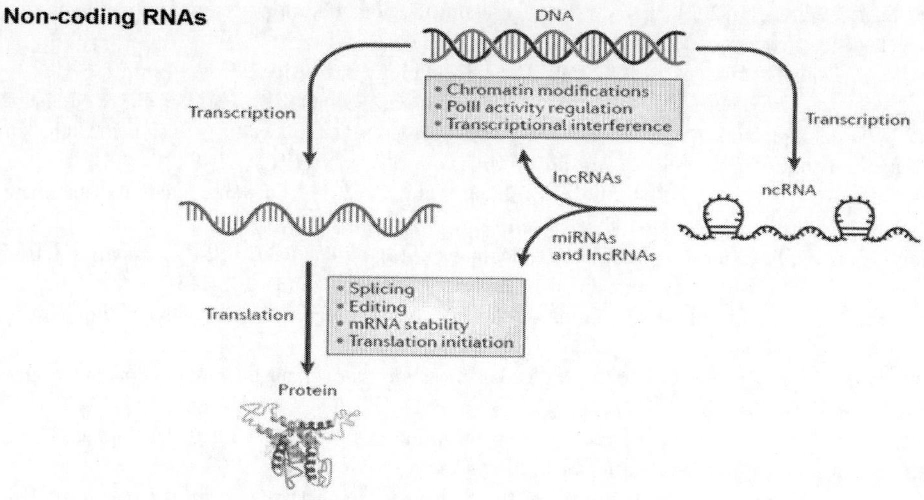

Figure 4. Transcriptional and post-transcriptional effect of non-coding RNAs (miRNA and lncRNA) (Gartstein and Skinner, 2018).

The heritability of obesity can be explained by identifying the role of ncRNAs such as miRNAs. It is known that miRNAs have an effect on the regulation of obesity, adipocyte differentiation, insulin resistance, and regulation of appetite. Therefore, dysregulation of miRNA expression potentially affects obesity susceptibility (Herrera and Lindgren, 2010).

Conclusion

Obesity is one of the most important health problems that is increasing in prevalence all over the world and threatening human life. Genetic and environmental factors known to cause obesity were not sufficient to explain the obesity pandemic. However, with the discovery of epigenetic mechanisms, the underlying causes of some diseases with a high incidence, such as obesity, have become clear. Epigenetic mechanisms are in a dynamic structure and interact with genotype, nutrition, and other environmental effects. This interaction causes individual differences in obesity susceptibility and appetite control. Nutrition has an important role in the epigenetic process. Nutritional disorders, especially during pregnancy, affect epigenetic mechanisms and increase the risk of obesity in the future of the offspring.

In conclusion, if the epigenetic mechanisms affecting obesity and the obesity susceptibility genes affected by these mechanisms are well determined, they can be used as biomarkers that can offer new personalized treatment options in the treatment of obesity. Because epigenetic mechanisms have an important place in explaining the pathogenesis of obesity, preventing it and improving treatment possibilities. In the future, epigenetic biomarkers may be beneficial in preventing the triggering or progression of obesity and many similar diseases.

References

Angers, B., Castonguay, E., & Massicotte, R. (2010). Environmentally induced phenotypes and DNA methylation: how to deal with unpredictable conditions until the next generation and after. *Molecular Ecology*, 19(7), 1283-1295.

Arslan, S., & Yıldıran, H. (2021). Effects of maternal nutrition on offspring: Fetal programming and epigenetic mechanisms. *Journal of Nutrition and Dietetics*, 49(1), 67-74.

Chooi, Y. C., Ding, C., & Magkos, F. (2019). The epidemiology of obesity. *Metabolism*, 92, 6-10.

Coco, C., Sgarra, L., Potenza, M. A., Nacci, C., Pasculli, B., Barbano, R., Parrella, P., & Montagnani, M. (2019). Can epigenetics of endothelial dysfunction represent the key to precision medicine in type 2 diabetes mellitus?. *International Journal of Molecular Sciences*, 20(12), 2949.

Cui, X., Jing, X., Wu, X., Yan, M., Li, Q., Shen, Y., & Wang, Z. (2016). DNA methylation in spermatogenesis and male infertility. *Experimental and Therapeutic Medicine*, 12(4), 1973-1979.

de Mello, V. D. F., Pulkkinen, L., Lalli, M., Kolehmainen, M., Pihlajamäki, J., & Uusitupa, M. (2014). DNA methylation in obesity and type 2 diabetes. *Annals of Medicine*, 46(3), 103-113.

Dönder, E., & Önalan, E. (2018). Definition of obesity, epidemiology and clinical evaluation. *Fırat Medical Journal*, 23, 1-4.

Fitz-James, M. H., & Cavalli, G. (2022). Molecular mechanisms of transgenerational epigenetic inheritance. *Nature Reviews Genetics*, 1-17.

Gartstein, M. A., & Skinner, M. K. (2018). Prenatal influences on temperament development: The role of environmental epigenetics. *Development and Psychopathology*, 30(4), 1269-1303.

Geyik, F. G., & Unaltuna, N. E. (2014). Epigenetic mechanisms in obesity. *Journal of Experimental Medicine*, 3(6), 7-16.

He, F., Berg, A., Imamura Kawasawa, Y., Bixler, E. O., Fernandez-Mendoza, J., Whitsel, E. A., & Liao, D. (2019). Association between DNA methylation in obesity-related genes and body mass index percentile in adolescents. *Scientific Reports*, 9(1), 1-8.

Herrera, B. M., & Lindgren, C. M. (2010). The genetics of obesity. *Current Diabetes Reports*, 10(6), 498-505.

Hjort, L., Jørgensen, S. W., Gillberg, L., Hall, E., Brøns, C., Frystyk, J., Vagg A. A., & Ling, C. (2017). 36 h fasting of young men influences adipose tissue DNA methylation of *LEP* and *ADIPOQ* in a birth weight-dependent manner. *Clinical Epigenetics*, 9(1), 1-12.

İnan, S. (2021). Going beyond the gene: Epigenetics in Biology education. *Inonu University Journal of the Graduate School of Education*, 8(15), 74-89.

Izquierdo, A. G., & Crujeiras, A. B. (2019). Obesity-related epigenetic changes after bariatric surgery. *Frontiers in Endocrinology*, 10, 232.

Kayar, H., & Utku, S. (2013). Disease of our time: Obesity and its treatment. *Mersin University Journal of Health Sciences*, 6(2).

Kim, S., & Kaang, B. K. (2017). Epigenetic regulation and chromatin remodeling in learning and memory. *Experimental & Molecular Medicine*, 49(1), e281-e281.

Koban, B. U., Vural, E. Z. T., Işıtmangil, G., & Gönenç, I. (2017). The effects of nutrition, other environmental factors and microbiota on the epigenetics of obesity. *The Journal of Turkish Family Physician,* 8(4), 108-117.

Kurt, A. K., Zoba, C. A., Ateş E., & Set, T. (2019). Primary care obesity management. *Klinik Tıp Aile Hekimliği*, 11(2), 55-60.

Liebers, R., Rassoulzadegan, M., & Lyko, F. (2014). Epigenetic regulation by heritable RNA. *PLoS Genetics*, 10(4), e1004296.

Ling, C., & Rönn, T. (2019). Epigenetics in human obesity and type 2 diabetes. *Cell Metabolism,* 29(5), 1028-1044.

Milagro, F. I., Mansego, M. L., De Miguel, C., & Martinez, J. A. (2013). Dietary factors, epigenetic modifications and obesity outcomes: progresses and perspectives. *Molecular Aspects of Medicine,* 34(4), 782-812.

Moore, L. D., Le, T., & Fan, G. (2013). DNA methylation and its basic function. *Neuropsychopharmacology*, 38(1), 23-38.

Nettore, I. C., Franchini, F., Palatucci, G., Macchia, P. E., & Ungaro, P. (2021). Epigenetic Mechanisms of Endocrine-Disrupting Chemicals in Obesity. *Biomedicines*, 9(11), 1716.

Obri, A., Serra, D., Herrero, L., & Mera, P. (2020). The role of epigenetics in the development of obesity. *Biochemical Pharmacology*, 177, 113973.

Ouni, M., & Schürmann, A. (2020). Epigenetic contribution to obesity. *Mammalian Genome,* 31(5), 134-145.

Özgür, E., Tığlı, H., & Tığlı, H. (2020). Clinical overview of the role of epigenetics in human diseases. *Istanbul Gelisim University Journal of Health Sciences*, (10), 107-122.

Şahin, Ö., Ayaz, G. B., & Ayaz, U. (2018). Plant epigenetics. *Madde, Diyalektik ve Toplum*, 1(2), 135-144.

Samblas, M., Milagro, F. I., & Martínez, A. (2019). DNA methylation markers in obesity, metabolic syndrome, and weight loss. *Epigenetics*, 14(5), 421-444.

Sayols-Baixeras, S., Subirana, I., Fernández-Sanlés, A., Sentí, M., Lluís-Ganella, C., Marrugat, J., & Elosua, R. (2017). DNA methylation and obesity traits: An epigenome-wide association study. The REGICOR study. *Epigenetics*, 12(10), 909-916.

Sırıken, B., Sırıken, F., Ünsal, C., & Çiftci, G. (2018). Nutrition and epigenetic. *Harran University Journal of the Faculty of Veterinary Medicine*, 7, 12-18.

Srijyothi, L., Ponne, S., Prathama, T., Ashok, C., & Baluchamy, S. (2018). *Roles of Non-Coding RNAs in Transcriptional Regulation* (Vol. 55). London, UK: IntechOpen.

van Dijk, S. J., Tellam, R. L., Morrison, J. L., Muhlhausler, B. S., & Molloy, P. L. (2015). Recent developments on the role of epigenetics in obesity and metabolic disease. *Clinical Epigenetics*, 7(1), 1-13.

Wang, S., Song, J., Yang, Y., Zhang, Y., Wang, H., & Ma, J. (2015). HIF3A DNA methylation is associated with childhood obesity and ALT. *PloS one*, 10(12), e0145944.

World Health Organization (2021). https://www.who.int/news-room/facts-in-pictures/detail/6-facts-on-obesity.

Yavari, M., & Borujeni, V. S. (2021). The importance of epigenetic modifications in cancer progression. *Laboratory & Diagnosis*, 13(53), 51-60.

Yaykaşlı, K. O., Hatipoğlu, Ö. F., Kaya, E., & Yaykaşlı, E. (2012). Epigenetic mechanisms and cancer. *Duzce Medical Journal*, 14(3), 58-68.

Chapter 18

Epigenetics and Diabetes

Zeynep Tüzün[1,*], MD and Serpil Çiftel[2], MD

[1]Department of Internal Medicine, Ataturk University, Erzurum, Turkey
[2]Department of Endocrinology, Erzurum City Hospital, Erzurum, Turkey

Abstract

Diabetes mellitus (DM) is a metabolic disease characterized by hyperglycemia resulting from a partial or absolute decrease in insulin secretion, with varying degrees of peripheral resistance to the impact of insulin. The prevalence of type 2 diabetes mellitus increases exponentially every day, along with an increase in obesity and bad eating habits. Prolonged hyperglycemia causes microvascular (retinopathy, nephropathy, neuropathy, and cardiovascular diseases) and macrovascular (cardiovascular diseases) complications and major morbidity and mortality in patients. The causes of disease in DM, which is such an important public health problem, are largely based on the interaction of genetic and environmental factors. Nevertheless, the etiopathogenesis of the disease has not been completely elucidated. Since epigenetics can provide a molecular link between genetic, environmental factors and diabetes and can be transmitted over generations, it is promising in elucidating the etiopathogenesis of diabetes and identifying new treatment options for its etiology. Even if hyperglycemia is corrected, epigenetic mechanisms are included in metabolic memory, and in the long term, complications secondary to DM persist. Furthermore, studies on epigenetics and metabolic memory demonstrate that diabetes and its complications can be prevented by changing environmental factors such as calorie control.

Keywords: diabetes mellitus, epigenetics, DNA methylation, histones

Introduction

The term "diabetes mellitus" defines diseases of abnormal carbohydrate metabolism characterized by hyperglycemia resulting from a partial or absolute decrease in insulin secretion, with varying degrees of peripheral resistance to the impact of insulin. Its prevalence in the world is increasing. The approximate prevalence of DM in adults was 366 million in 2011 and it is estimated to be 552 million in 2030 (Gouri and Dekaken, 2013). Its prevalence in Turkey also increases. According to the prevalence studies conducted in Turkey, the

[*] Corresponding Author's E-mail: zeynepdursuntuzun@gmail.com.

In: Epigenetics: Beyond the Genetics and Medicine
Editors: Sevgi Durna Daştan and Nazan Yurtcu
ISBN: 979-8-88697-228-3

frequency of DM was 7.2% in the 20-80 age group in 1997-1998, but the frequency of DM in 2010 increased to 13.7%, by showing a 90% increase (Satman et al., 2013).

Diabetes mellitus (DM) is divided into four main groups: type 1, type 2, gestational diabetes, and diabetes due to special causes (Tanriverdi et al., 2013). Type 1 diabetes mellitus (T1DM) is a severe chronic autoimmune disease caused by autoantibodies against pancreatic β cells. T1DM emerges when more than 70% of insulin-producing tissues are destroyed due to the interaction of the risk, protective, and neutral alleles of approximately 50 genes with the environment. There are three main statistically significant chromosomal regions associated with T1DM: the human leukocyte antigen (HLA) region on chromosome 6p21, the protein tyrosine-phosphatase non-receptor type 22 (PTPN22) gene on chromosome 1p13, and the d region of the insulin (INS) gene on chromosome 11p15 (Nyaga et al., 2018). Type 2 DM (T2DM) can occur through insulin resistance and insulin deficiency, genetic or environmental impacts. Additionally, hyperglycemia itself can impair pancreatic beta-cell function and exacerbate insulin resistance, called "glucotoxicity" (Li et al., 2004).

As a result, hyperglycemia is the main component of diabetes, regardless of its etiology. T2DM makes up more than 90 percent of DM cases in North America and Europe, and its prevalence increases every day due to the increasing obesity problem. Type 1 DM accounts for 5 to 10 percent, while the remaining part consists of gestational diabetes and diabetes due to special causes (Balasubramanyam, 2021). Prolonged hyperglycemia causes microvascular (retinopathy, nephropathy, neuropathy, and cardiovascular diseases) and macrovascular (cardiovascular diseases) complications and major morbidity and mortality in patients (Figure1) (Nathan et al., 1993; Reddy et al., 2015). The disease mechanism in DM, one of the most important public health problems, has not been well understood until the present day. Since epigenetics can provide a molecular link between genetic, environmental factors and diabetes, it is promising in elucidating the etiopathogenesis of diabetes (Mambia et al., 2019).

The Role of Epigenetic Changes in the Development of Diabetes Mellitus

Epigenetics is a concept that does not change the DNA sequence but includes modifications that result in changes in the function and regulation of DNA, proteins, and RNAs. Epigenetic mechanisms represent changes in gene expression that occur not by changing the DNA sequence but by changing DNA methylation or remodeling chromatin. Epigenetic factors have roles in various cellular processes, including cell differentiation, aging, DNA replication and repair (Mohn and Schübeler, 2019; Calvanese et al., 2009). Environmental factors, e.g., nutritional disorders and sedentary lifestyle, lead to the formation of DM through epigenetic mechanisms (Ding and Haung, 2014). Epigenetic changes persist for at least three generations after the exposure, causing the first change in the phenotype. Heredity can occur through the mother or father. A pregnant woman carries epigenetic information to the fetus, and fetal germ cells are also influenced by epigenetic changes while in the womb (Ding and Huang, 2014; Rissman and Adli, 2014). Early embryonic development and germ cell development stages are the periods when epigenetic coding is most sensitive and open to external impacts (Ding and Huang, 2014). Adverse environmental factors such as maternal stress, intrauterine malnutrition, smoking, or obesity during this period increase the risk of chronic diseases, such as DM, in the long term (Hajj et al., 2014). Paternal nutritional intake can also cause epigenetic changes in the sperm epigenome through DNA methylation. For example, paternal obesity impairs sperm count, concentration, motility, and morphology. These changes also cause DNA damage in sperm (Ding and Huang, 2014). Paternal impaired fasting glucose and glucose intolerance are indicators of prediabetes. This situation will change gene expression patterns in pancreatic islets by downregulating a number of genes in glucose metabolism and insulin signaling pathways. It will cause epigenetic changes in the sperm epigenome (Grayson et al., 2014).

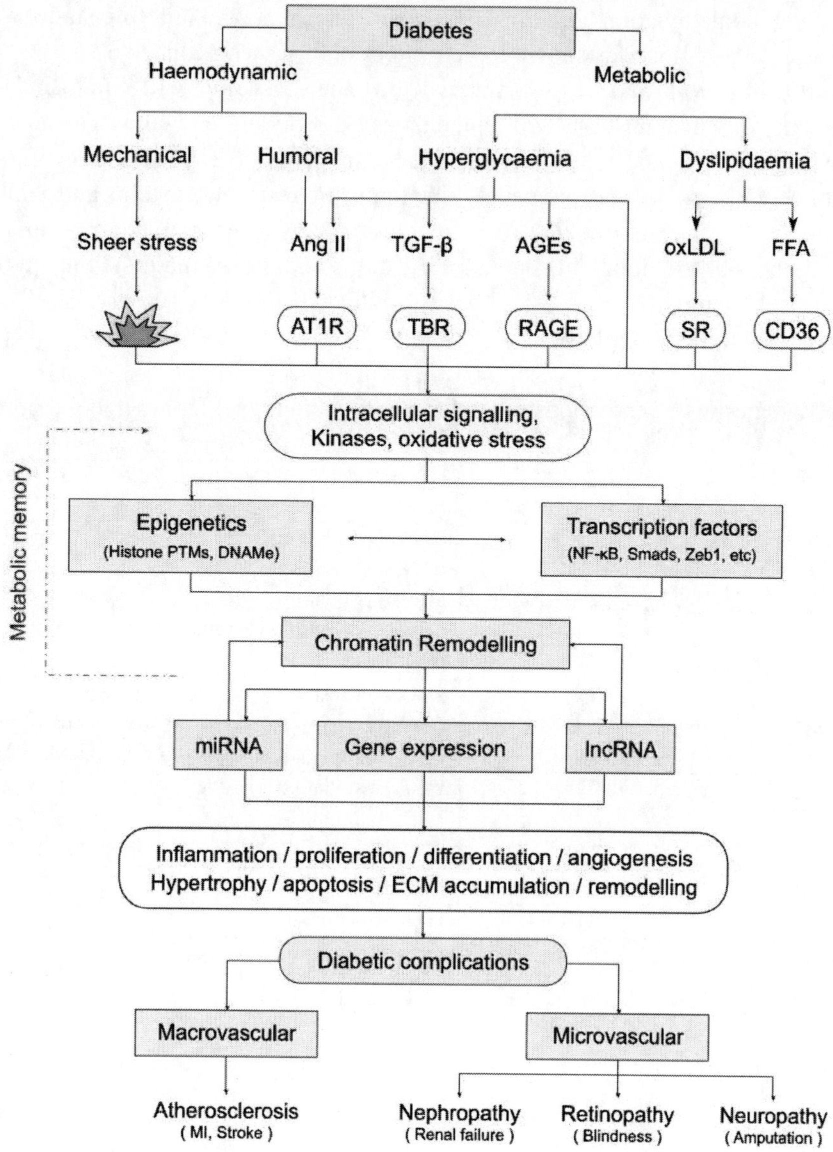

Figure 1. Potential metabolic pathways involved in the pathogenesis of diabetic complications and metabolic memory (Reddy et al., 2015)* (*Diabetes and its resulting metabolic disorders can regulate various growth factors and lipids by triggering receptors and multiple signaling pathways, transcription factors (TFs) and epigenetic networks. The persistence of such epigenetic abnormalities (including histone PTMs, DNAme, and ncRNAs) may lead to metabolic memory, which is associated with an increased risk of developing diabetic complications, even after hyperglycemia is normalized. AT1R, Ang II type 1 receptor; MI, myocardial infarction; oxLDL, Oxidized-LDL; RAGE, Receptor for AGEs; SR, scavenger receivers; TBR, TGF-β receptor).

Maternal obesity observed with gestational DM causes hyperinsulinemia in newborns and an increase in fat mass up to the sixth week. Maternal obesity during pregnancy is likely to initiate epigenetic processes for the newborn that will lead to chronic diseases in adulthood. Insulin Receptor Substrate-1 (IRS-1), regulated by the epigenetic mechanism through miRNA-126 (microRNA), mediates hyperinsulinemia due to maternal obesity (Grayson et al., 2014; Rehan, 2016). Maternal malnutrition during pregnancy also leads to epigenetic changes such as obesity. Hypomethylation in CpG (Cystosinephosphate-Guanine) islands within the important promoter region was shown to be present in those who conceived during the Dutch famine from 1944 to 1945 and was still observed up to 60 years afterward (Smith and Ryckman, 2016). Intrauterine malnutrition will epigenetically program newborns to survive in an environment with postnatal malnutrition. If they are exposed to high-energy foods in the postpartum period, they will become obese due to insulin resistance (Sterns and Smith, 2014).

Epigenetic mechanisms in DM may be impacted by gene activation, including DNA methylation, post-translational histone modification, and RNA methylation, and different epidemiological factors, such as age, obesity, nutrition, physical activity, and intrauterine environment (Table 1) (Villeneuve et al., 2011).

Table 1. Genes with expressions related to obesity and type 2 DM metabolic processes

Adipogenesis	CEBPA PPARA	Histone acetylation and methylation DNA methylation
Regulation of appetite	LEP MC4R NPY POMC	DNA methylation DNA methylation DNA methylation DNA methylation, Histone acetylation and methylation
Body weight regulation	FTO	DNA methylation
Glucose regulation	ADIPOQ GLUT4 INS	DNA methylation and Histone acetylation DNA methylation and Histone acetylation DNA methylation and Histone acetylation
Hypoxia	HIF1A	DNA methylation, Histone acetylation and methylation
Inflammation	IFNG TNF	DNA methylation DNA methylation
Lipid storage	FASN	DNA methylation
Stress	NR3C1	Histone acetylation
Thermogenesis	UCP1	DNA methylation

DNA Methylation

The conversion of the cytosine base of some regions on DNA to 5-methylcytosine is called DNA methylation (Klose and Bird, 2006). CpG islands are 500-2000 base pair long DNA regions where 5'-cytosine-phosphate-guanosine-3' dinucleotides are often found, and 5-methylcytosine (5-mC) modification is generally found in CpG islands. Most gene promoter regions contain CpG islands. Promoter regions are the part of DNA that initiates gene transcription and contain specific DNA fragments necessary for the transcription process and to which RNA polymerase can bind securely. Common epigenetic modifications in DNA occur in methylated-demethylated CpG islands in the promoter region. Disease processes and growth and developmental processes are related to the methylation of promoter regions and transcription arrest. DNA methylation can also be found in other parts of the genome outside of CpG islands (Hajj et al., 2014). The methyl group is attached to DNA by DNA methyltransferase (DNMT) enzymes. They consist of three isoforms, DNMT1, DNMT3a, and DNMT3b. Epigenetic modifications due to DNA methylation can be reversed by DNA demethylation. It has been demonstrated that intermediate products such as 5-hydroxymethylcytosine (5-hmC), 5-formylcytosine, and 5-carboxycytosine that develop during this process are also epigenetic markers on their own (Shen et al., 2014; Kohli and Zhang, 2013). Hyperglycemia can induce global demethylation in the whole genome, along with promoter, intergenic, and intragenic regions. A decrease occurs in methylation in methylated CpG sites (Li and Zhang, 2014). This may result from a decrease in DNMT1 activity during cell proliferation or a decrease in the activity of DNMT3a and 3b, which are responsible for methylation. Hyperglycemia leads to an increase in GADD45A protein, which causes demethylation in human pancreatic cells. A decrease in methyl donors may be another reason for the development of hypomethylation in hyperglycemia (Intine and Sarras, 2012). These changes are risk factors for DM and are kept in the metabolic memory state (Li and Zhang, 2014). As is seen, DM represents a disease that is impacted by epigenetic factors, and it is also an important epigenetic factor itself.

Post-Translational Histone Modifications

Histones (H1, H2A, H2B, H3, and H4) are globular proteins around DNA that are packaged to form chromatin. Post-translational histone modifications occur owing to enzymes that change the lysine and arginine residues at the amino terminus of histones. These modifications are acetylation and methylation. While methylation can increase or reduce DNA accessibility, acetylation reduces DNA accessibility (Fleisch et al., 2012; Choi and Friso, 2010).

RNA Methylation and Expression

The methylation of RNAs at carbon 6 on the adenine base is called RNA methylation (m6A) and is a significant epigenetic factor (Shen et al., 2015). m6A modification is the most frequently observed modification in mRNAs, and it has been revealed to be concentrated on coding sequences, especially near the stop codons (Liu and Pan, 2015; Xu et al., 2015). m6A modifications influence mRNAs in terms of splicing, stability, transport, and immunity (Xu et al., 2015). MicroRNAs (miRNAs), which are considered to be oncogenes and tumor suppressors, are among the major epigenetic regulators of the encoded genes of the genome. miRNA can function epigenetically by blocking or altering gene expression (Villeneuve et al., 2011). miRNA is a gene promoter and can reduce gene expression by maintaining histone deacetylation, histone methylation (H3K9 and H3K27), and DNA methylation (Handy et al., 2011).

Palmitate is the salt or ester of palmitic acid. Palmitic acid is the most common saturated fatty acid found in animals and plants. It is present in the oil of the palm tree and the palm kernel. It is also present in butter, cheese, milk, and meat. The exposure of pancreatic islet cells to palmitate may cause an increase in miR-34a and miR-146 (microRNAs) that activate p53 and reduce vesicle-associated membrane protein 2. This may cause the apoptosis of islet cells and reduced insulin secretion. miR-21, miR-34a, and miR-146 may be activated as a result of the exposure of proinflammatory cytokines to islet cells, which causes a decrease in insulin secretion and increased apoptosis of cells. Increased miR-29a and -29b levels in insulin target organs in hyperglycemia may lead to insulin resistance by reducing insulin-mediated glucose uptake (Joglekar et al., 2011). Different miRNAs contribute to the development of DM (Table 2).

Table 2. miRNAs targeting type 2 DM

miRNA	Target	Function
miR-375	myotrophin	Inhibition of insulin secretion
miR-9	OneCut2 transcription factor	Inhibition of glucose-stimulated insulin release
miR-192	E-box repressor	Matrix protein collagen col a-1 and -2 induced by miR-192 E-box repressor TGFb
miR-143	GLUT4, HSL, fatty acid-binding protein aP2, PPAR-m2	Adipocyte differentiation

Metabolic Memory

Hyperglycemia may reduce sirtuin1 (SIRT1) activity. This decreases the acetylation of histone 3 bound to p53, nuclear factor-kappa beta (NF-kβ), p65 subunit, and the p66shc promoter region. p53 becomes activated and causes the increased transcription of p66shc. Moreover, it may also cause the transcription of p66shc to decrease the role of GCN, an acetyltransferase, due to hyperglycemia. The p53 protein that increases P66shc levels perpetuates mitochondrial ROS production. Increased ROS production may lead to endothelial dysfunction, vascular inflammation, and the initiation of the apoptosis process in cells (Bender et al., 2013). High ROS production causes decreased insulin gene expression, insulin production, and insulin secretion by reducing the signaling process from IRS-1 to phosphatidylinositol 3 kinase (PI3K). Furthermore, high ROS production induces the degradation of mafA by activating c-jun N-terminal kinase, which moves pancreatic and duodenal homeobox-1 (PDX-1) from the nucleus to the cytoplasm. In this case, it causes decreased insulin gene expression, insulin production, and insulin secretion (Bender et al., 2013; Jia et al., 2013). Restricting daily calorie intake is useful for preventing DM and its complications. Calorie restriction delays the onset of degenerative diseases by stabilizing the genome through chromatin remodeling and epigenetic mechanisms. Thus, cardiovascular diseases, DM, and cancer can be delayed (Grayson et al., 2014).

Conclusion

DM represents a metabolic disease characterized by high blood sugar levels as a result of interactions between genes and the environment. There are three main epigenetic mechanisms in the development of DM. These are DNA methylation, post-translational histone modification, and microRNA transcription and methylation. Epigenetic changes are pre-existing in the mother and father and are inherited from the family. Epigenetic changes, which occur in the womb, at birth, and persist to adulthood, will be passed on through generations. Even in the case of a normal blood sugar level, the epigenetic mechanisms through which DM complications can occur are included in the metabolic memory. Calorie restriction may be useful in delaying the onset or progression of degenerative diseases, including DM, through epigenetic mechanisms to stabilize the genome.

References

Balasubramanyam A. (2021). Classification of diabetes mellitus and genetic diabetic syndromes In: *UpToDate*, Balasubramanyam A (Accessed on December, 2021).

Bender SB, McGraw AP, Jaffe IZ and Sowers JR. (2013). Mineralocorticoid receptor-mediated vascular insulin resistance: An early contributor to diabetes-related vascular disease? *Diabetes*, 62(2), 313-319. https://doi.org/10.2337/db12-0905.

Calvanese V, Lara E, Kahn A and Fraga MF. (2009). The role of epigenetics in aging and age-related diseases. *Ageing Research Reviews*, 8(4), 268-276. https://doi.org/10.1016/j.arr.2009.03.004.

Choi SW and Friso S. (2010). Epigenetics: A New Bridge between Nutrition and Health. *Advances in Nutrition*, (Bethesda, Md), 1(1), 8-16. https://doi.org/10.3945/an.110.1004.

Ding GL and Huang HF. (2014). Role for tet in hyperglycemia-induced demethylation: A novel mechanism of diabetic metabolic memory. *Diabetes*, 63(9), 2906-2908. https://doi.org/10.2337/db14-0675.

El Hajj N, Schneider E, Lehnen H and Haaf T. (2014). Epigenetics and life-long consequences of an adverse nutritional and diabetic intrauterine environment. *Reproduction*, (Cambridge, England), 148(6), R111-R120. https://doi.org/10.1530/REP-14-0334.

Fleisch AF, Wright RO and Baccarelli AA. (2012). Environmental epigenetics: A role in endocrine disease? *Journal of Molecular Endocrinology*, 49(2), R61-R67. https://doi.org/10.1530/JME-12-0066.

Gouri A, Dekaken A. (2013). Epigenetic pathways in type 2 diabetes and its complications. *iMedPub Journals*, 3(11),1-5. https://doi.org/ 10.3823/1400.

Grayson SE, Abel Ponce de Leon F and Muscoplat CC. (2014). Epigenetics: Understanding How our Choices Lead to our Diseases. *Journal of Clinical Case Reports*, 4:11 https://doi.org/10.4172/2165-7920.1000447.

Handy DE, Castro R and Loscalzo J. (2011). Epigenetic modifications: Basic mechanisms and role in cardiovascular disease. *Circulation*, 123(19), 2145-2156. https://doi.org/10.1161/CIRCULATIONAHA.110.956839.

Intine RV and Sarras MP Jr. (2012). Metabolic memory and chronic diabetes complications: Potential role for epigenetic mechanisms. *Current Diabetes Reports*, 12(5), 551-559. https://doi.org/10.1007/s11892-012-0302-7.

Jia L, Xing J, Ding Y, Shen Y, Shi X, Ren W, Wan M, Guo J, Zheng S, Liu Y, Liang X and Su D. (2013). Hyperuricemia causes pancreatic β-cell death and dysfunction through NF-κB signaling pathway. *PloS One*, 8(10), e78284. https://doi.org/10.1371/journal.pone.0078284.

Joglekar MV, Parekh VS and Hardikar AA. (2011). Islet-specific microRNAs in pancreas development, regeneration and diabetes. *Indian Journal of Experimental Biology*, 49(6), 401-408.

Klose RJ and Bird AP. (2006). Genomic DNA methylation: The mark and its mediators. *Trends in Biochemical Sciences*, 31(2), 89-97. https://doi.org/10.1016/j.tibs.2005.12.008.

Kohli RM and Zhang Y. (2013). TET enzymes, TDG and the dynamics of DNA demethylation. *Nature*, 502(7472), 472-479. https://doi.org/10.1038/nature12750.

Li E and Zhang Y. (2014). DNA methylation in mammals. *Cold Spring Harbor Perspectives in Biology*, 6(5), a019133. https://doi.org/10.1101/cshperspect.a019133.

Li Y, Xu W, Liao Z, Yao B, Chen X, Huang Z, Hu G and Weng J. (2004). Induction of long-term glycemic control in newly diagnosed type 2 diabetic patients is associated with improvement of beta-cell function. *Diabetes Care,* 27(11), 2597-2602. https://doi.org/10.2337/diacare.27.11.2597.

Liu N and Pan T. (2015). RNA epigenetics. *Translational Research: The Journal of Laboratory and Clinical Medicine,* 165(1), 28-35. https://doi.org/10.1016/j.trsl.2014.04.003.

Mambiya M, Shang M, Wang Y, Li Q, Liu S, Yang L, Zhang Q, Zhang K, Liu M, Nie F, Zeng F and Liu W. (2019). The Play of Genes and Non-genetic Factors on Type 2 Diabetes. *Frontiers in Public Health,* 7, 349. https://doi.org/10.3389/fpubh.2019.00349.

Mohn F and Schübeler D. (2009). Genetics and epigenetics: Stability and plasticity during cellular differentiation. *Trends in Genetics: TIG,* 25(3), 129-136. https://doi.org/10.1016/j.tig.2008.12.005.

Nathan DM, Genuth S, Lachin J, Cleary P, Crofford O, Davis M, Rand L and Siebert C. (1993). The effect of intensive treatment of diabetes on the development and progression of long-term complications in insulin-dependent diabetes mellitus. *Diabetes Control and Complications Trial Research Group, The New England Journal of Medicine*, 329(14), 977-986. https://doi.org/10.1056/NEJM199309303291401.

Nyaga DM, Vickers MH, Jefferies C, Perry JK and O'Sullivan JM. (2018). The genetic architecture of type 1 diabetes mellitus. *Molecular and Cellular Endocrinology*, 477, 70-80. https://doi.org/10.1016/j.mce. 2018.06.002.

Reddy MA, Zhang E and Natarajan R. (2015). Epigenetic mechanisms in diabetic complications and metabolic memory. *Diabetologia,* 58(3), 443-455. https://doi.org/10.1007/s00125-014-3462-y.

Rehan MK. (2016). Epigenetics and diabetes mellitus. *Egypt J Intern Med*, 28, 39-51. https://doi.org/10.4103/ 1110-7782.193890.

Rissman EF and Adli M. (2014). Minireview: Transgenerational epigenetic inheritance: Focus on endocrine disrupting compounds. *Endocrinology*, 155(8), 2770-2780. https://doi.org/10.1210/en.2014-1123.

Satman I, Omer B, Tutuncu Y, Kalaca S, Gedik S, Dinccag N, Karsidag K, Genc S, Telci A, Canbaz B, Turker F, Yilmaz T, Cakir B, Tuomilehto J and TURDEP-II Study Group. (2013). Twelve-year trends in the prevalence and risk factors of diabetes and prediabetes in Turkish adults. *European Journal of Epidemiology,* 28(2), 169-180. https://doi.org/10.1007/s10654-013-9771-5.

Shen F, Huang W, Huang JT, Xiong J, Yang Y, Wu K, Jia GF, Chen J, Feng YQ, Yuan BF and Liu SM. (2015). Decreased N(6)-methyladenosine in peripheral blood RNA from diabetic patients is associated with FTO expression rather than ALKBH5. *The Journal of Clinical Endocrinology and Metabolism,* 100(1), E148-E154. https://doi.org/10.1210/jc.2014-1893.

Shen L, Song CX, He C and Zhang Y. (2014). Mechanism and function of oxidative reversal of DNA and RNA methylation. *Annual Review of Biochemistry,* 83, 585-614. https://doi.org/10.1146/annurev-biochem-060 713-035513.

Smith CJ and Ryckman KK. (2015). Epigenetic and developmental influences on the risk of obesity, diabetes, and metabolic syndrome. *Diabetes, Metabolic Syndrome and Obesity: Targets and Therapy,* 8, 295-302. https://doi.org/10.2147/DMSO.S61296.

Sterns JD, Smith CB, Steele JR, Stevenson KL and Gallicano GI. (2014). Epigenetics and type II diabetes mellitus: underlying mechanisms of prenatal predisposition. *Frontiers in Cell and Developmental Biology,* 2, 15. https://doi.org/10.3389/fcell.2014.00015.

Tanrıverdi MH, Çelepkolu T and Aslanhan H. (2013). Diabetes mellitus and primary healthcare. *Journal of Clinical and Experimental Investigations,* 4(4), 562-567. https://doi.org/10.5799/ahinjs.01.2013.04.0347.

Villeneuve LM, Reddy MA and Natarajan R. (2011). Epigenetics: Deciphering its role in diabetes and its chronic complications. *Clinical and Experimental Pharmacology and Physiology,* 38(7), 451-459. https://doi.org/10.1111/j.1440-1681.2011.05497.x.

Xu C, Liu K, Tempel W, Demetriades M, Aik W, Schofield CJ and Min J. (2014). Structures of human ALKBH5 demethylase reveal a unique binding mode for specific single-stranded N6-methyladenosine RNA demethylation. *Journal of Biological Chemistry,* 289(25), 17299-17311. https://doi.org/10.1074/ jbc.M114.550350.

Chapter 19

The Role of Epigenetics in Osteoporosis

Öner Kılınç*, MD
Department of Orthopaedics and Traumatology,
Mersin City Hospital, Mersin, Turkey

Abstract

Osteoporosis is a disease that is more common in old age nowadays, significantly reduces bone quality and causes severe morbidity with fractures and in the development of which many factors have a role. It has extensive etiopathogenesis, and it has been investigated for many years. Along with the increasing knowledge of genes, the evolving technological developments open new windows, and the adventure that starts with this small window turns into a large world. New approaches, new possible drugs, and new etiopathogenesis for osteoporosis are present in this new world of epigenetic science. Determining this cycle of bone tissue, which starts with gene sequences and turns into the most robust tissue of people, through genetic, epigenetic, and molecular mechanisms has still been discussed in studies. The fact that epigenetic factors are modifiable, editable, and recyclable causes this world to be much more interesting.

Keywords: epigenetics, osteoporosis, bone metabolism, osteoporotic fracture

Introduction

Nowadays, osteoporosis impacts many more people and significantly reduces the quality of life of people along with increasing life expectancy and multidirectional life variables. It makes bones more fragile with the low bone mineral density it causes. It shapes both the conservative and surgical treatment protocols of the resulting fracture patterns according to itself. It manifests itself with hip and spinal fractures, especially in the elderly population, and maintains its importance with its morbidities. A large number of old and new studies on the pathogenesis of osteoporosis are available. The secrets of the human genome are uncovered with the increasing technological infrastructures, and by going further, the etiopathogenesis of osteoporosis is becoming deeper. It has been demonstrated that bone mineral density is a highly inherited condition and leads to osteoporosis and osteoporotic fractures with the accompanying changing factors.

---

* Corresponding Author's Email: dronerkilinc@hotmail.com.

In: Epigenetics: Beyond the Genetics and Medicine
Editors: Sevgi Durna Daştan and Nazan Yurtcu
ISBN: 979-8-88697-228-3

Osteoporosis, the most common bone disease worldwide, is a multifactorial disease characterized by low bone mineral density (BMD) and the increased risk of osteoporotic fractures caused by it (Kanis, 2002). According to the WHO, osteoporosis is defined as a BMD that is 2.5 standard deviations or more below the mean value measured for young healthy women (T-score $\leq$ 2.5) ("Assessment of fracture risk and its application to screening for postmenopausal osteoporosis. Report of a WHO Study Group," 1994). In conclusion, clinical diagnosis and evaluation of osteoporosis are primarily based on the measurements of the bone mineral density (Johnell et al., 2005). Of the variation in BMD, 60-80% is inherited from parents, and the rest is shaped by the factors from the environment (Urano and Inoue, 2014). Furthermore, the heritability of osteoporotic fracture, the clinical consequence of osteoporosis, is 50-70% (Deng et al., 2002).

Considering the internal structure of the bone tissue, it is observed that it needs to respond quickly to internal dynamics and keep the balance of calcium and phosphate ions. The bone tissue performs this cycle with numerous and complex functions and epigenetic rearrangements that are effective on genes. Epigenetics is composed of changes in the expression of genes without changes in their basic structure. Its basic mechanisms are histone-containing protein expressions/modifications, DNA methylation, and regulation with non-coding RNAs, which are independent of the inherited DNA nucleotide sequences.

All epigenetic modifications are reversible and highly dynamic. They are age-, cell-, and tissue-specific and highly responsive to endogenous signals and environmental stimulation. With all these aspects, it is possible to reveal epigenetic features, the determination of an individual's osteoporosis, and the related fracture risks. On the other hand, it is possible to develop therapeutic molecules that are effective on these mechanisms, protecting them from osteoporosis.

DNA Methylation

DNA methylation, which is an epigenetic modification, is associated with transcriptional silencing and is necessary for normal development. It is catalyzed by DNA methyltransferases (DNMTs), including DNMT1, DNMT3a, and DNMT3b (Bestor, 2000; Chen and Li, 2004).

Abnormal patterns of DNA methylation affect the disease processes and have significant roles, especially in human tumors (Esteller, 2008; Feinberg and Tycko, 2004). Some studies have argued that DNA methylation has an important role in the differentiation of osteoblasts, and it has been demonstrated that methylation changes are observed during the osteogenic differentiation of mesenchymal cells. The transcription factor (RUNX2) has a key role at this stage (Kang et al., 2007).

Furthermore, DNA methylation has a role in the separation of osteoblasts and osteoclasts. Osteoblasts have RANKL receptors on their cell surfaces, and conversion into osteoclasts occurs with this receptor-stimulus relationship (Delgado-Calle et al., 2012). On the other hand, DNA methylation is also closely associated with many factors that have important functions in bone cells and are related to the expression of genes. They are alkaline phosphatase (ALP), sclerostin (SOST), OSX, DLX5, estrogen receptor alpha (ESR1), OPN, RANKL, osteoprotegerin (OPG), secreted frizzled-related protein 1 (SFRP1), and leptin (LEP) (Vrtacnik et al., 2014).

A recent study on DNMT3a, one of the enzymes of DNA methylation, demonstrated that the DNMT3a inhibitor administered to mice had a positive effect on bones, caused an increase in bone mass and had protective effects from postmenopausal osteoporosis (Nishikawa et al., 2015).

Histone Modifications

Another epigenetic mechanism that regulates gene expression is provided by histones. The main components of chromatin and the nucleosome are histone proteins that cause the compaction and assembly of DNA. They have a role in important tasks such as transcription, replication, and repair of cells. They do most of these processes by changing the structure of chromatin (Arnsdorf et al., 2010). In studies on bone cells, it was observed that histone proteins were closely associated with the structure of RANKL receptors and the use of histone inhibitors reduced RANKL-induced osteoclast formation (Kim et al., 2009). The structure of histones is modified by histone acetyltransferases (HAT) and histone deacetylases (HDAC), and their activity is controlled (Pu et al., 2019). Osteoblastic activity and bone mineralization were observed to increase in the increased activities of special class III HDAC molecules, which have a role in bone metabolism; however, there was a shift from inhibition to adipogenic tissue (Backesjo et al., 2006; Wang et al., 2021).

Non-Coding RNAs

Although 90% of the human genome is transcribed into RNA, protein can be synthesized from only 1-2% of these gene sequences. The remaining structures are an end product not used in protein production. These products are ncRNAs with a regulatory role in gene expression during and after the transcription. With regard to bone homeostasis and bone diseases, ncRNAs and miRNAs have been mostly studied. The varying expression levels of miRNAs affect osteoblasts and osteoclasts and take an important place in bone metabolism and osteoporosis (Garmilla-Ezquerra et al., 2015). It has been demonstrated that they significantly regulate the RUNX2 gene, which controls osteoblast differentiation (Huang et al., 2010). The RUNX2 gene is a central transcription factor that regulates osteogenesis, especially in osteoblasts. Their effects on osteoporosis were investigated in detail, and they were divided into subgroups and acted with inhibitory/activator mechanisms (Kagiya, 2015). The size of mature miRNAs varies between 21-23 nucleotides. Their role is to modulate gene expression via post-transcriptional silencing.

Osteoporosis with its Epigenetic Aspect

Bones in the human body are important structures that not only support the body but also protect the internal organs. The bone tissue has many metabolic functions to keep the mineral balance. This situation, which occurs in a very dynamic way, includes the cycles of bone destruction and bone formation in balance. The main cause of osteoporosis is the disruption of this balance in the direction of its destruction. DNA methylations, histone modifications, chromatin remodeling, and ncRNAs, which are epigenetic mechanisms that affect gene expression, are closely associated with osteoporosis.

The etiopathogenesis of osteoporosis has been discussed in studies for many years. Osteoporosis is a multifactorial and polygenic skeletal disease that is shaped by hormonal, environmental, lifestyle (such as smoking, physical exercise) and nutritional factors (calcium intake, alcohol consumption) (Ferrari and Rizzoli, 2005; Giguere and Rousseau, 2000; Ralston, 2002). Studies have demonstrated that genetic factors are responsible for 50-85% of changes in bone phenotype, in addition to being multifactorial (Baldock and Eisman, 2004; Gencosmanoglu B E, 2001).

Studies on the genomic basis of the disease have revealed that many genes are closely associated with osteoporosis. The genes that are considered to be associated with osteoporosis are Vitamin D Receptor Gene (VDR), Estrogen Receptor Gene (ESR), Interleukin Receptor Gene (IL-R), Type 1 Collagen Alpha A1 Chain Gene (COL1A1), Androgen Receptor Gene (AR), Progesterone Receptor Gene (PR), Transforming Growth Factor β (TGF β), Apolipoprotein E Gene (Apo E), Parathyroid Hormone (PTH), Low-Density Lipoprotein (LDL)-Like Protein 5 (LRP5 Parathyroid Hormone Receptor Gene (PTHR1) (Aerssens et al., 2000; Gennari et al., 2002).

Epigenetic studies are relatively more up-to-date than these studies, and they seem to continue to be up-to-date because there are studies revealing that silencing or activating the factors that have a role in the expression of genes causes the existing infrastructural problems to dampen or further exacerbate (Jintaridth et al., 2013; Reppe et al., 2015).

The osteoprotegerin (OPG)/RANKL system is important in the balance between bone formation and bone loss. The relationship between both of them has a role in bone loss in osteoporotic patients (Giner et al., 2009). Furthermore, there are studies revealing that the balance between both of them and DNA methylation are associated with osteoporotic fractures ("DNA methylation and its role in bone formation and resorption," 2012). It is well known that estrogen deficiency leads to osteoporosis. The methylation of the ERa (Estrogen receptor alpha) gene reduces the amount of mERa bound to it, which reduces the amount of estrogen (Lv et al., 2011).

Nevertheless, histone modifications lead to osteogenic or catabolic effects by affecting bone cell differentiation. During osteoporosis, the imbalance between bone mass and fat increases, which increases the risk of fractures. KDM4B and KDM6B, which are histone demethylases, significantly reduce osteogenic differentiation and increase adipogenic differentiation (Ye et al., 2012). On the other hand, it was also demonstrated that H3K27me and H3K9me, which are histone proteins, increased the osteogenic activity (Jing et al., 2016). Furthermore, histone modifications have a role in the transformation of cells into adipose tissue and thus in the transformation of bone marrow cells into adipose tissue with increasing age (McGee-Lawrence et al., 2016). Since the structures of histone proteins are modifiable and have a reversible effect, they have the potential to form the treatment step in bone diseases such as osteoporosis.

There is published evidence indicating that miRNAs have a critical role in regulating various diseases. They play an active role in the differentiation of bone cells and the regulation of bone resorption. It was observed that the concentration of miRNAs increased in the blood serum levels of patients with osteoporosis who presented with osteoporotic fractures (Seeliger et al., 2014; Weilner et al., 2015). These circulating miRNA species can be used as biomarkers for diagnostic purposes and be identified as targets for drug development (Panach et al., 2015).

miRNAs are now being studied in clinical experiments to treat cancer and type II diabetes (Trajkovski et al., 2011; Wiggins et al., 2010). In a recent study, the resveratrol molecule suppressed a microRNA called miR-338-3p, had osteogenic and osteoinductive effects, and increased the Runx2 ratio. All of them prevent the progression and development of osteoporosis (Guo et al., 2015).

Osteoporosis and Epigenetic Drugs

Along with the developing epigenetic knowledge, it has become inevitable that drugs that directly and indirectly affect bone metabolism come to the fore. In the last few decades, HDAC inhibitors and bromodomain (BRD) inhibitors have been developed. They serve as anticancer drugs by inhibiting the deacetylation of histones or the recognition of acetyl-lysine (He and Lomberk, 2021; Wang et al., 2021). It was also shown that these molecules increased the osteoblastic effect and decreased the osteoclastic effect by acting on HDACs, which are involved in the regulation of bone metabolism (Baertschi et al., 2014). It was revealed that histone methyltransferase DOT1L inhibition delayed osteoporosis and stimulated mesenchymal cells in an osteogenic direction (Gao and Ge, 2018).

On the other hand, microRNAs were investigated in order to slow down osteoporosis. An anabolic effect was achieved in bone tissue by regulating microRNA on recombinant adeno-associated virus and reducing the formation of osteoblasts through RANK (Yang et al., 2020). In another study, the intravenous injection of the miR-338 inhibitor administered to mice reduced the risk of osteoporosis-related fractures by improving the bone mass and trabecular structure (Lin et al., 2019).

The DNA methylation inhibitor 5-aza-20-deoxycytidine led to increased density and mineralization in osteopenic bone (Li et al., 2018).

Conclusion

The etiopathogenesis, diagnosis, and treatment of a disease, which exists in a very large groups of people and reduces the quality of life, especially due to the fractures it causes, such as osteoporosis, have been investigated for many years. Despite a consensus on certain issues, the science of genetics and epigenetics can make new information out of the ordinary. The interaction and regulation of gene-defined sequences by external factors seem awesome. This effect has a much deeper voice on the parameters that form the disease, and this effect seems to persist existentially. Currently, understanding epigenetics goes beyond the tables and data set in laboratory rooms. Although most clinical studies have been conducted on animals, it is obvious with the strong data obtained that much more effective studies will be conducted on humans in the near future. A much closer relationship has been established, especially with the emergence of therapeutic drugs effective on osteoporosis. New drugs are very promising and may radically change clinical perspectives.

References

Aerssens J, Dequeker J, Peeters J, Breemans S, Broos P and Boonen S. (2000). Polymorphisms of the VDR, ER and COLIA1 genes and osteoporotic hip fracture in elderly postmenopausal women. *Osteoporos Int*, 11(7), 583-591. https://doi.org/10.1007/s001980070079.

Arnsdorf EJ, Tummala P, Castillo AB, Zhang F and Jacobs CR. (2010). The epigenetic mechanism of mechanically induced osteogenic differentiation. *J Biomech*, 43(15), 2881-2886. https://doi.org/10.1016/j.jbiomech.2010.07.033.

Assessment of fracture risk and its application to screening for postmenopausal osteoporosis. Report of a WHO Study Group. (1994). *World Health Organ Tech Rep Ser*, 843, 1-129. https://www.ncbi.nlm.nih.gov/pubmed/7941614.

Backesjo CM, Li Y, Lindgren U and Haldosen LA. (2006). Activation of Sirt1 decreases adipocyte formation during osteoblast differentiation of mesenchymal stem cells. *J Bone Miner Res*, 21(7), 993-1002. https://doi.org/10.1359/jbmr.060415.

Baertschi S, Baur N, Lueders-Lefevre V, Voshol J and Keller H. (2014). Class I and IIa histone deacetylases have opposite effects on sclerostin gene regulation. *J Biol Chem*, 289(36), 24995-25009. https://doi.org/10.1074/jbc.M114.564997.

Baldock PA and Eisman JA. (2004). Genetic determinants of bone mass. *Curr Opin Rheumatol*, 16(4), 450-456. https://doi.org/10.1097/01.moo.0000127828.34643.b4.

Bestor TH. (2000). The DNA methyltransferases of mammals. *Hum Mol Genet*, 9(16), 2395-2402. https://doi.org/10.1093/hmg/9.16.2395.

Chen T and Li E. (2004). Structure and function of eukaryotic DNA methyltransferases. *Curr Top Dev Biol*, 60, 55-89. https://doi.org/10.1016/S0070-2153(04)60003-2.

Delgado-Calle J, Sanudo C, Fernandez AF, Garcia-Renedo R, Fraga MF and Riancho JA. (2012). Role of DNA methylation in the regulation of the RANKL-OPG system in human bone. *Epigenetics*, 7(1), 83-91. https://doi.org/10.4161/epi.7.1.18753.

Deng HW, Mahaney MC, Williams JT, Li J, Conway T, Davies KM, Li JL, Deng H and Recker RR. (2002). Relevance of the genes for bone mass variation to susceptibility to osteoporotic fractures and its implications to gene search for complex human diseases. *Genet Epidemiol*, 22(1), 12-25. https://doi.org/10.1002/gepi.1040.

DNA methylation and its role in bone formation and resorption. (2012). *Bonekey Rep*, *1*, 45. https://doi.org/10.1038/bonekey.2012.45.

Esteller M. (2008). Epigenetics in cancer. *N Engl J Med*, 358(11), 1148-1159. https://doi.org/10.1056/NEJMra072067.

Feinberg AP and Tycko B. (2004). The history of cancer epigenetics. *Nat Rev Cancer*, 4(2), 143-153. https://doi.org/10.1038/nrc1279.

Ferrari SL and Rizzoli R. (2005). Gene variants for osteoporosis and their pleiotropic effects in aging. *Mol Aspects Med*, 26(3), 145-167. https://doi.org/10.1016/j.mam.2005.01.002.

Gao Y and Ge W. (2018). The histone methyltransferase DOT1L inhibits osteoclastogenesis and protects against osteoporosis. *Cell Death Dis*, 9(2), 33. https://doi.org/10.1038/s41419-017-0040-5.

Garmilla-Ezquerra P, Sanudo C, Delgado-Calle J, Perez-Nunez MI, Sumillera M and Riancho JA. (2015). Analysis of the bone microRNome in osteoporotic fractures. *Calcif Tissue Int*, 96(1), 30-37. https://doi.org/10.1007/s00223-014-9935-7.

Gencosmanoglu BE EM. (2001). *Genetic of Osteoporosis,* (Vol. 7).

Gennari L, Becherini L, Falchetti A, Masi L, Massart F and Brandi ML. (2002). Genetics of osteoporosis: Role of steroid hormone receptor gene polymorphisms. *J Steroid Biochem Mol Biol*, 81(1), 1-24. https://doi.org/10.1016/s0960-0760(02)00043-2.

Giguere Y and Rousseau F. (2000). The genetics of osteoporosis: 'complexities and difficulties'. *Clin Genet,* 57(3), 161-169. https://doi.org/10.1034/j.1399-0004.2000.570301.x.

Giner M, Rios MA, Montoya MA, Vazquez MA, Naji L and Perez-Cano R. (2009). RANKL/OPG in primary cultures of osteoblasts from post-menopausal women. Differences between osteoporotic hip fractures and osteoarthritis. *J Steroid Biochem Mol Biol*, 113(1-2), 46-51. https://doi.org/10.1016/j.jsbmb.2008.11.005.

Guo DW, Han YX, Cong L, Liang D and Tu GJ. (2015). Resveratrol prevents osteoporosis in ovariectomized rats by regulating microRNA-338-3p. *Mol Med Rep*, 12(2), 2098-2106. https://doi.org/10.3892/mmr.2015.3581.

He L and Lomberk G. (2021). Collateral Victim or Rescue Worker?-The Role of Histone Methyltransferases in DNA Damage Repair and Their Targeting for Therapeutic Opportunities in Cancer. *Front Cell Dev Biol*, 9, 735107. https://doi.org/10.3389/fcell.2021.735107.

Huang J, Zhao L, Xing L and Chen D. (2010). MicroRNA-204 regulates Runx2 protein expression and mesenchymal progenitor cell differentiation. *Stem Cells*, 28(2), 357-364. https://doi.org/10.1002/stem.288.

Jing H, Liao L, An Y, Su X, Liu S, Shuai Y, Zhang X and Jin Y. (2016). Suppression of EZH2 Prevents the Shift of Osteoporotic MSC Fate to Adipocyte and Enhances Bone Formation During Osteoporosis. *Mol Ther*, 24(2), 217-229. https://doi.org/10.1038/mt.2015.152.

Jintaridth P, Tungtrongchitr R, Preutthipan S and Mutirangura A. (2013). Hypomethylation of Alu elements in post-menopausal women with osteoporosis. *PLoS One*, 8(8), e70386. https://doi.org/10.1371/journal.pone.0070386.

Johnell O, Kanis JA, Oden A, Johansson H, De Laet C, Delmas P, Eisman JA, Fujiwara S, Kroger H, Mellstrom D, Meunier PJ, Melton LJ 3rd, O'Neill T, Pols H, Reeve J, Silman A and Tenenhouse A. (2005). Predictive value of BMD for hip and other fractures. *J Bone Miner Res*, 20(7), 1185-1194. https://doi.org/10.1359/JBMR.050304.

Kagiya T. (2015). MicroRNAs and Osteolytic Bone Metastasis: The Roles of MicroRNAs in Tumor-Induced Osteoclast Differentiation. *J Clin Med*, 4(9), 1741-1752. https://doi.org/10.3390/jcm4091741.

Kang MI, Kim HS, Jung YC, Kim YH, Hong SJ, Kim MK, Baek KH, Kim CC and Rhyu MG. (2007). Transitional CpG methylation between promoters and retroelements of tissue-specific genes during human mesenchymal cell differentiation. *J Cell Biochem*, 102(1), 224-239. https://doi.org/10.1002/jcb.21291.

Kanis JA. (2002). Diagnosis of osteoporosis and assessment of fracture risk. *Lancet*, 359(9321), 1929-1936. https://doi.org/10.1016/S0140-6736(02)08761-5.

Kim HN, Ha H, Lee JH, Jung K, Yang D, Woo KM and Lee ZH. (2009). Trichostatin A inhibits osteoclastogenesis and bone resorption by suppressing the induction of c-Fos by RANKL. *Eur J Pharmacol*, 623(1-3), 22-29. https://doi.org/10.1016/j.ejphar.2009.09.025.

Li B, Zhao J, Ma JX, Li GM, Zhang Y, Xing GS, Liu J and Ma XL. (2018). Overexpression of DNMT1 leads to hypermethylation of H19 promoter and inhibition of Erk signaling pathway in disuse osteoporosis. *Bone*, 111, 82-91. https://doi.org/10.1016/j.bone.2018.03.017.

Lin C, Yu S, Jin R, Xiao Y, Pan M, Pei F, Zhu X, Huang H, Zhang Z, Chen S, Liu H and Chen Z. (2019). Circulating miR-338 Cluster activities on osteoblast differentiation: Potential Diagnostic and Therapeutic Targets for Postmenopausal Osteoporosis. *Theranostics*, 9(13), 3780-3797. https://doi.org/10.7150/thno.34493.

Lv H, Ma X, Che T and Chen Y. (2011). Methylation of the promoter A of estrogen receptor alpha gene in hBMSC and osteoblasts and its correlation with homocysteine. *Mol Cell Biochem*, 355(1-2), 35-45. https://doi.org/10.1007/s11010-011-0836-z.

McGee-Lawrence ME, Carpio LR, Schulze RJ, Pierce JL, McNiven MA, Farr JN, Khosla S, Oursler MJ and Westendorf JJ. (2016). Hdac3 Deficiency Increases Marrow Adiposity and Induces Lipid Storage and Glucocorticoid Metabolism in Osteochondroprogenitor Cells. *J Bone Miner Res*, 31(1), 116-128. https://doi.org/10.1002/jbmr.2602.

Nishikawa K, Iwamoto Y, Kobayashi Y, Katsuoka F, Kawaguchi S, Tsujita T, Nakamura T, Kato S, Yamamoto M, Takayanagi H and Ishii M. (2015). DNA methyltransferase 3a regulates osteoclast differentiation by coupling to an S-adenosylmethionine-producing metabolic pathway. *Nat Med*, 21(3), 281-287. https://doi.org/10.1038/nm.3774.

Panach L, Mifsut D, Tarin JJ, Cano A and Garcia-Perez MA. (2015). Serum Circulating MicroRNAs as Biomarkers of Osteoporotic Fracture. *Calcif Tissue Int*, 97(5), 495-505. https://doi.org/10.1007/s00223-015-0036-z.

Pu M, Chen J, Tao Z, Miao L, Qi X, Wang Y and Ren J. (2019). Regulatory network of miRNA on its target: coordination between transcriptional and post-transcriptional regulation of gene expression. *Cell Mol Life Sci*, 76(3), 441-451. https://doi.org/10.1007/s00018-018-2940-7.

Ralston SH. (2002). Genetic control of susceptibility to osteoporosis. *J Clin Endocrinol Metab*, 87(6), 2460-2466. https://doi.org/10.1210/jcem.87.6.8621.

Reppe S, Noer A, Grimholt RM, Halldorsson BV, Medina-Gomez C, Gautvik VT, Olstad OK, Berg JP, Datta H, Estrada K, Hofman A, Uitterlinden AG, Rivadeneira F, Lyle R, Collas P and Gautvik KM. (2015). Methylation of bone SOST, its mRNA, and serum sclerostin levels correlate strongly with fracture risk in postmenopausal women. *J Bone Miner Res*, 30(2), 249-256. https://doi.org/10.1002/jbmr.2342.

Seeliger C, Karpinski K, Haug AT, Vester H, Schmitt A, Bauer JS and van Griensven M. (2014). Five freely circulating miRNAs and bone tissue miRNAs are associated with osteoporotic fractures. *J Bone Miner Res*, 29(8), 1718-1728. https://doi.org/10.1002/jbmr.2175.

Trajkovski M, Hausser J, Soutschek J, Bhat B, Akin A, Zavolan M, Heim MH and Stoffel M. (2011). MicroRNAs 103 and 107 regulate insulin sensitivity. *Nature*, 474(7353), 649-653. https://doi.org/10.1038/nature10112.

Urano T and Inoue S. (2014). Genetics of osteoporosis. *Biochem Biophys Res Commun*, 452(2), 287-293. https://doi.org/10.1016/j.bbrc.2014.07.141.

Vrtacnik P, Marc J and Ostanek B. (2014). Epigenetic mechanisms in bone. *Clin Chem Lab Med*, 52(5), 589-608. https://doi.org/10.1515/cclm-2013-0770.

Wang JS, Yoon SH and Wein MN. (2021). Role of histone deacetylases in bone development and skeletal disorders. *Bone*, 143, 115606. https://doi.org/10.1016/j.bone.2020.115606.

Weilner S, Skalicky S, Salzer B, Keider V, Wagner M, Hildner F, Gabriel C, Dovjak P, Pietschmann P, Grillari-Voglauer R, Grillari J and Hackl M. (2015). Differentially circulating miRNAs after recent osteoporotic fractures can influence osteogenic differentiation. *Bone*, 79, 43-51. https://doi.org/10.1016/j.bone.2015.05.027.

Wiggins JF, Ruffino L, Kelnar K, Omotola M, Patrawala L, Brown D and Bader AG. (2010). Development of a lung cancer therapeutic based on the tumor suppressor microRNA-34. *Cancer Res*, 70(14), 5923-5930. https://doi.org/10.1158/0008-5472.CAN-10-0655.

Yang YS, Xie J, Chaugule S, Wang D, Kim JM, Kim J, Tai PWL, Seo SK, Gravallese E, Gao G and Shim JH. (2020). Bone-Targeting AAV-Mediated Gene Silencing in Osteoclasts for Osteoporosis Therapy. *Mol Ther Methods Clin Dev*, 17, 922-935. https://doi.org/10.1016/j.omtm.2020.04.010.

Ye L, Fan Z, Yu B, Chang J, Al Hezaimi K, Zhou X, Park NH and Wang CY. (2012). Histone demethylases KDM4B and KDM6B promotes osteogenic differentiation of human MSCs. *Cell Stem Cell*, 11(1), 50-61. https://doi.org/10.1016/j.stem.2012.04.009.

Chapter 20

The Role of Epigenetics in Osteoarthritis

Fatih Günaydın*, MD

Department of Orthopaedic Surgery, Mersin City Hospital, Mersin, Turkey

Abstract

Osteoarthritis (OA) is a common degenerative joint disease worldwide. Considering the large number of people it affects, it creates serious limitations on patients and creates a serious burden on the healthcare system. Obesity, gender, genetic predisposition, trauma, and some systemic diseases can be listed as the most common causes of OA. However, in recent years, with the research on the concept of epigenetics and its relationship with various diseases, there have been serious changes in the view of the etiology of OA. The imbalance of anabolic and catabolic events that have a role in cartilage physiology is the most important element in the pathogenesis of OA. Epigenetic factors are also blamed for the disruption of this balance. DNA methylation, Histone modification, and non-coding RNAs are the most widely accepted epigenetic mechanisms in OA. Many published studies have revealed the relationship of each of these mechanisms with the pathogenesis of OA. New doors will likely be opened in the prevention and treatment of OA with the studies that have been conducted and will be conducted in this regard.

Keywords: epigenetics, osteoarthritis, articular cartilage, chondrocyte

Introduction

Osteoarthritis (OA) is a common degenerative joint disease worldwide. Women are more predominantly affected. The joints most commonly affected by OA are the knees, hips, hands, and spine and less commonly, OA develops in the feet, wrists, shoulders, and ankles (Newman et al., 2003). OA treatment has been studied for years and millions of people apply to health institutions every year because of OA. Considering the large number of people it affects, it creates serious limitations on patients and creates a serious burden on the healthcare system. In the USA, Canada, UK, France, and Australia approximately 1.0-2.5% of the gross domestic product is spent on the treatment of these diseases (March & Bachmeier, 1997). Therefore, understanding the etiology of OA will be the most important milestone in the prevention of the disease. In the past, OA was seen as a natural consequence of aging rather than a disease. However, it was realized that OA is a disease and its pathophysiology is not as simple as it was

* Corresponding Author's E-mail: drfatihgunaydin@gmail.com.

In: Epigenetics: Beyond the Genetics and Medicine
Editors: Sevgi Durna Daştan and Nazan Yurtcu
ISBN: 979-8-88697-228-3

thought over time. Many studies on the etiology of OA have been published in the past decades. Obesity, gender, genetic predisposition, trauma, and some systemic diseases can be listed as the most common causes of OA. However, in recent years, with the research on the concept of epigenetics and its relationship with various diseases, there have been serious changes in the view of the etiology of OA.

Pathogenesis of Osteoarthritis

Synovial joints are formed by the articulation of two or more bones. It consists of a synovial membrane surrounding the joint, joint cavity, joint fluid within the cavity, and joint cartilage. The joint capsule has an inner layer called the synovial membrane. The synovial membrane also has layers; the internal synovial intima and subsynovial layer are the outer layer (Fathollahi et al., 2019). The synovial membrane contains the vasculature, lymphatics, and nerves. Synovocytes, mostly formed by macrophages, dendritic cells, and fibroblasts, are also found in this layer. Since the articular cartilage is avascular, it is nourished by synovial fluid. Glucosaminoglycan hyaluronate (HA), produced by synoviocytes, is the most important component of joint fluid and contributes to the lubrication and protection of articular cartilage surfaces (Schurz & Ribitsch, 1987). Articular cartilage consists of hyaline cartilage. Articular cartilage does not contain vascular, neural, or lymphatic structures (Bora Jr & Miller, 1987). Although it is hypocellular and has low access to oxygen and glucose, it is metabolically active (Mobasheri et al., 2008). Articular cartilage contains the extracellular matrix (ECM), which is almost composed of a single type of cell called chondrocytes. Chondrocytes are involved in both anabolic and catabolic processes. Chondrocytes are stimulated by cytokines and growth factors to synthesize and degrade the ECM (Van den Berg, 1999). These cytokines basically act by three different mechanisms: anabolic (Growth factors, IGF, COMPs, TGF b), regulatory and enzyme inhibitory (IL-6, Il-8, IL-4, IL-10, IFNg), and catabolic (IL1a, IL1b, TNFa) (Goldring, 2000). The balance of these mechanisms is disturbed in osteoarthritis. These cytokines are mostly found in macrophages and partly in other synoviocytes, and when they are released into the synovial fluid, they initiate the catabolic process in chondrocytes (Mathiessen & Conaghan, 2017). A disinterring and metalloprotease with thrombospondin motifs (ADAMTS) and Matrix metalloproteinases (MMPs) are enzymes that are effective in cartilage degradation and their release is associated with these cytokines (Kevorkian et al., 2004). ADAMTs and MMTs released from chondrocytes after pathological stimulation initiate the catabolic process and then the process following cartilage destruction continues. At the end of all these cellular events; ECM disruption, articular cartilage destruction, subchondral bone sclerosis, and osteophyte formations occur (Sandell, 2012).

Role of Epigenetics in OA

Arthur Riggs et al. defined the term epigenetics as "the study of mitotically and/or meiotically heritable changes in gene function that cannot be explained by changes in DNA sequence." (Russo et al., 1996). In other words, epigenetics refers to heritable changes that are not transmitted by DNA. When we consider this concept in terms of OA, the question arises of whether there are reasons that predispose to OA other than heredity transmitted by DNA. While OA was previously seen as a natural consequence of aging, in recent years it has been understood that OA is a disease and has a very complex pathophysiology. As studies on epigenetics have increased, the role of epigenetic mechanisms on the etiology of OA has often been questioned. DNA methylation, Histone modification, and non-coding RNAs are the most widely accepted epigenetic mechanisms in OA.

DNA Methylation in OA

DNA methylation is a biochemical process which occurs mostly in the CpG dinucleotide, through the conversion of cytosine to 5-methyl cytosine. DNA methyltransferase (DNMTs) enzyme is required for DNA methylation and at least four have been identified: DNMT1, DNMT2, NMT3A, DNMT3B (Jin & Robertson, 2013). After DNA methylation, transcription is repressed because the binding site of some transcription factors is blocked and it also facilitates the binding of transcription inhibitor proteins to DNA (Prokhortchouk & Defossez, 2008). The ten-eleven translation (TET) family of enzymes converts methylcytosine to hydroxymethylcytosine. This is a hypomethylation process and is associated with transcription activation (Jaenisch & Bird, 2003). In other words, while DNA methylation regulates transcription at the physiological level, disruption of this process due to various reasons such as environmental factors and nutrition may lead to disruptions in the expression of tissue-specific genes. In the case of hypermethylation, genes that affect the anabolic process in cartilage metabolism can be suppressed. In the opposite case of hypomethylation, the expression of genes involved in the catholic process may increase and the balance of cartilage metabolism may be disturbed. In recent years, many articles have been published investigating the relationship between OA and DNA methylation.

In a study by Zimmermann et al., they found that COL10A1 gene silencing due to DNA methylation was found in articular cartilage and human articular chondrocytes from donors with OA (Zimmermann et al., 2008). They showed that after demethylation in the 2 CpG regions of the COL10A1 gene in MSCs, there is COL10A1 gene induction, which facilitates *in vitro* chondrogenesis.

In another study, hypermethylation of the COL9A1 gene is associated with down-regulation of gene expression, thus it has been shown that OA formation can be triggered by suppressing the anabolic process (Imagawa et al., 2014).

In the two studies mentioned above, DNA methylation samples that have a role in the formation of OA by influencing ECM synthesis were mentioned. There are also studies showing that protease activity increases in OA through an increase in the expression of genes such as MMP 13 and ADAMTS 4 after hypomethylation (Hashimoto et al., 2013; Roach et al., 2005).

The influence of epigenetic factors on inflammatory processes is blamed on the etiology of OA. Studies are showing that the expression of the IL1B, IL8, and SOCS2 genes is increased in OA (de Andrés et al., 2011; Hashimoto et al., 2009; Hashimoto et al., 2013; Takahashi et al., 2015). Also decreased LEP gene expression has been associated with OA (Iliopoulos et al., 2007).

While studies show that chondrogenesis is affected by the methylation of genes such as SOX9, SOX4, and RUNX2 (Ezura et al., 2009), studies show that methylation of growth factors such as BMP7, SOST, and GDF5 plays a role in OA (Loeser et al., 2009; Papathanasiou et al., 2015; Reynard et al., 2011).

Histon Modifications in OA

Enzymatic post-translational modification of histones is also one of the mechanisms regulating gene expression. These modifications occur primarily in the amino-terminal tails of histone proteins, which regulate gene expression by altering the chromatin structure (Cosgrove et al., 2004). Acetylation, methylation, phosphorylation, ubiquitination, sumoylation, ADP-ribosylation, deamination, and proline isomerization are examples of such modifications (Fathollahi et al., 2019). The most common modifications are acetylation and methylation of lysine residues in the amino-terminal of histone 3 (H3) and histone 4 (H4) (Yan & Boyd, 2006). Although cancer and epigenetic regulations by histone modification are important research topics, the relationship between OA and histone modification has not been much investigated yet. Most studies have focused on acetylation and deacetylation, which are mediated by histone acetyltransferases (HATs) and histone deacetylases (HDACs). HDAC1 and HDAC2 levels are elevated in both chondrocytes and synovium in patients with OA compared with controls (Hong et al., 2009; Huber et al., 2007). These studies also showed that the carboxy-terminal domain of HDAC1 and HDAC2 have an important role in suppressing the expression of the collagen gene COL2A1 by binding to the transcriptional repressor Snail.

Trichostatin (TSA) is an HDAC inhibitor that reduces the induction of MMP expression (Wang et al., 2009). TSA was also shown to suppress synovial inflammation and cartilage breakdown in a mouse model of arthritis induced by a collagen antibody (Nasu et al., 2008). There are promising studies on the use of TSA in the prevention and treatment of OA. For example, a study reported that TSA inhibited IL1β-induced matrix metalloproteinase upregulation in human chondrocyte cultures *in vitro* (Wang et al., 2009). Another study by Culley et al., along with similar results, also found that inhibition of Class I HDACs by valproic acid and MS275 was sufficient to prevent IL1β-induced upregulation of the matrix metalloproteinase MMP-13 (Culley et al., 2013).

The change in the expression of a gene can be by more than one epigenetic mechanism. For example, the SOX9 gene, whose expression is altered by DNA methylation, has also been shown in OA chondrocytes, with increased methylation of histone residues H3K9 and H3K27 at the SOX9 promoter and decreased histone acetylation at H3K9, 15, 18, 23, and 27 (Kim et al., 2013).

Proinflammatory cytokines regulate the expression of many genes involved in OA through histone modifications. As a result of H3K4 di- and tri-methylation in their promoter, cyclooxygenase-2 (COX-2), and iNOS expression are induced by IL-1 (El Mansouri et al., 2011).

As mentioned before, an increase in catabolic activity and a decrease in the synthesis of ECM proteins are observed in the pathogenesis of OA. An association has been shown between increased expression of HDAC1 and HDAC2 and suppression of transcription of genes encoding COL2A1 and ACAN matrix proteins (Goldring & Marcu, 2012).

Sirtuin 1 (SirT1) is a protein that increases chondrocyte survival by inhibiting apoptosis (Horio et al., 2011). SirT1 levels decrease in chondrocytes of OA cartilage (Fujita et al., 2011). SirT1 can directly deacetylate and thereby activate HIF-2a66, resulting in upregulation of metalloproteinases and cartilage destruction when hypoxic conditions occur (Dioum et al., 2009). Besides its task of reducing apoptosis, SirT1 inhibits ADAMTS5 expression while promoting cartilage matrix gene expression such as ACAN, COL2A1, COL9A1, and COMP, potentially by deacetylation of SOX962 (Dvir-Ginzberg et al., 2008; Fujita et al., 2011).

Non-Coding RNAs in OA

The non-coding RNAs, including micro ribonucleic acids (miRNAs; miRs) and long non-coding RNAs (lncRNAs), are involved in another epigenetic mechanism in OA. miRs are found in both healthy and damaged cartilage in OA.

miRs are single-stranded non-coding RNAs of 20-30 nucleotides in length. It is thought that they are involved in the post-transcriptional regulation of genes by interacting with mRNA (D'Adamo et al., 2017). The studies of many researchers show that miRs have an active role in normal cartilage hemostasis and OA. In addition, transforming growth factor-ß (TGF-β)/SMA and Drosophila MADs (SMADs)/Bone Morphogenetic Proteins (BMPs), MMPs, ADAMTS, inducible nitric acid synthase miRs have been found to have a role in the regulation of cartilage signaling pathways such as (iNOS) IL-1, and TNF-α (Ping Li et al., 2015). The expression of the aggrecanase ADAMTS-5 gene, which is directly regulated by miR-140, increases in OA (Miyaki et al., 2010). Abnormal expression of microRNAs such as miR-9, miR-27, miR-34a, miR-140, miR-146a, miR-558, and miR-602 in OA led to the association between OA pathology and miRs (Cong et al., 2017).

miRs may have a role in OA pathology by various mechanisms. One of them is by affecting chondrocyte signaling pathways. NF-κB, SOX9, bone morphogenetic protein (BMP), transforming growth factor β (TGF-β), and insulin-like growth factor (IGF) are some of these pathways responsible for the development of OA (Xu et al., 2016). TGF-β has been shown to have a critical role in the pathogenesis of OA (Shen et al., 2014). There is evidence that some miRs are involved in the pathology of OA by the TGF-β signaling pathway. miRNA-140 and miRNA-455 are microRNAs that affect the formation of OA in this way (Swingler et al., 2012). In an experimental study on rats, the effect of miR-210 on cartilage hemostasis was demonstrated through the relationship between miR-210 and the NF-kB signaling pathway (Zhang et al., 2015). In many similar studies, the relationship between chondrocyte signaling pathways and miRs, thus the effect of miRs on OA through this mechanism has been shown.

Another mechanism in which miRs are implicated in the pathogenesis of OA is their effect on apoptosis. Studies have demonstrated that miR-146a, miR-34a, and miR-181 cause OA by increasing chondrocyte apoptosis (Jin et al., 2014; Wu et al., 2017; Yan et al., 2016).

In addition to the signaling pathways mentioned above, microRNAs can also cause the disease by affecting inflammatory mediators that have a role in the pathogenesis of OA. *In vitro* studies have shown that miR-9, miR-98, and miR-146 microRNAs reduce the production of tumor necrosis factor (TNF)-α (Jones et al., 2009). There are also studies showing the relationship of these microRNAs with other inflammatory mediators such as monocyte chemotactic protein (MCP)-induced protein 1 (MCPIP1), IL-6, and NF-κB1 (Makki & Haqqi, 2015; Makki et al., 2015; Matsushita et al., 2009).

The role of ECM in the pathophysiology of OA has been mentioned before. Factors that directly or indirectly affect the production and destruction of the ECM may also be responsible for the formation of OA. There are many studies investigating the role of miRs in this regard.

In one of these studies, it was shown that miR-27a has a role in OA pathogenesis by decreasing mRNA expression of IGFBP-5 and MMP13 genes (Tardif et al., 2009). miR-27a has also been reported to down-regulate MMP13 (Akhtar et al., 2010). There is evidence that miR-29b from the miR-29 family disrupts the collagen structure through COL2A1 and COL1A2 (Moulin et al., 2017). As examples of which are briefly mentioned, there are many articles on the role of miRs in the pathogenesis of OA with different mechanisms, and studies on this subject are gaining momentum day by day.

As with miRs, many studies investigate the effect of lncRNAs on OA formation. lncRNAs such as GAS5, PMS2L2, RP11-445H22.4, H19, CTD-2574D22.4, and HOTAIR are upregulated in AC tissues of OA patients (Xing et al., 2014). lncRNA-CIR, Growth arrest specific 5 (GAS5) lncRNA, LncRNA PVT1, and lncRNA-MSR, some of the lncRNAs upregulated in OA (Li et al., 2017; Liu et al., 2016; Liu et al., 2014; Song et al., 2014). On the other hand, LncRNA UFC1 is one of the down-regulated lncRNAs (Zhang et al., 2016).

Conclusion

Epigenetic factors and their relationship with diseases have been one of the popular fields in recent years. Although there are many studies on this subject, it must be admitted that what we know yet is much less than what we do not know. Epigenetic factors and their roles in the pathogenesis of OA have also received their share of interest in this topic. Undoubtedly, understanding the pathogenesis of OA is very important both in the prevention and treatment of the disease. Considering the incidence of OA, its effect on the life quality of individuals, and the resources spent on its treatment, it is seen how appropriate the studies on this subject are.

Since OA is a chronic and slow-progressing disease, most of the time, when clinical findings appear, permanent pathological changes in the articular cartilage have already occurred. Therefore, understanding the epigenetic mechanisms and environmental factors involved in disease formation and preventing the disease is as important as treating it. Many published articles have been proven that cartilage hemostasis is impaired by multiple mechanisms in the pathogenesis of OA and that there are many epigenetic inheritance elements in each mechanism. In this context, it is an issue that needs to be considered whether the treatment developed for a single mechanism or an epigenetic factor will cure the disease satisfactorily. Maybe in the future, this problem will be eliminated with individual epigenetic heredity assessment and treatment. Although that point is not yet close, studies and results on this subject are promising.

References

Akhtar, N., Rasheed, Z., Ramamurthy, S., Anbazhagan, A. N., Voss, F. R., & Haqqi, T. M. (2010). MicroRNA-27b regulates the expression of matrix metalloproteinase 13 in human osteoarthritis chondrocytes. *Arthritis & Rheumatism*, *62*(5), 1361-1371.

Bora Jr, F. W., & Miller, G. (1987). Joint physiology, cartilage metabolism, and the etiology of osteoarthritis. *Hand Clinics*, *3*(3), 325-336.

Cong, L., Zhu, Y., & Tu, G. (2017). A bioinformatic analysis of microRNAs role in osteoarthritis. *Osteoarthritis and Cartilage*, *25*(8), 1362-1371.

Cosgrove, M. S., Boeke, J. D., & Wolberger, C. (2004). Regulated nucleosome mobility and the histone code. *Nature Structural & Molecular Biology*, *11*(11), 1037-1043.

Culley, K. L., Hui, W., Barter, M. J., Davidson, R. K., Swingler, T. E., Destrument, A. P., Rowan, A. D. (2013). Class I histone deacetylase inhibition modulates metalloproteinase expression and blocks cytokine-induced cartilage degradation. *Arthritis & Rheumatism*, *65*(7), 1822-1830.

D'Adamo, S., Cetrullo, S., Minguzzi, M., Silvestri, Y., Borzì, R. M., & Flamigni, F. (2017). MicroRNAs and autophagy: fine players in the control of chondrocyte homeostatic activities in osteoarthritis. *Oxidative Medicine and Cellular Longevity*, *2017*.

de Andrés, M. C., Imagawa, K., Hashimoto, K., Gonzalez, A., Goldring, M. B., Roach, H. I., & Oreffo, R. O. (2011). Suppressors of cytokine signalling (SOCS) are reduced in osteoarthritis. *Biochemical and Biophysical Research Communications*, *407*(1), 54-59.

Dioum, E. M., Chen, R., Alexander, M. S., Zhang, Q., Hogg, R. T., Gerard, R. D., & Garcia, J. A. (2009). Regulation of hypoxia-inducible factor 2α signaling by the stress-responsive deacetylase sirtuin 1. *Science*, *324*(5932), 1289-1293.

Dvir-Ginzberg, M., Gagarina, V., Lee, E.-J., & Hall, D. J. (2008). Regulation of cartilage-specific gene expression in human chondrocytes by SirT1 and nicotinamide phosphoribosyltransferase. *Journal of Biological Chemistry*, *283*(52), 36300-36310.

El Mansouri, F. E., Chabane, N., Zayed, N., Kapoor, M., Benderdour, M., Martel-Pelletier, J., Fahmi, H. (2011). Contribution of H3K4 methylation by SET-1A to interleukin-1–induced cyclooxygenase 2 and inducible nitric oxide synthase expression in human osteoarthritis chondrocytes. *Arthritis & Rheumatism*, *63*(1), 168-179.

Ezura, Y., Sekiya, I., Koga, H., Muneta, T., & Noda, M. (2009). Methylation status of CpG islands in the promoter regions of signature genes during chondrogenesis of human synovium–derived mesenchymal stem cells. *Arthritis & Rheumatism*, *60*(5), 1416-1426.

Fathollahi, A., Aslani, S., Jamshidi, A., & Mahmoudi, M. (2019). Epigenetics in osteoarthritis: novel spotlight. *Journal of Cellular Physiology*, *234*(8), 12309-12324.

Fujita, N., Matsushita, T., Ishida, K., Kubo, S., Matsumoto, T., Takayama, K., Kuroda, R. (2011). Potential involvement of SIRT1 in the pathogenesis of osteoarthritis through the modulation of chondrocyte gene expressions. *Journal of Orthopaedic Research*, *29*(4), 511-515.

Goldring, M. B. (2000). Osteoarthritis and cartilage: the role of cytokines. *Current Rheumatology Reports*, *2*(6), 459-465.

Goldring, M. B., & Marcu, K. B. (2012). Epigenomic and microRNA-mediated regulation in cartilage development, homeostasis, and osteoarthritis. *Trends in Molecular Medicine*, *18*(2), 109-118.

Hashimoto, K., Oreffo, R. O., Gibson, M. B., Goldring, M. B., & Roach, H. I. (2009). DNA demethylation at specific CpG sites in the IL1B promoter in response to inflammatory cytokines in human articular chondrocytes. *Arthritis & Rheumatism: Official Journal of the American College of Rheumatology*, *60* (11), 3303-3313.

Hashimoto, K., Otero, M., Imagawa, K., De Andrés, M. C., Coico, J. M., Roach, H. I., Goldring, M. B. (2013). Regulated transcription of human matrix metalloproteinase 13 (MMP13) and interleukin-1β (IL1B) genes in chondrocytes depends on methylation of specific proximal promoter CpG sites. *Journal of Biological Chemistry*, *288*(14), 10061-10072.

Hong, S., Derfoul, A., Pereira-Mouries, L., & Hall, D. J. (2009). A novel domain in histone deacetylase 1 and 2 mediates repression of cartilage-specific genes in human chondrocytes. *The FASEB Journal*, *23*(10), 3539-3552.

Horio, Y., Hayashi, T., Kuno, A., & Kunimoto, R. (2011). Cellular and molecular effects of sirtuins in health and disease. *Clinical Science*, *121*(5), 191-203.

Huber, L. C., Brock, M., Hemmatazad, H., Giger, O. T., Moritz, F., Trenkmann, M., Moch, H. (2007). Histone deacetylase/acetylase activity in total synovial tissue derived from rheumatoid arthritis and osteoarthritis patients. *Arthritis & Rheumatism*, *56*(4), 1087-1093.

Iliopoulos, D., Malizos, K. N., & Tsezou, A. (2007). Epigenetic regulation of leptin affects MMP-13 expression in osteoarthritic chondrocytes: possible molecular target for osteoarthritis therapeutic intervention. *Annals of the Rheumatic Diseases*, *66*(12), 1616-1621.

Imagawa, K., De Andrés, M. C., Hashimoto, K., Itoi, E., Otero, M., Roach, H. I., Oreffo, R. O. (2014). Association of reduced type IX collagen gene expression in human osteoarthritic chondrocytes with epigenetic silencing by DNA hypermethylation. *Arthritis & Rheumatology*, *66*(11), 3040-3051.

Jaenisch, R., & Bird, A. (2003). Epigenetic regulation of gene expression: how the genome integrates intrinsic and environmental signals. *Nature Genetics*, *33*(3), 245-254.

Jin, B., & Robertson, K. D. (2013). DNA methyltransferases, DNA damage repair, and cancer. *Epigenetic Alterations in Oncogenesis*, 3-29.

Jin, L., Zhao, J., Jing, W., Yan, S., Wang, X., Xiao, C., & Ma, B. (2014). Role of miR-146a in human chondrocyte apoptosis in response to mechanical pressure injury *in vitro*. *International Journal of Molecular Medicine*, *34*(2), 451-463.

Jones, S., Watkins, G., Le Good, N., Roberts, S., Murphy, C., Brockbank, S., Newham, P. (2009). The identification of differentially expressed microRNA in osteoarthritic tissue that modulate the production of TNF-α and MMP13. *Osteoarthritis and Cartilage*, *17*(4), 464-472.

Kevorkian, L., Young, D. A., Darrah, C., Donell, S. T., Shepstone, L., Porter, S., Clark, I. M. (2004). Expression profiling of metalloproteinases and their inhibitors in cartilage. *Arthritis & Rheumatism: Official Journal of the American College of Rheumatology*, *50*(1), 131-141.

Kim, K. I., Park, Y. S., & Im, G. I. (2013). Changes in the epigenetic status of the SOX-9 promoter in human osteoarthritic cartilage. *Journal of Bone and Mineral Research*, *28*(5), 1050-1060.

Li, Y., Li, S., Luo, Y., Liu, Y., & Yu, N. (2017). LncRNA PVT1 regulates chondrocyte apoptosis in osteoarthritis by acting as a sponge for miR-488-3p. *DNA and cell biology*, *36*(7), 571-580.

Liu, Q., Hu, X., Zhang, X., Dai, L., Duan, X., Zhou, C., & Ao, Y. (2016). The TMSB4 pseudogene LncRNA functions as a competing endogenous RNA to promote cartilage degradation in human osteoarthritis. *Molecular Therapy*, *24*(10), 1726-1733.

Liu, Q., Zhang, X., Dai, L., Hu, X., Zhu, J., Li, L., Ao, Y. (2014). Long noncoding RNA related to cartilage injury promotes chondrocyte extracellular matrix degradation in osteoarthritis. *Arthritis & Rheumatology*, *66*(4), 969-978.

Loeser, R., Im, H.-J., Richardson, B., Lu, Q., & Chubinskaya, S. (2009). Methylation of the OP-1 promoter: potential role in the age-related decline in OP-1 expression in cartilage. *Osteoarthritis and Cartilage*, *17*(4), 513-517.

Makki, M. S., & Haqqi, T. M. (2015). miR-139 modulates MCPIP1/IL-6 expression and induces apoptosis in human OA chondrocytes. *Experimental & molecular medicine*, *47*(10), e189-e189.

Makki, M. S., Haseeb, A., & Haqqi, T. M. (2015). MicroRNA-9 promotes IL-6 expression by inhibiting MCPIP1 expression in IL-1β-stimulated human chondrocytes. *Arthritis & rheumatology (Hoboken, NJ)*, *67*(8), 2117.

March, L. M., & Bachmeier, C. J. (1997). 10 Economics of osteoarthritis: a global perspective. *Bailliere's Clinical Rheumatology*, *11*(4), 817-834.

Mathiessen, A., & Conaghan, P. G. (2017). Synovitis in osteoarthritis: current understanding with therapeutic implications. *Arthritis Research & Therapy*, *19*(1), 1-9.

Matsushita, K., Takeuchi, O., Standley, D. M., Kumagai, Y., Kawagoe, T., Miyake, T., Nakamura, H. (2009). Zc3h12a is an RNase essential for controlling immune responses by regulating mRNA decay. *Nature*, *458*(7242), 1185-1190.

Miyaki, S., Sato, T., Inoue, A., Otsuki, S., Ito, Y., Yokoyama, S., Yamashita, S. (2010). MicroRNA-140 plays dual roles in both cartilage development and homeostasis. *Genes & Development*, *24*(11), 1173-1185.

Mobasheri, A., Bondy, C. A., Moley, K., Mendes, A. F., Rosa, S. C., Richardson, S., Shakibaei, M. (2008). Facilitative glucose transporters in articular chondrocytes: expression, distribution and functional regulation of GLUT isoforms by hypoxia, hypoxia mimetics, growth factors and pro-inflammatory cytokines. *Adv Anat Embryol Cell Biol*, 200(1), 1-84.

Moulin, D., Salone, V., Koufany, M., Clément, T., Behm-Ansmant, I., Branlant, C., Jouzeau, J.-Y. (2017). MicroRNA-29b contributes to collagens imbalance in human osteoarthritic and dedifferentiated articular chondrocytes. *BioMed Research International*, *2017*.

Nasu, Y., Nishida, K., Miyazawa, S., Komiyama, T., Kadota, Y., Abe, N., Ozaki, T. (2008). Trichostatin A, a histone deacetylase inhibitor, suppresses synovial inflammation and subsequent cartilage destruction in a collagen antibody-induced arthritis mouse model. *Osteoarthritis and Cartilage*, *16*(6), 723-732.

Newman, A. B., Haggerty, C. L., Goodpaster, B., Harris, T., Kritchevsky, S., Nevitt, M., Visser, M. (2003). Strength and muscle quality in a well-functioning cohort of older adults: the Health, Aging and Body Composition Study. *Journal of the American Geriatrics Society*, *51*(3), 323-330.

Papathanasiou, I., Kostopoulou, F., Malizos, K. N., & Tsezou, A. (2015). DNA methylation regulates sclerostin (SOST) expression in osteoarthritic chondrocytes by bone morphogenetic protein 2 (BMP-2) induced changes in Smads binding affinity to the CpG region of SOST promoter. *Arthritis Research & Therapy*, *17*(1), 1-10.

Ping Li, Y., Chun Wei, X., Cui Li, P., Wei Chen, C., Hu Wang, X., Jiao, Q., Wei, L. (2015). The role of miRNAs in cartilage homeostasis. *Current Genomics*, *16*(6), 393-404.

Prokhortchouk, E., & Defossez, P.-A. (2008). The cell biology of DNA methylation in mammals. *Biochimica et Biophysica Acta (BBA)-Molecular Cell Research*, *1783*(11), 2167-2173.

Reynard, L. N., Bui, C., Canty-Laird, E. G., Young, D. A., & Loughlin, J. (2011). Expression of the osteoarthritis-associated gene GDF5 is modulated epigenetically by DNA methylation. *Human Molecular Genetics*, *20*(17), 3450-3460.

Roach, H. I., Yamada, N., Cheung, K. S., Tilley, S., Clarke, N. M., Oreffo, R. O., Bronner, F. (2005). Association between the abnormal expression of matrix-degrading enzymes by human osteoarthritic chondrocytes and demethylation of specific CpG sites in the promoter regions. *Arthritis & Rheumatism: Official Journal of the American College of Rheumatology*, *52*(10), 3110-3124.

Russo, V. E., Martienssen, R. A., & Riggs, A. D. (1996). *Epigenetic Mechanisms of Gene Regulation*. Cold Spring Harbor Laboratory Press.

Sandell, L. J. (2012). Etiology of osteoarthritis: genetics and synovial joint development. *Nature Reviews Rheumatology*, *8*(2), 77-89.

Schurz, J., & Ribitsch, V. (1987). Rheology of synovial fluid. *Biorheology*, *24*(4), 385-399.

Shen, J., Li, S., & Chen, D. (2014). TGF-β signaling and the development of osteoarthritis. *Bone Research*, *2*(1), 1-7.

Song, J., Ahn, C., Chun, C. H., & Jin, E. J. (2014). A long non-coding RNA, GAS5, plays a critical role in the regulation of miR-21 during osteoarthritis. *Journal of Orthopaedic Research*, *32*(12), 1628-1635.

Swingler, T. E., Wheeler, G., Carmont, V., Elliott, H. R., Barter, M. J., Abu-Elmagd, M., Münsterberg, A. (2012). The expression and function of microRNAs in chondrogenesis and osteoarthritis. *Arthritis & Rheumatism*, *64*(6), 1909-1919.

Takahashi, A., De Andrés, M., Hashimoto, K., Itoi, E., & Oreffo, R. (2015). Epigenetic regulation of interleukin-8, an inflammatory chemokine, in osteoarthritis. *Osteoarthritis and Cartilage*, *23*(11), 1946-1954.

Tardif, G., Hum, D., Pelletier, J.-P., Duval, N., & Martel-Pelletier, J. (2009). Regulation of the IGFBP-5 and MMP-13 genes by the microRNAs miR-140 and miR-27a in human osteoarthritic chondrocytes. *BMC Musculoskeletal Disorders*, *10*(1), 1-11.

Van den Berg, W. (1999). The role of cytokines and growth factors in cartilage destruction in osteoarthritis and rheumatoid arthritis. *Zeitschrift für Rheumatologie*, *58*(3), 136-141.

Wang, X., Song, Y., Jacobi, J. L., & Tuan, R. S. (2009). Inhibition of histone deacetylases antagonized FGF2 and IL-1β effects on MMP expression in human articular chondrocytes. *Growth Factors*, *27*(1), 40-49.

Wu, X.-F., Zhou, Z.-H., & Zou, J. (2017). MicroRNA-181 inhibits proliferation and promotes apoptosis of chondrocytes in osteoarthritis by targeting PTEN. *Biochemistry and Cell Biology*, *95*(3), 437-444.

Xing, D., Liang, J. q., Li, Y., Lu, J., Jia, H. B., Xu, L. Y., & Ma, X. l. (2014). Identification of long noncoding RNA associated with osteoarthritis in humans. *Orthopaedic Surgery*, *6*(4), 288-293.

Xu, B., Li, Y. Y., Ma, J., & Pei, F. X. (2016). Roles of microRNA and signaling pathway in osteoarthritis pathogenesis. *Journal of Zhejiang University-SCIENCE B*, *17*(3), 200-208.

Yan, C., & Boyd, D. D. (2006). Histone H3 acetylation and H3 K4 methylation define distinct chromatin regions permissive for transgene expression. *Molecular and Cellular Biology*, *26*(17), 6357-6371.

Yan, S., Wang, M., Zhao, J., Zhang, H., Zhou, C., Jin, L., Fan, Q. (2016). MicroRNA-34a affects chondrocyte apoptosis and proliferation by targeting the SIRT1/p53 signaling pathway during the pathogenesis of osteoarthritis. *International Journal of Molecular Medicine*, *38*(1), 201-209.

Zhang, D., Cao, X., Li, J., & Zhao, G. (2015). MiR-210 inhibits NF-κB signaling pathway by targeting DR6 in osteoarthritis. *Scientific Reports*, *5*(1), 1-7.

Zhang, G., Wu, Y., Xu, D., & Yan, X. (2016). Long noncoding RNA UFC1 promotes proliferation of chondrocyte in osteoarthritis by acting as a sponge for miR-34a. *DNA and Cell Biology*, *35*(11), 691-695.

Zimmermann, P., Boeuf, S., Dickhut, A., Boehmer, S., Olek, S., & Richter, W. (2008). Correlation of COL10A1 induction during chondrogenesis of mesenchymal stem cells with demethylation of two CpG sites in the COL10A1 promoter. *Arthritis & Rheumatism*, *58*(9), 2743-2753.

Chapter 21

Effect of Epigenetic Factors on Degenerative Disc Disease

Uğur Özdemir*, MD

Orthopedics and Traumatology Clinic,
Simav Doç. Dr. İsmail Karakuyu State Hospital, Kütahya, Turkey

Abstract

Degenerative disc disease (DDD) is one of the most common spine-related diseases. Its etiology is not exactly known, but recent studies have elucidated that this disease is a complex and multifactorial disease resulting from the interaction of genetic and environmental factors. In general terms, these studies focus on changes in genes encoding the structural components of the intervertebral disc.

Keywords: epigenetic, polymorphism, methylation, disc degeneration

Introduction

Degenerative disc disease (DDD) is one of the most common spine-related diseases, and it is a complex and multifactorial disease resulting from the interaction of genetic and environmental factors (Chan et al., 2006) Pathological changes at molecular and cellular levels, which develop in the annulus fibrosus and nucleus pulposus, are regarded as degeneration. Disc degeneration, mostly occurring in the lower lumbar region, is the most common cause of low back pain.

Structure of the Intervertebral Disc

The intervertebral disc mainly consists of chondrocytes and fibroblasts in the matrix comprised of collagen and proteoglycans. It has a few cells and many extracellular matrices (Buckwalter, 1995).

It comprises two main parts: The nucleus pulposus inside and the lamellar annulus outside. The structure that helps the disc attach to the vertebral body is the cartilage endplate. The nucleus pulposus and annulus fibrosus distribute the load on the disc equally to the vertebral

* Corresponding Author's E-mail: ugurozdemir.md@gmail.com.

In: Epigenetics: Beyond the Genetics and Medicine
Editors: Sevgi Durna Daştan and Nazan Yurtcu
ISBN: 979-8-88697-228-3

endplates and resist compressive loads on the spine (Goupille et al., 1998). The avascular disc tissue is nourished by diffusion from the cartilage endplates.

The fibrogelatinous nucleus pulposus in the center of the disc constitutes about 40% of the cross-sectional area of the disc. It is mainly composed of proteoglycans, water, and a loose network of type 2 collagen and elastin fibers. Aggrecan is the main proteoglycan of the disc. Aggrecan contains chondroitin sulfate and keratan sulfate, which are highly anionic glycosaminoglycan (GAG) chains. These GAGs attract positively charged ions, enabling water to enter the tissue and increasing the volume of the nucleus (Comper and Laurent, 1978). Accordingly, the osmotic pressure required for the compressive resistance of the disc is created (Adams and Roughley, 2006). A study investigating the proteoglycan contents of normal and degenerated disc tissues revealed that the amount of aggrecan decreased and, instead, proteoglycans such as decorin and biglycan, which retain less water, increased (Inkinen et al., 1998). This indicates that the hydrodynamic and viscoelastic characteristics of the disc tissue depend on aggrecan.

The annulus fibrosus is the peripheral structure surrounding the nucleus pulposus with 12 concentric lamellae. It helps to maintain the shape and integrity of the disc. The lamellae of the annulus fibrosus contain type 1 collagen fibers and extend obliquely at an angle of around 30 degrees between the vertebral bodies. In each lamella, collagen fibers have reverse orientation. All these ensure the compression, torsion, and flexion capabilities of the disc (Adams and Roughley, 2006).

Pathogenesis

Disc cells balance the construction and destruction of the matrix by synthesizing matrix molecules and matrix metalloproteinases (MMPs). The impairment of this balance leads to loss of density in the matrix, and disc degeneration develops with the impact of mechanical stresses (Roberts et al., 2000).

The degenerative process in the disc tissue is assumed to start as a result of the impairment in the cartilage endplates (Schmorl and Junghanns, 1971). As a result of the impaired diffusion, lactic acid accumulates in the disc, and the pH value decreases. A low pH value leads to denser inflammation cells within the disc. With increased protease activation, the amount of proteoglycan in the nucleus decreases, and type 2 collagen is denatured and is usually replaced by type 1 collagen. As a result, the density of the matrix decreases, and the scar tissue appears. The migration of the scar tissue impairs the fibrocartilaginous structure of the annulus, resulting in tears in the annulus and the development of disc hernias (Herkowitz et al., 2004).

Developing in the annulus fibrosus and nucleus pulposus at the molecular and cellular levels, the degenerative process is mostly observed in the lower lumbar region. Segmental instability resulting from lumbar disc degeneration is the most common cause of low back pain. To control this instability-related pain, the lumbar lordosis increases, and hypertrophy of the posterior elements occurs in patients. This situation leads to stenosis in the spinal canal and foramina and results in radiculopathy complaints (Kirkaldy-Willis et al., 1974, Kirkaldy-Willis and McIvor, 1976).

Etiology

The etiology of intervertebral disc degeneration is not exactly known. In addition to some biomechanical and biochemical changes, some environmental and genetic factors also have a role in its etiology. Environmental factors such as aging, overloading, compression on the spine and torsional injuries, smoking, and obesity are the most frequent causes of disc degeneration. Moreover, some recent studies have revealed that genetic and epigenetic factors have an important effect on disc degeneration (Ala-Kokko, 2002, Ikuno et al., 2019). Studies on changes in genes that encode the structural components of the disc constitute a basis for the genetics of disc degeneration (Kawaguchi et al., 1999, Videman et al., 2001).

The genome structures of any two individuals in society are approximately 99.9% identical. Phenotypic differences between individuals emerge because of environmental factors and changes in DNA structure. Nucleotide changes in the exon or intron regions of DNA may influence individuals' predisposition to intervertebral disc degeneration. Meanwhile, in epigenetic events such as gene activation, suppression, and chromatin formation, a correlation is observed between the methylation mechanism, which regulates gene expression, and disc degeneration.

In this chapter, gene polymorphisms and epigenetic methylation mechanisms will be elaborated to reveal the effect of genetic factors on the formation of disc degeneration.

Gene Polymorphism

Polymorphism refers to the different phenotypic allele variations in the same gene region (Sherry et al., 1999). Examples of polymorphism are mostly seen in the non-coded regions of DNA. They are sometimes found in or remarkably close to a gene responsible for the disease, causing a predisposition to certain diseases in societies. More than 90% of the polymorphisms in the human genome are single nucleotide polymorphisms (SNPs) (Collins et al., 1998). Many studies on the genetic factors associated with degenerative disc disease (DDD) have reported some phenotypic variations (Ala-Kokko, 2002). Particularly studies on genes encoding the structural components of the disc constitute a basis for the genetics of disc degeneration (Kawaguchi et al., 1999, Videman et al., 2001).

Collagen Gene Polymorphisms

Collagen is the most plentiful protein in humans and has 28 different types. It acts in the formation of the extracellular matrix with different structural characteristics in different parts of the body. Types 1, 2, 9, and 11 are the collagen types responsible for intervertebral disc degeneration with changes in the genetic chain.

Type 1 collagen is the main collagen of the annulus fibrosus. This type increases the tensile strength of the annulus fibrosus and enables it to resist spinal compression and intra-nucleus hydrostatic pressure. Accordingly, the shape and integrity of the disc are maintained (Ricard-Blum, 2011). Type 2 collagen is the main collagen of the nucleus pulposus, and type 2 collagen binds to each other and increases tissue elasticity (Kadow et al., 2015).

Type 9 collagen enhances structural durability by creating cross-links between different collagen types. Type 11 collagen improves durability by supporting the link between type 2 collagen, proteoglycan, and other collagen types (Kepler et al., 2013).

Type 1 Collagen Gene Polymorphism

Type 1 collagen is created by the binding of two α1 chains and one α2 chain in a helix form. The α1 chain is encoded with the COL1A1 gene, and the α2 chain is encoded with the COL1A2 gene. Many polymorphisms associated with these genes encoding the chains of type 1 collagen have been defined (Martirosyan et al., 2016). The nucleotide polymorphism of thymine (T) in the Sp-1 binding region of the COL1A1 gene has been shown to be associated with intervertebral disc degeneration (Toktaş et al., 2015). Nucleotide polymorphisms increase the synthesis of mRNA and proteins that have a role in the production of the COL1A1 gene. This leads to an imbalance in the synthesis of α1 and α2 chains and weakens the link between type 1 collagen fibers (Pluijm et al., 2004). In a study involving 966 patients over 65 years of age, a 3.6 times higher incidence of disc degeneration was identified in patients with the TT sequence than in those with GT or GG sequences (Pluijm et al., 2004). In another study on 24 soldiers with disc degeneration, it was stated that the TT genotype was observed by 33%, and this sequence was never seen in the control group. The remaining patients were found to have a GT sequence, and this sequence was reported in 41.7% of the control group (Tilkeridis et al., 2005).

Type 9 Collagen Gene Polymorphism

Type 9 collagen is a heterotrimer consisting of the α1, α2, and α3 chains encoded by the COL9A1, COL9A2, and COL9A3 genes (Toktaş et al., 2015). Changes in the structure and function of type 9 collagen influence all three parts of the disc and lead to the development of disc degeneration (Jim et al., 2005). In many studies, nucleotide gene polymorphisms of the COL9A2 and COL9A3 genes were observed to increase the risk of intervertebral disc degeneration (IVDD). In a study conducted on Southern European patients, the COL9A3 Trp3 polymorphism increased the risk of IVDD, but the COL9A2 Trp2 polymorphism had no association with IVDD (Toktaş et al., 2015). A study conducted on 105 patients under 60 years of age revealed that the COL9A2 Trp2 polymorphism did not increase the risk of IVDD (Kales et al., 2004). However, in another study on the Finnish population, patients with the COL9A2 polymorphism were observed to have a 4.5 times higher risk of IVDD compared to the control group (Annunen et al., 1999). In a similar study conducted on the Finnish population, the risk of IVDD was found to be 2.7 times higher in patients with the Trp3 allele. (Paassilta et al., 2001). Accordingly, the Trp2 and Trp3 gene polymorphisms can cause different results in terms of risk factors related to degenerative disc disease in different communities.

Type 11 Collagen Gene Polymorphism

Type 11 collagen in the nucleus pulposus and annulus fibrosus in the disc contributes to the structural integrity of the disc by linking type 2 collagen with proteoglycans and other types of collagen (Kepler et al., 2013). It is a heterotrimer composed of the α1, α2, and α3 chains (Kepler et al., 2013). In a study conducted on the Finnish population, the change in the Guanine-Adenine nucleotide in the 9th intron of the COL11A2 gene was observed to cause a 2.1 times higher increase in the risk of disc bulging (Solovieva et al., 2006). In another study on the genetics of disc degeneration, COL11A2 gene polymorphisms were found to be associated with reduced disc signaling on MRI, whereas COL11A1 gene polymorphisms increased the risk of disc bulging (Videman et al., 2009). In a similar study conducted on 308 patients in Indian society, the COL11A1 gene polymorphism was reported to cause a 1.55 times higher increased risk of disc degeneration (Rajasekaran et al., 2015).

Aggrecan Gene Polymorphism

A proteoglycan consists of a protein nucleus and glycosaminoglycan chains linked to it. Aggrecan is the main proteoglycan of the disc, and its main function is to retain water in the tissue. Aggrecan contains chondroitin sulfate (CS) and keratan sulfate (KS), which are highly anionic glycosaminoglycan (GAG) chains. The KS/CS ratio is high in the nucleus and low in the annulus. These GAGs attract positively charged ions, enabling water to enter the tissue and increasing the volume of the nucleus (Comper and Laurent, 1978). Accordingly, the osmotic property required for the compressive resistance of the disc is formed (Adams and Roughley, 2006). In a study comparing the experimental disc degeneration model and intact disc tissue from histological aspects, the synthesis of aggrecan was observed to decrease significantly (Melrose et al., 1997). This shows that the hydrodynamic and viscoelastic characteristics of the intervertebral disc are associated with aggrecan.

The CS chain contains two binding regions: CS1 and CS2. CS1 contains repetitive sequences (VNTR-variable number tandem repeats), and the number of repeats varies between 13-33. The more VNTR sequences aggrecan has, the higher its ability to retain water and compressive resistance will be (Kawaguchi et al., 1999). Short alleles lead to a decrease in compressive resistance and increased tissue degeneration. In a study reviewing the proteoglycan contents of normal and degenerated intervertebral disc tissues, it was revealed that the amounts of shorter decorin and biglycan, which also retain less water, increased in the degenerated disc tissue, whereas longer chondroitin sulfate chains decreased or disappeared completely (Inkinen et al., 1998).

In studies on aggrecan gene polymorphism, differences have been observed in the allele types and lengths in different societies. The most common types of alleles are A27 (27%), A28 (21.8%), and A26 (18.7%), respectively (Eser et al., 2010). In a study on VNTR polymorphism, the risk of IVDD was higher in people with short alleles containing 18-21 sequences. Meanwhile, it has been reported that these people experience a more severe degeneration process compared to disk degeneration in people with a long VNTR sequence (Kawaguchi et al., 1999). A similar study revealed that people with 13-20 VNTR sequences had a high risk of IVDD, and more than one level of disc degeneration was observed in these people compared to people with long alleles (Eser et al., 2010). There are similar studies on different societies which support this result (Xu et al., 2012, Gu et al., 2013).

Carbohydrate sulfotransferase 3 enzyme (CHST-3) is an important enzyme that enables the sulfation of aggrecan chains and hence contributes indirectly to disc hydration. It is coded by CHST3. In a study conducted on 4043 patients with lumbar disc herniation, the rs4148941 nucleotide polymorphism of CHST3 was found to be a genetic risk factor for IVDD. The study reported that people with the AA or AC genotype had a 1.48 times higher risk of IVDD. In these people with the risk allele A, the low CHST-3 enzyme level observed due to the decrease in CHST3 mRna expression is held responsible for disc degeneration (Song et al., 2013).

Vitamin D Receptor (VDR) Gene Polymorphism

Vitamin D is biologically inactive and has different forms because of differences in its side chain. Vitamin D3 is of animal origin and is synthesized in the skin by ultraviolet rays. Vitamin D2 is obtained from plants and fungi. Vitamin D has 25 hydroxy and 1,25 dihydroxy metabolites, and 1α, 25 dihydroxycholecalciferol (1,25 (OH)2 D3) is its active form. Vitamin D metabolites circulate in the blood by binding to the vitamin D-binding protein (DBP). 1,25 (OH)2 D3, a steroid, enters the cell and acts through the VDR protein, a nuclear receptor. While binding to vitamin D with its hormone-binding region, VDR binds to different nucleotide sequences, called vitamin D response elements, in the target gene with its DNA-binding region and starts functioning.

It is known that VDR has a role in normal bone mineralization and remodeling by acting in Ca+2 and 1,25 (OH)2 D3 metabolism (Haussler et al., 1998). Studies have revealed that VDR is associated not only with bone structure but also with degeneration of nonmineralized connective tissue (Keen et al., 1997, Riggs 1997, Videman et al., 1998). In addition to bone and Ca+2 metabolism, Vitamin D is also important for the sulfation of glycosaminoglycans in the synthesis of proteoglycans (Fernandes et al., 1997, Bolt et al., 2004).

Sulfate homeostasis is regulated by the kidneys. A large part of the sulfate filtered from the renal glomerulus is reabsorbed through the proximal tubules, and only 5-10% is excreted in the urine. Sulfate is transferred from the proximal tubule to the blood through the sodium-sulfate cotransporter (NaSi-1) protein. There are studies suggesting that Vitamin D affects serum sulfate levels, renal sulfate mechanism, and NaSi-1 expression (Fernandes et al., 1997, Bolt et al., 2004). In the study by Fernandes et al., low serum sulfate levels and reduced NaSi-1 expression were observed in mice with vitamin D deficiency (Fernandes et al., 1997). In another study showing the effect of vitamin D amount in the body on sulfate metabolism, a 72% reduction in NaSi-1 expression in the kidney, a 42% increase in urine sulfate excretion, a 50% reduction in serum sulfate concentration, and a 45% reduction in sulfated proteoglycan levels in the skeleton were observed in lack of VDR (Bolt et al., 2004).

For the normal functioning of proteoglycans, which are the most important extracellular matrix components of bone and cartilage, the sulfation mechanism and VDR need to be intact. Therefore, vitamin D deficiency resulting from the polymorphisms of the VDR gene has been asserted to contribute to the emergence of IVDD by causing structural defects in proteoglycans (Chan et al., 2006).

In the *VDR* gene, more than 25 polymorphisms have been reported (Uitterlinden et al., 2004). Nucleotide polymorphisms in DNA and ligand-binding regions are the most common form (Malloy et al., 1997). Nucleotide polymorphisms are often observed in the FokI, TaqI, and ApaI regions. T-C change in exon 2 forms the FokI (ATG>ACG) polymorphism, and T-C change in exon 9 forms the TaqI (ATT>ATC) polymorphism (Zmuda et al., 2000, Park et al., 2006). The FokI polymorphism changes the structure of the DNA binding region, and the TaqI polymorphism changes the structure of the ligand-binding region, influencing the function of VDR for binding to DNA and Vitamin D3 hormone.

FokI and TaqI polymorphisms are the most researched polymorphic regions among the VDR gene polymorphisms. In a study on the FokI polymorphism, disc degeneration was mentioned to be more severe (grade 3-4) in patients with the ff genotype (Eser et al., 2010). In another study on 85 Finnish twins, a low disc signal was observed on MRI in people with Ff and ff genotypes (Videman et al., 1998). A similar study stated that people with the "f" genotype had a 1.58 times higher possibility of developing IVDD (Vieira et al., 2014). In a study on the TaqI polymorphism, another important polymorphic region, disc degeneration was reported to have a milder course (grade 1-2) in patients with the TT genotype compared to the tt genotype (Eser et al., 2010). In the study by Toktaş et al., similar results were obtained and the tt genotype was found to be associated with more severe disc degeneration (Toktaş et al., 2015).

Matrix Metalloproteinase Gene Polymorphisms

Many enzymes are responsible for extracellular matrix destruction of the intervertebral disc. Matrix metalloproteinase (MMP) and ADAMTS are the two most important enzymes responsible for extracellular matrix destruction. Disc cells balance the construction and destruction of the matrix by synthesizing matrix molecules and matrix metalloproteinases (MMPs). The impairment of this balance leads to a loss of density in the matrix, and disc degeneration develops with the impact of mechanical stresses (Roberts et al., 2000). Different MMPs are responsible for the destruction of matrix molecules. MMP-1,8 and 13 are mainly responsible for the destruction of collagens 1, 2, and 3, whereas MMP-2 and MMP-9 are responsible for destroying denatured collagens (Ricard-Blum, 2011).

MMP-1 Gene Polymorphism

In their study on the Chinese population, Song et al., revealed that Guanine and Deoxyribose nucleotide polymorphisms in the MMP-1 gene increased the risk of IVDD. They reported that the risk of IVDD was 1.41 times higher, particularly in people with the D allele, and the main risk allele was the D allele, unlike previous studies (Song et al., 2008).

MMP-2 (Gelatinase-A) Gene Polymorphism

Increased MMP-2 expression in the disc tissue is associated with degenerative lesions (Crean et al., 1997). In their study, Dong et al., observed that the risk of IVDD increased as a result of the 1306C/T polymorphism of the MMP-2 gene, and this risk was 3 times higher in patients with CC genotype. On the other hand, it was suggested that people with the CC genotype had more severe degeneration compared to people with the CT and TT genotypes (Dong et al., 2007). Zhang et al., determined that the 735C/T polymorphism of the MMP-2 gene increased the risk of disc degeneration. They stated that patients with the CC genotype had 2.5 times higher risk of IVDD compared to the TT genotype (Zhang et al., 2013).

MMP-3 (Stromelysin 1) Gene Polymorphism

MMP-3 is the enzyme responsible for the destruction of proteoglycan and collagen contents in the extracellular matrix (Haro et al., 2000). Moreover, it contributes to indirect destruction by activating other MMP enzymes (Takahashi et al., 2001). Studies mostly focus on the 5A allele polymorphism in the promoter region of the MMP-3 gene. In their study on the Japanese population, Takahashi et al., observed that the risk of IVDD increased in elderly patients with 5A/5A or 5A/6A genotype. Likewise, Zawilla et al., reported that patients with the short 5A variant had a 2.5 times higher risk of IVDD, and degeneration was more severe in the 5A variant (Zawilla et al., 2014). Yuan et al., obtained similar results in their study on the Chinese population (Yuan et al., 2010).

MMP-9 Gene Polymorphism

In their study on the Chinese population, Sun et al., found that the 1562C/T polymorphism of the MMP-9 gene increased the risk of IVDD in patients. The risk of IVDD was suggested to be 2.14 times higher in patients with the TT and CT genotypes than in patients with the CC genotype (Sun et al., 2009).

MMP-14 Gene Polymorphism

The MMP-14 enzyme is connected to the cell surface membrane and is responsible for the destruction of small collagen fragments. It also enables the activation of the MMP-2 enzyme. The effect of MMP-14 on disc degeneration is assumed to be caused by the increase in MMP-2 enzyme activity as a result of its overexpression (Zhang et al., 2015). In their study involving 908 patients, Zang et al., found that the 378T/C polymorphism of the MMP-14 gene increased the risk of IVDD. They reported that patients with the TT genotype developed disc degeneration 1.59 times more often than patients with the CC genotype.

ADAMTS (Aggrecanase) Gene Polymorphism

The reduction of aggrecan, which is the main proteoglycan of the intervertebral disc, is associated with the development of disc degeneration. Therefore, the effect of ADAMTS on disc degeneration depends on aggrecan destruction. Studies have mostly concentrated on the relationship between the ADAMTS-4 and ADAMTS-5 enzymes and disc degeneration. In their study involving 482 patients, Liu et al., reported that the 1877C/T polymorphism of the ADAMTS-4 gene increased the risk of IVDD, and this rate was higher in patients with the TT genotype compared to the CC genotype (Liu et al., 2016). Hatano et al., revealed that ADAMTS-4 gene expression increased in herniated discs (Hatano et al., 2006). On the other hand, Rajasekaran et al., found that the risk of IVDD increased 1.28 times in ADAMTS-5 gene polymorphism (Rajasekaran et al., 2015).

Epigenetic Mechanism

The methylation mechanism is the best-known epigenetic mechanism. Methylation refers to the addition of the methyl group (CH3) to a chemical compound. It occurs in two ways: DNA methylation and protein (histone) methylation. In the organism, gene expression and protein functions are regulated accordingly (Weaver 2007).

Protein methylation takes place by adding the methyl group to arginine and lysine amino acids, which are among the amino acids that form the protein. Protein methylation is a system that has been studied mostly for histone proteins and is often referred to as histone methylation. This methylation occurs with the addition of 1, 2, or 3 methyl groups (mono, di, tri-methylation) to the histone protein by histone methyltransferases (HMTs). Methylation of histones checks whether the gene product is formed by activating or repressing the gene expression (Grewal and Rice, 2004).

DNA methylation typically occurs when a methyl group binds to CpG (C; cytosine - P; phosphate - G; Guanine) regions with the DNA methyltransferase enzyme. CpG regions are more observed in the gene promoter regions, in other words, at the beginning of the gene. DNA methyltransferase (DNMT) adds the methyl group to the CpG islands in DNA. In mammals, there are three DNA methyltransferases, called DNMT1, DNMT3A, and DNMT3B (Baylin et al., 1998). Methylation in the promoter region of DNA causes the inactivation of DNA, and methylation in the center leads to increased gene expression (Jones, 2012).

DNA methylation is the most studied epigenetic mechanism whose effect has been investigated. However, there are few studies indicating its association with disc degeneration. Disc degeneration is mainly observed due to deterioration of the anabolic and catabolic balance in the nucleus pulposus. Therefore, Ikuno et al., reviewed different (hypo/hyper) methylation profiles of nucleus pulposus genes in patients with disc degeneration. There were no methylation changes in the genes encoding the matrix components (collagen, proteoglycan) and the genes encoding the molecules that manage the anabolic (TGF-β, IGF-1, BMP) and catabolic (MMP, ADAMTS, proinflammatory cytokines) processes of these components (Ikuno et al., 2019). However, they stated that changes in the methylation profiles of some important molecules in the anabolic and catabolic pathways were responsible for disc degeneration.

In the study, CARD14, WNT5A, YAP1, MAPKAPK5, PRKCZ, SMAD3, IGFBP4, and FGFBP2, among the nucleic genes with changes in methylation profiles, were mainly held responsible for early and advanced disc degeneration.

They stimulate the synthesis of MMP and ADAMTS, which are the enzymes responsible for collagen and proteoglycan destruction of proinflammatory cytokines such as TNF-α, IL-1β, IL-6 and IL-8, during the inflammation (Le Maitre et al., 2007). The activation of nuclear factor-β (NF-β), which induces the transcription of these proinflammatory cytokines, plays a role in disc degeneration. The study reported that the hypermethylation of CARD14, which was observed in advanced disc degeneration, led to disc degeneration by enabling the activation of NF-β (Ikuno et al., 2019). Likewise, EFHD2 and RTKN2 are the other genes observed to cause NF-β activation as a result of hypermethylation and thus disc degeneration (Myouzen et al., 2012). As a result of MAPKAP5 hypermethylation, the MAPK pathway is activated, and the synthesis of catabolic molecules increases. Hence, matrix destruction and degeneration are observed (Ni et al., 1998).

An immunohistochemical study performed by Li et al., stated that Wnt-5a expression increased in degenerated nucleus pulposus tissue (Li et al., 2018). Wnt-5a is an important protein that allows the activation of β-catenin in the Wnt pathway (Li et al., 2018). WNT5A hypermethylation leads to disc degeneration by activating this pathway, which regulates the inflammatory process (De Santis et al., 2018). In the study, WNT5A and YAP1 hypermethylation observed in advanced disc degeneration was reported to result in disc degeneration by intensifying the activation of the Wnt/β-catenin pathway (Ikuno et al., 2019).

TGF-β and IGF-1 are basically the molecules responsible for the anabolic regulation of disc cells (Masuda and An, 2004). TGF-β creates an anabolic effect in disc cells by increasing the synthesis of aggrecan and sulfated glycosaminoglycans (De Santis et al., 2018). The SMAD proteins, which function as signal regulators at TGF-β receptors, have a role in regulating the metabolism of the disc matrix (Li et al., 2005). In the study by Ikuno et al., different methylation changes were noticed in the SMAD3 gene in advanced disc degeneration (Ikuno et al., 2019). In the study, methylation changes were also seen in the CHST1, EXTL3, and SLC26A2 genes that catalyze the synthesis of sulfated glycosaminoglycans (Ikuno et al., 2019).

Hedgehog (Hh) genes are responsible for cell growth and differentiation. The signal protein Sonic Hedgehog (Shh) is secreted in nucleus pulposus cells and is essentially responsible for the growth and differentiation of the intervertebral disc. Ikuno et al., identified methylation differences in the SUFU, TTCIB, and IQCTH genes, which regulate the Hedgehog signaling pathway, and thought this was primarily responsible for disc degeneration (Ikuno et al., 2019).

Conclusion

Degenerative disc disease with complex etiopathogenesis is a multifactorial disease affected by many genes and environmental factors. In addition to the effect of specific genes and some environmental factors, gene-gene, gene-environment, and gene-age interactions may also be effective in the mechanism of this disease. It is important to determine the risk factors of the degenerative disc disease, which is a serious health problem, in order to plan treatment strategies.

References

Adams, M. A., & Roughley, P. J. (2006). What is intervertebral disc degeneration, and what causes it?. *Spine*, *31*(18), 2151-2161.

Ala-Kokko, L. (2002). Genetic risk factors for lumbar disc disease. *Annals of Medicine*, *34*(1), 42-47.

Annunen, S., Paassilta, P., Lohiniva, J., Perala, M., Pihlajamaa, T., Karppinen, J., & Ala-Kokko, L. (1999). An allele of COL9A2 associated with intervertebral disc disease. *Science*, *285*(5426), 409-412.

Baylln, S. B., Herman, J. G., Graff, J. R., Vertino, P. M., & Issa, J. P. (1997). Alterations in DNA methylation: a fundamental aspect of neoplasia. *Advances in Cancer Research*, *72*, 141-196.

Bolt, M. J., Liu, W., Qiao, G., Kong, J., Zheng, W., Krausz, T., & Li, Y. C. (2004). Critical role of vitamin D in sulfate homeostasis: regulation of the sodium-sulfate cotransporter by 1, 25-dihydroxyvitamin D3. *American Journal of Physiology-Endocrinology and Metabolism*, *287*(4):E744-9. doi: 10.1152/ajpendo.00151.2004. PMID: 15165995.

Buckwalter, J. A. (1995). Aging and degeneration of the human intervertebral disc. *Spine*, *20*(11), 1307-1314.

Chan, D., Song, Y., Sham, P., & Cheung, K. (2006). Genetics of disc degeneration. *European spine journal*, *15*(3), 317-325. doi: 10.1007/s00586-006-0171-3. Epub 2006 Jul 4. PMID: 16819621; PMCID: PMC2335375.

Collins, F. S., Brooks, L. D., & Chakravarti, A. (1998). A DNA polymorphism discovery resource for research on human genetic variation. *Genome research*, *8*(12), 1229-1231. PMID: 9872978.

Comper, W. D., & Laurent, T. C. (1978). Physiological function of connective tissue polysaccharides. *Physiological reviews*, *58*(1), 255-315. doi: 10.1152/physrev.1978.58.1.255. PMID: 414242.

Crean, J. K., Roberts, S., Jaffray, D. C., Eisenstein, S. M., & Duance, V. C. (1997). Matrix metalloproteinases in the human intervertebral disc: role in disc degeneration and scoliosis. *Spine*, *22*(24), 2877-2884. doi: 10.1097/00007632-199712150-00010. PMID: 9431623.

De Santis, M., Di Matteo, B., Chisari, E., Cincinelli, G., Angele, P., Lattermann, C., & Kon, E. (2018). The role of Wnt pathway in the pathogenesis of OA and its potential therapeutic implications in the field of regenerative medicine. *BioMed Research International*, *2018*. doi: 10.1155/2018/7402947. PMID: 30410938; PMCID: PMC6205317.

Dong, D. M., Yao, M., Liu, B., Sun, C. Y., Jiang, Y. Q., Wang, Y. S. (2007). Association between the -1306C/T polymorphism of matrix metalloproteinase-2 gene and lumbar disc disease in Chinese young adults. *Eur Spine J.*, *16*(11):1958-61. doi: 10.1007/s00586-007-0454-3. Epub 2007 Aug 7. PMID: 17680282; PMCID: PMC2223336.

Eser, B., Cora, T., Eser, O., Kalkan, E., Haktanır, A., Erdogan, M. O., & Solak, M. (2010). Association of the polymorphisms of vitamin D receptor and aggrecan genes with degenerative disc disease. *Genetic Testing and Molecular Biomarkers*, *14*(3), 313-317. doi: 10.1089/gtmb.2009.0202. PMID: 20367178.

Fernandes, I., Hampson, G., Cahours, X., Morin, P., Coureau, C., Couette, S., & Silve, C. (1997). Abnormal sulfate metabolism in vitamin D-deficient rats. *The Journal of Clinical Investigation*, *100*(9), 2196-2203.

Goupille, P., Jayson, M. I., Valat, J. P., & Freemont, A. J. (1998). Matrix metalloproteinases: the clue to intervertebral disc degeneration?. *Spine*, *23*(14), 1612-1626. doi: 10.1097/00007632-199807150-00021. PMID: 9682320.

Grewal, S. I., & Rice, J. C. (2004). Regulation of heterochromatin by histone methylation and small RNAs. *Current Opinion in Cell Biology*, *16*(3), 230-238. doi: 10.1016/j.ceb.2004.04.002. PMID: 15145346.

Gu, J., Guan, F., Guan, G., Xu, G., Wang, X., Zhao, W., & Yan, J. (2013). Aggrecan variable number of tandem repeat polymorphism and lumbar disc degeneration: a meta-analysis. *Spine*, *38*(25), E1600-E1607. doi: 10.1097/BRS.0000000000000012. PMID: 24296484.

Haro, H., Crawford, H. C., Fingleton, B., MacDougall, J. R., Shinomiya, K., Spengler, D. M., & Matrisian, L. M. (2000). Matrix metalloproteinase-3–dependent generation of a macrophage chemoattractant in a model of herniated disc resorption. *The Journal of Clinical Investigation*, *105*(2), 133-141. doi: 10.1172/JCI7090. PMID: 10642591; PMCID: PMC377425.

Hatano, E., Fujita, T., Ueda, Y., Okuda, T., Katsuda, S., Okada, Y., & Matsumoto, T. (2006). Expression of ADAMTS-4 (aggrecanase-1) and possible involvement in regression of lumbar disc herniation. *Spine*, *31*(13), 1426-1432. doi: 10.1097/01.brs.0000219954.67368.be. PMID: 16741450.

Haussler, M. R., Whitfield, G. K., Haussler, C. A., Hsieh, J. C., Thompson, P., Selznick, S. H., & Jurutka, P. W. (1998). The nuclear vitamin D receptor: biological and molecular regulatory properties revealed. *Journal of Bone and Mineral Research*, *13*(3), 325-349. doi: 10.1359/jbmr.1998.13.3.325. PMID: 952 5333.

Herkowitz, H. N., Jiri Dvorak, Gordon R. Bell, Margareta Nordin, Dieter Grob, International Society for the Study of the Lumbar Spine; (2004). *The Lumbar Spine. (3rd ed)*, Philadelphia, Lippincott Williams and Wilkins.

Ikuno, A., Akeda, K., Takebayashi, S. I., Shimaoka, M., Okumura, K., & Sudo, A. (2019). Genome-wide analysis of DNA methylation profile identifies differentially methylated loci associated with human intervertebral disc degeneration. *PLoS One*, *14*(9), e0222188. doi: 10.1371/journal.pone.0222188. PMID: 31513634; PMCID: PMC6742346.

Inkinen, R. I., Lammi, M. J., Lehmonen, S., Puustjärvi, K., Kääpä, E., & Tammi, M. I. (1998). Relative increase of biglycan and decorin and altered chondroitin sulfate epitopes in the degenerating human intervertebral disc. *The Journal of Rheumatology*, *25*(3), 506-514. PMID: 9517772.

Jim, J. J., Noponen-Hietala, N., Cheung, K. M., Ott, J., Karppinen, J., Sahraravand, A., & Chan, D. (2005). The TRP2 allele of COL9A2 is an age-dependent risk factor for the development and severity of intervertebral disc degeneration. *Spine*, *30*(24), 2735-2742. doi: 10.1097/01.brs.0000190828.85331.ef. PMID: 16371896.

Jones, P. A. (2012). Functions of DNA methylation: islands, start sites, gene bodies and beyond. *Nature Reviews Genetics*, *13*(7), 484-492. doi: 10.1038/nrg3230. PMID: 22641018.

Kadow, T., Sowa, G., Vo, N., & Kang, J. D. (2015). Molecular basis of intervertebral disc degeneration and herniations: what are the important translational questions?. *Clinical Orthopaedics and Related Research*, *473*(6), 1903-1912. PMID: 25024024; PMCID: PMC4418989.

Kales, S. N., Linos, A., Chatzis, C., Sai, Y., Halla, M., Nasioulas, G., & Christiani, D. C. (2004). The role of collagen IX tryptophan polymorphisms in symptomatic intervertebral disc disease in Southern European patients. *Spine*, *29*(11), 1266-1270. doi: 10.1097/00007632-200406010-00017. PMID: 15167667.

Kawaguchi, Y., Osada, R., Kanamori, M., Ishihara, H., Ohmori, K., Matsui, H., & Kimura, T. (1999). Association between an aggrecan gene polymorphism and lumbar disc degeneration. *Spine*, *24*(23), 2456. doi: 10.1097/00007632-199912010-00006. PMID: 10626307.

Keen, R. W., Hart, D. J., Lanchbury, J. S., & Spector, T. D. (1997). Association of early osteoarthritis of the knee with a Taq I polymorphism of the vitamin D receptor gene. *Arthritis & Rheumatism: Official Journal of the American College of Rheumatology*, *40*(8), 1444-1449. doi: 10.1002/art.1780400812. PMID: 9259424.

Kepler, C. K., Ponnappan, R. K., Tannoury, C. A., Risbud, M. V., & Anderson, D. G. (2013). The molecular basis of intervertebral disc degeneration. *The Spine Journal*, *13*(3), 318-330. doi: 10.1016/j.spinee.2012.12.003. Epub 2013 Feb 8. PMID: 23537454.

Kirkaldy-Willis, W. H., McIvor, G. W. (1976). Editorial: Lumbar spinal stenosis. *Clin Orthop Relat Res.*, (115):2-3. PMID: 1253483.

Kirkaldy-Willis, W. H., Paine, K. W., Cauchoix, J., McIvor, G. (1974). Lumbar spinal stenosis. *Clin Orthop Relat Res.,* (99):30-50. doi: 10.1097/00003086-197403000-00004. PMID: 4274946.

Le Maitre, C. L., Hoyland, J. A., & Freemont, A. J. (2007). Catabolic cytokine expression in degenerate and herniated human intervertebral discs: IL-1β and TNFα expression profile. *Arthritis Research & Therapy*, *9*(4), 1-11. doi: 10.1186/ar2275. PMID: 17688691; PMCID: PMC2206382.

Li, T. F., O'Keefe, R. J., & Chen, D. (2005). TGF-β signaling in chondrocytes. *Frontiers in Bioscience: A Journal and Virtual Library*, *10*, 681. PMID: 15569609; PMCID: PMC2647990.

Li, Z., Zhang, K., Li, X., Pan, H., Li, S., Chen, F., & Liu, H. (2018). Wnt5a suppresses inflammation-driven intervertebral disc degeneration via a TNF-α/NF-κB–Wnt5a negative-feedback loop. *Osteoarthritis and Cartilage*, *26*(7), 966-977. doi: 10.1016/j.joca.2018.04.002. Epub 2018 Apr 12. PMID: 29656141.

Liu, S., Wu, N., Liu, J., Liu, H., Su, X., Liu, Z., & Wu, Z. (2016). Association between ADAMTS-4 gene polymorphism and lumbar disc degeneration in Chinese Han population. *Journal of Orthopaedic Research*, *34*(5), 860-864. doi: 10.1002/jor.23081. Epub 2015 Nov 23. PMID: 26495885.

Malloy, P. J., Eccleshall, T. R., Gross, C., Van Maldergem, L., Bouillon, R., & Feldman, D. (1997). Hereditary vitamin D resistant rickets caused by a novel mutation in the vitamin D receptor that results in decreased affinity for hormone and cellular hyporesponsiveness. *The Journal of Clinical Investigation*, *99*(2), 297-304. doi: 10.1172/JCI119158. PMID: 9005998; PMCID: PMC507797.

Martirosyan, N. L., Patel, A. A., Carotenuto, A., Kalani, M. Y. S., Belykh, E., Walker, C. T., & Theodore, N. (2016). Genetic alterations in intervertebral disc disease. *Frontiers in Surgery*, *3*, 59. doi: 10.3389/fsurg.2016.00059. PMID: 27917384; PMCID: PMC5116693.

Masuda, K., & An, H. S. (2004). Growth factors and the intervertebral disc. *The Spine Journal*, *4*(6), S330-S340. doi: 10.1016/j.spinee.2004.07.028. PMID: 15541686.

Melrose, J., Ghosh, P., Taylor, T. K., Latham, J., & Moore, R. (1997). Topographical variation in the catabolism of aggrecan in an ovine annular lesion model of experimental disc degeneration. *Journal of Spinal Disorders*, *10*(1), 55-67. PMID: 9041497.

Myouzen, K., Kochi, Y., Okada, Y., Terao, C., Suzuki, A., Ikari, K., & Yamamoto, K. (2012). Functional variants in NFKBIE and RTKN2 involved in activation of the NF-κB pathway are associated with rheumatoid arthritis in Japanese. *PLoS Genet*, 8(9). doi: 10.1371/journal.pgen.1002949. Epub 2012 Sep 13. PMID: 23028356; PMCID: PMC3441678.

Ni, H., Wang, X. S., Diener, K., & Yao, Z. (1998). MAPKAPK5, a novel mitogen-activated protein kinase (MAPK)-activated protein kinase, is a substrate of the extracellular-regulated kinase (ERK) and p38 kinase. *Biochemical and Biophysical Research Communications*, *243*(2), 492-496. doi: 10.1006/bbrc.1998.8135. PMID: 9480836.

Paassilta, P., Lohiniva, J., Göring, H. H., Perälä, M., Räinä, S. S., Karppinen, J., & Ala-Kokko, L. (2001). Identification of a novel common genetic risk factor for lumbar disk disease. *Jama*, *285*(14), 1843-1849. doi: 10.1001/jama.285.14.1843. PMID: 11308397.

Park, K., Woo, M., Nam, J., & Kim, J. C. (2006). Start codon polymorphisms in the vitamin D receptor and colorectal cancer risk. *Cancer Letters*, *237*(2), 199-206. doi: 10.1016/j.canlet.2005.05.048. Epub 2005 Jul 12. PMID: 16019132.

Pluijm, S. M. F., Van Essen, H. W., Bravenboer, N., Uitterlinden, A. G., Smit, J. H., Pols, H. A. P., & Lips, P. (2004). Collagen type I α1 Sp1 polymorphism, osteoporosis, and intervertebral disc degeneration in older men and women. *Annals of the Rheumatic Diseases*, *63*(1), 71-77. doi: 10.1136/ard.2002.002287. PMID: 14672895; PMCID: PMC1754707.

Rajasekaran, S., Kanna, R. M., Senthil, N., Raveendran, M., Ranjani, V., Cheung, K., & Shetty, A. P. (2015). Genetic susceptibility of lumbar degenerative disc disease in young Indian adults. *European Spine Journal*, *24*(9), 1969-1975. doi: 10.1007/s00586-014-3687-y. Epub 2014 Nov 22. PMID: 25416170.

Ricard-Blum, S. (2011). The collagen family. *Cold Spring Harb Perspect Biol* *3*(1): a004978. doi: 10.1101/cshperspect.a004978. PMID: 21421911; PMCID: PMC3003457.

Riggs, B. L. (1997). Vitamin D–Receptor Genotypes and Bone Density. *New England Journal of Medicine*, *337*(2), 125-126.. doi: 10.1056/NEJM199707103370210. PMID: 9211684.

Roberts, S., Caterson, B., Menage, J., Evans, E. H., Jaffray, D. C., & Eisenstein, S. M. (2000). Matrix metalloproteinases and aggrecanase: their role in disorders of the human intervertebral disc. *Spine*, *25*(23), 3005-3013. doi: 10.1097/00007632-200012010-00007. PMID: 11145811.

Schmorl, G. (1971). The human spine in health and disease. In *The Human Spine in Health and Disease* (pp. xi-504). (2nd ed), New York, Grune and Stratton.

Sherry, S. T., Ward, M., & Sirotkin, K. (1999). dbSNP—database for single nucleotide polymorphisms and other classes of minor genetic variation. *Genome Research*, *9*(8), 677-679. PMID: 10447503.

Solovieva, S., Lohiniva, J., Leino-Arjas, P., Raininko, R., Luoma, K., Ala-Kokko, L., & Riihimäki, H. (2006). Intervertebral disc degeneration in relation to the COL9A3 and the IL-1ss gene polymorphisms. *European Spine Journal*, *15*(5), 613-619.. doi: 10.1007/s00586-005-0988-1.

Song, Y. Q., Ho, D. W., Karppinen, J., Kao, P. Y., Fan, B. J., Luk, K. D., & Cheung, K. (2008). Association between promoter-1607 polymorphism of MMP1 and lumbar disc disease in Southern Chinese. *BMC Medical Genetics*, *9*(1), 1-6. doi: 10.1186/1471-2350-9-38. PMID: 18439317; PMCID: PMC2386444.

Song, Y. Q., Karasugi, T., Cheung, K. M., Chiba, K., Ho, D. W., Miyake, A., & Chan, D. (2013). Lumbar disc degeneration is linked to a carbohydrate sulfotransferase 3 variant. *The Journal of Clinical Investigation*, *123*(11), 4909-4917. doi: 10.1172/JCI69277. PMID: 24216480; PMCID: PMC3809787.

Sun, Z. M., Miao, L., Zhang, Y. G., & Ming, L. (2009). Association between the-1562 C/T polymorphism of matrix metalloproteinase-9 gene and lumbar disc disease in the young adult population in North China. *Connective Tissue Research*, *50*(3), 181-185. doi: 10.1080/03008200802585630. PMID: 19444758.

Takahashi, M., Haro, H., Wakabayashi, Y., Kawa-Uchi, T., Komori, H., & Shinomiya, K. (2001). The association of degeneration of the intervertebral disc with 5a/6a polymorphism in the promoter of the human matrix metalloproteinase-3 gene. *The Journal of Bone and Joint Surgery. British volume*, *83*(4), 491-495. doi: 10.1302/0301-620x.83b4.11617. PMID: 11380116.

Tilkeridis, C., Bei, T., Garantziotis, S., & Stratakis, C. A. (2005). Association of a COL1A1 polymorphism with lumbar disc disease in young military recruits. *Journal of Medical Genetics*, *42*(7), e44-e44. doi: 10.1136/jmg.2005.033225. PMID: 15994869; PMCID: PMC1736100.

Toktaş, Z. O., Ekşi, M. Ş., Yılmaz, B., Demir, M. K., Özgen, S., Kılıç, T., & Konya, D. (2015). Association of collagen I, IX and vitamin D receptor gene polymorphisms with radiological severity of intervertebral disc degeneration in Southern European Ancestor. *European Spine Journal*, *24*(11), 2432-2441. doi: 10.1007/s00586-015-4206-5. Epub 2015 Sep 5. PMID: 26342701.

Uitterlinden, A. G., Fang, Y., Van Meurs, J. B., Pols, H. A., & Van Leeuwen, J. P. (2004). Genetics and biology of vitamin D receptor polymorphisms. *Gene*, *338*(2), 143-156. doi: 10.1016/j.gene.2004.05.014. PMID: 15315818.

Videman, T., Gibbons, L. E., Battié, M. C., Maravilla, K., Vanninen, E., Leppävuori, J., & Peltonen, L. (2001). The relative roles of intragenic polymorphisms of the vitamin D receptor gene in lumbar spine degeneration and bone density. *Spine*, *26*(3), A1-A6. doi: 10.1097/00007632-200102010-00003. PMID: 11224872.

Videman, T., Leppävuori, J., Kaprio, J., Battie, M. C., Gibbons, L. E., Peltonen, L., & Koskenvuo, M. (1998). Intragenic polymorphisms of the vitamin D receptor gene associated with intervertebral disc degeneration. *Spine*, *23*(23), 2477-2485. doi: 10.1097/00007632-199812010-00002. PMID: 9854746.

Videman, T., Saarela, J., Kaprio, J., Näkki, A., Levälahti, E., Gill, K., & Battié, M. C. (2009). Associations of 25 structural, degradative, and inflammatory candidate genes with lumbar disc desiccation, bulging, and height narrowing. *Arthritis & Rheumatism: Official Journal of the American College of Rheumatology*, *60*(2), 470-481. doi: 10.1002/art.24268. PMID: 19180518.

Vieira, L. A., De Marchi, P. L., dos Santos, A. A., Christofolini, D. M., Barbosa, C. P., Fonseca, F. L. A., & Rodrigues, L. M. R. (2014). Analysis of FokI polymorphism of vitamin D receptor gene in intervertebral disc degeneration. *Genetic Testing and Molecular Biomarkers*, *18*(9), 625-629. doi: 10.1089/gtmb.2014.0030. Epub 2014 Jul 9. PMID: 25006683; PMCID: PMC4150369.

Weaver, I. C. (2007). Epigenetic programming by maternal behavior and pharmacological intervention Nature versus nurture: let's call the whole thing off. *Epigenetics*, *2*(1), 22-28. doi: 10.4161/epi.2.1.3881. Epub 2007 Jan 15. PMID: 17965624.

Xu, G., Mei, Q., Zhou, D., Wu, J., & Han, L. (2012). Vitamin D receptor gene and aggrecan gene polymorphisms and the risk of intervertebral disc degeneration—a meta-analysis. *PLoS One*, *7*(11), e50243. doi: 10.1371/journal.pone.0050243. Epub 2012 Nov 28. PMID: 23209686; PMCID: PMC 3509154.

Yuan, H. Y., Tang, Y., Liang, Y. X., Lei, L., Xiao, G. B., Wang, S., & Xia, Z. L. (2010). Matrix metalloproteinase-3 and vitamin d receptor genetic polymorphisms, and their interactions with occupational exposure in lumbar disc degeneration. *Journal of Occupational Health*, 0912140108-0912140108. doi: 10.1539/joh.l8149. Epub 2009 Dec 16. PMID: 20009418.

Zawilla, N. H., Darweesh, H., Mansour, N., Helal, S., Taha, F. M., Awadallah, M., & El Shazly, R. (2014). Matrix metalloproteinase-3, vitamin D receptor gene polymorphisms, and occupational risk factors in lumbar disc degeneration. *Journal of Occupational Rehabilitation*, *24*(2), 370-381. doi: 10.1007/s10926-013-9472-7. PMID: 23975061.

Zhang, J., Sun, X., Liu, J., Liu, J., Shen, B., & Nie, L. (2015). The role of matrix metalloproteinase 14 polymorphisms in susceptibility to intervertebral disc degeneration in the Chinese Han population. *Archives of Medical Science*, *11*(4), 801-806. doi: 10.5114/aoms.2015.53301. Epub 2015 Aug 11. PMID: 26322093; PMCID: PMC4548033.

Zhang, Y., Gu, Z., & Qiu, G. (2013). Association of the polymorphism of MMP2 with the risk and severity of lumbar disc degeneration in the Chinese Han population. *Eur Rev Med Pharmacol Sci*, *17*(13), 1830-4. PMID: 23852912.

Zmuda, J. M., Cauley, J. A., & Ferrell, R. E. (2000). Molecular epidemiology of vitamin D receptor gene variants. *Epidemiologic Reviews*, *22*(2), 203-217. doi: 10.1093/oxfordjournals.epirev.a018033. PMID: 11218372.

Chapter 22

Epigenetics in Scoliosis

Ömer Bozduman[1,*], MD and Selim Görgün[2], MD

[1]Department of Orthopedics and Traumatology,
Samsun Training and Research Hospital, Samsun University, Samsun, Turkey
[2]Department of Microbiology and Clinical Microbiology,
Samsun Training and Research Hospital, Samsun University, Samsun, Turkey

Abstract

Spinal deformity in neuromuscular scoliosis is the result of various neurological or muscular pathologies. Loss of muscle tone and weakness, which are often the main symptoms. Sometimes in addition to the clinical picture of muscle retraction, sensitivity disorder, accompanied by mental retardation, and digestive, heart, or respiratory problems. DNA modifications are thought to have a role in epigenetic deterioration and disease formation in congenital scoliosis (CS) that occurs with congenital deformity of the vertebrae. When DNA is extracted from the hemivertebra and spinal process during surgical correction operations, aberrant DNA methylation has been found to be associated with the development of hemivertebrae and congenital scoliosis. In studies conducted in recent years, TGFR1, EGFR, IGF1R, and GHR are in spinal growth stages; Chondrogenic alteration of the SOX9, PAX1, PAX9, and IHH genes and during differentiation; In the cartilage matrix structure of the ACAN, LUM, VCAN, COL1A1, COL2A1, and HAPLN1 genes; It has been shown that the SLC26A2, CHST1, and CHST3 genes are involved in the formation of the extracellular matrix in vivo. In a different study, it has been observed that there is a predisposition to spinal pathologies in the CALM1 gene polymorphism, which is involved in muscle contraction and bone synthesis. Statistical differences were found in the polymorphic distribution of the rs2234693 region of the ER1 gene in patients with double curve, Cobb angle $\geq 40°$, and thoracic curve. In addition, it was determined that there was a difference in the polymorphic distribution of the rs12885713 region in the CALM1 gene in patients with double curves and in the polymorphic distribution of the same gene in patients with thoracic curves.

Keywords: scoliosis, epigenetics, spinal deformity

Introduction

The definition of scoliosis clinically refers to curvature in the coronal plane and radiologically, curvatures exceeding 10 degrees on posteroanterior radiography (Cobb, 1948). Scoliosis is not

[*] Corresponding Author's E-mail: omerbozduman@gmail.com.

In: Epigenetics: Beyond the Genetics and Medicine
Editors: Sevgi Durna Daştan and Nazan Yurtcu
ISBN: 979-8-88697-228-3

only in the coronal plane, but also in all three planes may cause deformities. Scoliosis is etiologically evaluated in 3 groups as idiopathic, congenital, and neuromuscular.

Congenital scoliosis (CS) and Adolescent Idiopathic Scoliosis (AIS) are serious clinical conditions that affect the life standards of patients with its cosmetic effects as well as additional complications. The disease is a spine pathology that has been observed since ancient times and has been the subject of research, followed by different treatment methods. Today, the pathogenesis and origins of the disease, in which successful surgical results are obtained, have been the subject of many studies in the literature.

Idiopathic Scoliosis may affect approximately 80% of the coronal region structure of the spine (Horton, 2002). Idiopathic scoliosis is examined in 3 stages according to age, infantile (0-3 years), juvenile (4-9 years), and adolescent (10 years-maturity).

Although there are over a thousand articles on the etiology of idiopathic scoliosis in the literature, no proven cause has been found yet and the search for the cause continues.

Main hypotheses include genetic factors, hormonal factors, bone and connective tissue abnormalities, and the autonomic nervous system. All the reasons mentioned above were related to their mutual influence on each other.

Spinal deformity in neuromuscular scoliosis is the result of various neurological or muscular pathologies. Loss of muscle tone and weakness, which are often the main symptoms. Sometimes in addition to the clinical picture of muscle retraction, sensitivity disorder, accompanied by mental retardation, and digestive, heart, or respiratory problems.

Neuromuscular scoliosis is classified by the Scoliosis Research Society (SRS) as having central or peripheral motor involvement, or both, or as myopathic (McCarthy, 1999).

Since many neuromuscular pathologies can cause scoliosis, they all have different etiological genetic backgrounds.

Historical Development in Scoliosis Clinic

Hippocrates, in the fifth century BC is considered the first person to describe spinal deformities in the history of medicine and to state that these pathologies can cause back pain. Posture changes and muscle exercises were recommended for the treatment of patients with this clinical condition. In the period of Galen (131-201), different spinal deformity terms such as lordosis, kyphosis and scoliosis entered the literature. In the period of the Dark Ages (400-1000), curvature of the spine was considered a divine punishment. Congenital scoliosis was first described by Ambrosio Paré (1510 -1590) and it was emphasized that this pathology could cause plegia. However, it was necessary to wait until the mid of the 19th century for surgical treatment trials in the treatment of scoliosis (Moen and Nachemson, 1999). After the 1960s, both fusion and rod insertion became the standard treatment method in spinal surgery (Zaydman et al., 2021).

Nowadays, Adolescent Idiopathic Scoliosis (AIS) is a serious spinal pathology that causes spinal deformities in the form of a S-shaped spine, rib hump, and chest curvature. This disease, which affects 2-3% of the general population in the society, is not only a cosmetic defect, but also an important cause of morbidity, especially with serious complications in the cardiovascular and respiratory systems (Zaydman et al., 2021).

DNA modifications are thought to have a role in epigenetic deterioration and disease formation in congenital scoliosis (CS) that occurs with congenital deformity of the vertebrae.

When DNA is extracted from the hemivertebra and spinal process during surgical correction operations, aberrant DNA methylation has been found to be associated with the development of hemivertebrae and congenital scoliosis (Liu et al., 2021).

Biomechanical Causes in Scoliosis

The spine has a vectorially fixed direction of rotation (Stagnara et al., 1982). In a normal spine, the axis of rotation passes through the front of the rib cage. This prevents bending of the thoracic region when compressed. However, if lordosis develops, this forces the vertebrae to overcome the rotational motion, which makes the spine susceptible to bending. This is the reason why the deformity increases in the patient who bends forward, as in the Adams forward bending test (Adams, 1865, Millner and Dickson, 1996).

Anatomical studies have shown that axial deformity in the t4-t9 vertebrae due to the descending thoracic aorta results in rightward bending (Farkas, 1941). Treatment of idiopathic scoliosis depends on age and degree of curvature. Conservative methods used in treatment include corset and physical exercise. Growth-preserving surgery and fusion methods are frequently used surgically. Preop and postop scoliosis surgery pictures Figure 1a-Figure 1b.

Genetic Studies for Scoliosis Pathogenesis

After the millennium and the completion of the draft Human Genome Project (HGP) in 2000, many studies have been conducted on the existence of candidate gene or genes causing AIS. As a result of these studies, the etiology and pathogenesis of AIS were tried to be clarified. In addition, different candidate genes related to connective tissue, bone, and skeletal system development that may cause clinical picture in patients are emphasized. In addition, the effects of adolescence and growth periods on scoliosis were investigated (Cheng et al., 2007; Hawes and O'Brien, 2008).

In the literature on type I collagen A1 and A2 (COL1A1, COL1A2) and type II collagen A1 (COL2A1), fibrillin (FBN1), elastin (ELN), collagen COL1A1, COL1A2 and COL2A1 genes emphasizing the connection between AIS and connective tissue structural proteins. Many studies appear and yet there was no consensus on the effect in these studies. In different studies, the connection of the matrilin-1 gene (MATN1), which encodes a non-collagen protein in the skeletal system, also known as cartilage matrix protein, with scoliosis has been emphasized. In addition, it was determined that there was no relationship between AIS and LOX, LOX1, LOX2, LOX3, and LOX4 genes encoding lysyl oxidase enzymes seen in the collagen and elastin synthesis steps. Although TIMP2 gene promoter polymorphism is not associated with the severity of lumbar spine deformity in scoliosis pathology, it has been shown to increase the clinical picture of thoracic deformity. The effect of the MMP3 gene in the pathogenesis of scoliosis was not found to be compatible in different publications (Zaydman et al., 2021).

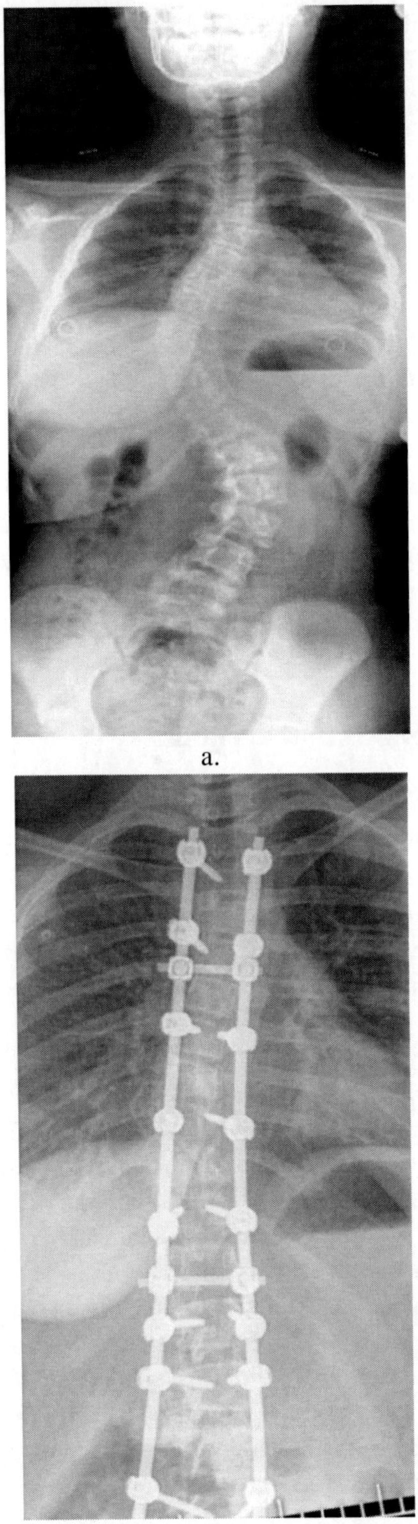

a.

b.

Figure 1. (a) Preop scoliosis fusion surgery; (b) Postop scoliosis fusion surgery.

In the studies, it was found that the deficiency of the (BMP4) gene, which has a role in the synthesis of bone and cartilage, is associated with scoliosis. In this study, it was also stated that the detected promoter polymorphisms of BMP4, IL6, leptin, MMP3, and MTNR1B may have a synergistic effect in the formation of the pathogenesis of scoliosis (Mórocz et al., 2011). In a different study, it has been observed that there is a predisposition to spinal pathologies in the CALM1 gene polymorphism, which is involved in muscle contraction and bone synthesis. Statistical differences were found in the polymorphic distribution of the rs2234693 region of the ER1 gene in patients with double curve, Cobb angle ≥ 40°, and thoracic curve. In addition, it was determined that there was a difference in the polymorphic distribution of the rs12885713 region in the CALM1 gene in patients with double curves and in the polymorphic distribution of the same gene in patients with thoracic curves (Zhao et al., 2009).

In studies conducted in recent years, TGFR1, EGFR, IGF1R and GHR are in spinal growth stages; Chondrogenic alteration of the SOX9, PAX1, PAX9 and IHH genes and during differentiation; In the cartilage matrix structure of the ACAN, LUM, VCAN, COL1A1, COL2A1 and HAPLN1 genes; It has been shown that SLC26A2, CHST1, and CHST3 genes are involved in the formation of extracellular matrix in vivo (Zaydman et al., 2021).

Conclusion

Spinal deformity in neuromuscular scoliosis is the result of various neurological or muscular pathologies. In addition, new studies are needed to show possible relationships between the coding of genes involved in the construction of connective tissue in the organism and the etiopathogenesis of scoliosis.

References

Adams, W. (1882). *Lectures on the Pathology and Treatment of Lateral and Other Forms of Curvature of the Spine*. J. & A. Churchill.

Cheng, J. C., Tang, N. L., Yeung, H. Y., & Miller, N. (2007). Genetic association of complex traits: using idiopathic scoliosis as an example. *Clinical Orthopaedics and Related Research*, 462, 38–44.

Cobb, J. R. (1948). Outline for the study of scoliosis. *Instr. Course Lect. AAOS*, 5, 261-275.

Farkas, A. (1941). Physiological scoliosis. *JBJS*, 23(3), 607-627.

Hawes, M. C., & O'Brien, J. P. (2008). Scoliosis and the human genome project. *Studies in Health Technology and informatics*, 135, 97–111.

Horton, W. A. (2013). Common skeletal deformities. In *Emery and Rimoin's Principles and Practice of Medical Genetics* (pp. 1-10). Academic Press.

Liu, G., Zhao, H., Yan, Z., Zhao, S., Niu, Y., Li, X., Wang, S., Yang, Y., Liu, S., Zhang, T. J., Wu, Z., & Wu, N. (2021). Whole-genome methylation analysis reveals novel epigenetic perturbations of congenital scoliosis. *Molecular Therapy: Nucleic Acids*, 23, 1281–1287. https://doi.org/10.1016/j.omtn.2021.02.002.

McCarthy, R. E. (1999). Management of neuromuscular scoliosis. *Orthopedic Clinics of North America*, 30(3), 435-449.

Millner, P. A., & Dickson, R. A. (1996). Idiopathic scoliosis: biomechanics and biology. *European Spine Journal*, 5(6), 362-373.

Moen, K. Y., & Nachemson, A. L. (1999). Treatment of scoliosis. An historical perspective. *Spine*, 24(24), 2570–2575.

Mórocz, M., Czibula, A., Grózer, Z. B., Szécsényi, A., Almos, P. Z., Raskó, I., & Illés, T. (2011). Association study of BMP4, IL6, Leptin, MMP3, and MTNR1B gene promoter polymorphisms and adolescent idiopathic scoliosis. *Spine*, 36(2), E123–E130. https://doi.org/10.1097/BRS.0b013e318a511b0e.

Stagnara, P. E. I. R. R. E., De Mauroy, J. C., Dran, G., Gonon, G. P., Costanzo, G. I. U. S. E. P. P. E., Dimnet, J., & Pasquet, A. (1982). Reciprocal angulation of vertebral bodies in a sagittal plane: approach to references for the evaluation of kyphosis and lordosis. *Spine*, 7(4), 335-342.

Zaydman, A. M., Strokova, E. L., Pahomova, N. Y., Gusev, A. F., Mikhaylovskiy, M. V., Shevchenko, A. I., Zaidman, M. N., Shilo, A. R., & Subbotin, V. M. (2021). Etiopathogenesis of adolescent idiopathic scoliosis: Review of the literature and new epigenetic hypothesis on altered neural crest cells migration in early embryogenesis as the key event. *Medical Hypotheses*, 151, 110585. https://doi.org/10.1016/j.mehy.2021.110585.

Zhao, D., Qiu, G. X., Wang, Y. P., Zhang, J. G., Shen, J. X., & Wu, Z. H. (2009). Association between adolescent idiopathic scoliosis with double curve and polymorphisms of calmodulin1 gene/estrogen receptor-α gene. *Orthopaedic Surgery*, 1(3), 222–230. https://doi.org/10.1111/j.1757-7861.2009.00038.x.

Chapter 23

Epigenetics in Endometriosis and Endometrial Cancer

Neşe Yeldir*, **MD**
Department of Pathology, Cumhuriyet University, Sivas, Turkey

Abstract

The endometrium is a functional tissue under the control of ovarian steroid hormones. The endometrium shows cyclic changes including biochemical and morphological. These cyclic changes occur with the growth, proliferation, and death of endometrial stromal and glandular cells. Cyclic changes of endometrial tissue are regulated by levels and nuclear receptors of ovarian steroid hormones. During the normal menstrual cycle, epigenetic mechanisms, especially DNA methylation, have important roles in gene expression regulation and influence functional changes.

Epigenetic mechanisms affect gene expression with transcriptional regulation and control endometrial cell proliferation, angiogenesis, desidualization, and embryo implantation. DNA methylation is an essential modification for the normal cell cycle. Abnormal DNA methylation can be associated with abortus and other endometrial pathologies. Recent studies focus also on the combination of epigenetic changes with genetic changes in the development of endometrial pathologies such as endometriosis and endometrial cancer.

The most known epigenetic mechanisms are DNA methylation, post-translational modifications, and non-coding RNAs. Understanding the epigenetic mechanisms and identifying the methylation profile can help create personalized treatment for each patient.

Keywords: proliferative endometrium, secretory endometrium, epigenetic, endometrial cancer, endometriosis, DNA methylation, non-coding RNAs, histon modifications

Introduction

The endometrium, which shows cyclic changes through the effect of ovarian steroid hormones, is a highly dynamic tissue. The endometrial cycle consists of the proliferative phase, secretory phase, and menstrual phase accompanied by cell growth, proliferation, differentiation, apoptosis, and angiogenesis in the endometrial tissue. These phases that are regulated by estradiol, progesterone, and other hormones, include many biochemical and morphological

* Corresponding Author's E-mail: nese.yeldir@gmail.com.

In: Epigenetics: Beyond the Genetics and Medicine
Editors: Sevgi Durna Daştan and Nazan Yurtcu
ISBN: 979-8-88697-228-3

changes. The cellular changes are provided by specific transcriptional regulation, which is controlled by epigenetic mechanisms.

The epigenetic is heritable changes in gene expression that are not caused by alterations in the primary DNA sequence (Waddington, 1942). The basic epigenetic mechanisms are DNA methylation, histone modifications, nucleosome positioning, and non-coding RNAs. Epigenetic changes affect both the normal endometrial cycle and endometrial pathologies. Especially, abnormal epigenetic changes have important role in the development of endometrial pathologies such as endometriosis and endometrial cancer.

Endometrial Cycle

The endometrium is a hormone-sensitive tissue. This tissue is composed of basal and functional layers. The endometrium includes cyclical changes involving cell regeneration, growth, differentiation, regression, and apoptosis on average every 28 days (21-35 days) and undergoes menstrual cycle under control of the ovarian steroid hormones estradiol and progesterone. The menstrual cycle is divided into proliferative, secretory, and menstrual phases. These phases coordinate with phases of the ovulation. The follicular phase of the ovulation cycle corresponds to the endometrial proliferative phase and the ovarian luteal phase corresponds to the endometrial secretory phase.

Menstrual Cycle

Table 1. Menstrual cycle

Menstrual phase — Proliferative phase — Secretory phase

day 0 — 4 — ovulation 14 — 28

Increased hormone	Estrogens	Progesterone
Ovarian cycle	Follicular phase	Luteal phase

The proliferative phase, characterized by proliferation of endometrial glands and stroma, occurs between 4th day and 14th day of the cycle. During proliferative phase, plasma levels of estradiol increase and reach the highest level before ovulation. After ovulation, plasma estradiol levels start to decrease, and progesterone levels increase. The secretory phase occurs between 14th day and 28th day after ovulation. In this phase, the endometrium includes increased vascularity and secretion, as well as the desidualization in endometrial stromal cells. An important feature of the secretory phase is to provide an appropriate environment for embryo implantation. If the embryo does not hold on to the endometrium, endometrial functional layer is shed, and the menstrual phase occurs (Figure 1).

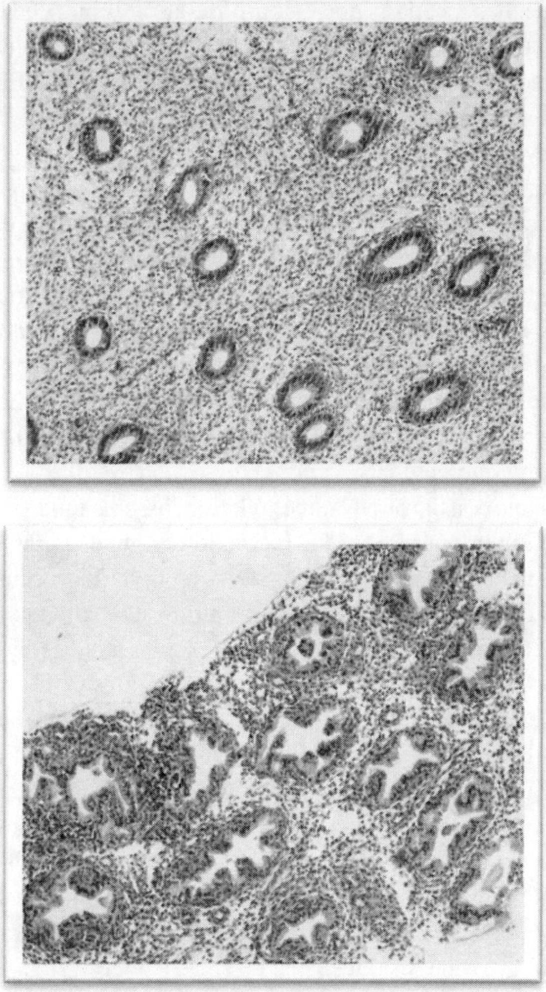

(a)

(b)

Figure 1. (a) Histopathological imaging of the proliferative endometrium. It is seen that proliferate the endometrial tubular glands with columnar cells and dense stroma surrounding these glands; (b) Histopathological imaging of the secretory endometrium. There are larger tortuous glands with secretions.

Epigenetic modifications are defined as any heritable changes in genomic DNA causing transcriptional silencing of DNA. These modifications do not alter the DNA sequence and can be essential or harmful. The cellular processes are regulated by specific transcriptional networks associated with estrogens and progesterone in the endometrial cycle. Epigenetic mechanisms regulate these transcriptional networks and gene expression. Epigenetic changes are involved in fundamental processes such as cell growth, proliferation, differantiation, and diseases in the endometrial tissue (Egger et al., 2004). During the endometrial cycle, chromatin remodeling is crucial for inducing specific transcriptional networks by the hormones.

Different genomic and epigenomic changes occur in different phases of the endometrial cycle. The gene products such as estrogen receptor 1 (ESR1) and insulin-like growth factor 1 (IGF-1) mediate cellular processes during the proliferative phase of the endometrial cycle. The highest levels of expressions of these genes are reached in the proliferative phase. These products bind to their specific receptors and cell proliferation is induced (Zelenko et al., 2012). In addition, genes included in tissue remodeling (MMP26), cell differentiation (HOXA10, HOXA11), vasculogenesis (HOXB7), angiogenesis (CXCR4, ENG, PECAM1) are upregulated in this phase.

During the secretory phase, the endometrium is prepared for the survival of the embryo and most of the gene expression occurs around implantation, which is a progesterone-dependent event. Progesterone affects the estrogen response during the embryo implantation and regulates the inflammatory response, cell death, epithelial, and stromal regulation related to this process (Chi et al., 2020). Several genes of growth factors, such as transforming growth factor alfa (TGFα) and placental growth factor (PIGF), mediate the cellular process and embryo implantation. In the menstrual phase of the endometrial cycle, the genes expressions associated with inflammatory cytokines, angiogenic mediators, cysteine-rich angiogenic inducer 61 (CYR61), hypoxia-induced proteins, vascular endothelial growth factor (VEGF), and matrix metalloproteases are highly increased.

Eginetenic mechanisms consist of DNA methylation, histone modification, and non-coding RNAs and they have an important role for the regulation of gene expression during the normal endometrial cycle (Deans and Maggert, 2015). DNA methylation occurs in cytosines within CpG dinucleotides called CpG islands and is catalyzed by DNA methyltransferase (DNMT). In the human genome, about 80% of all cytosine residues are methylated. However, their patterns vary in different cell types. The human genome contains CpG rich and CpG poor sites. DNA methyl-transferases (DNMT) enzym transfers a methyl group to the fifth carbon of the cytosine for producing 5-methylcytosine. Several DNMT were identified such as DNMT1, DNMT3A, and DNMT3B. Another important components of the DNA methylation mechanism are the DNA methyl-binding protein (MBD) family and TET enzymes. Enzymes of the DNA methylation mechanism can be divided into three groups: writers (DNMT), readers (MBD) and, eraser (TET). The writer enzymes resume the DNA metyhlation pattern, and the reader enzymes recognize and bind to the methylated CpG sites. Also, eraser enzymes remove methylation groups from cytosine residues.

It is known that different endometrial phases show changes in the DNA methylation pattern throughout the endometrial cycle. The changes in DNA methylation patterns are associated with changes in expression levels of DNMT. These expression levels are controlled with ovarian steroid hormones and nuclear receptors of hormones. It has been shown that the expression of enzymes in the endometrium is differantially regulated (upregulated or downregulated) in each endometrial phase and by in vitro hormonal treatment (Yamagata et al., 2009, Retis-Resendiz et al., 2011).

Post translational histone modifications are another epigenetic changes. The chromatin is formed by the nucleosome structures consisting of DNA wrapped around histone proteins. Histone proteins are H2A, H2B, H3, and H4. Acetylation of some histone proteins is regulated by steroid hormones in stromal cells of endometrial tissue. The amino acids in the N-terminal tails of histone proteins that interact with DNA undergo post translational modifications. Acetylation, methylation, phosphorylation, and ubiquitination are some of these modifications. Histone deacetylases associated with gene silencing and reverse these modifications. Different methylations in the same histon can also cause gene activation or silencing.

The histone acetylation levels in the endometrial tissue change during the endometrial cycle. The increase in acetylation can induce several genes and pathways associated with the endometrial epithelial growth, angiogenesis, and cell differentiation. For example, it has been showed that the enrichment of H3K27me3 on the HOXA10 promoter is higher in the proliferative phase compared to the secretory phase. HOXA10 is essential for endometrial embryogenesis and endometrial cycle regulation (Taylor et al., 1998, Munro et al., 2010).

Non-coding RNAs, which are another epigenetic change, are functional RNA structures without protein-coding ability. Non-coding RNAs include small interfering RNAs (siRNAs), microRNAs (miRNAs), PIWI-interacting RNAs (piRNAs), and long non-coding RNAs (lncRNAs). Non-coding RNAs influence histone remodeling complexes and DNMTs for regulating gene expression. In addition, they can regulate gene expression by interacting directly with other RNA molecules (Fang and Fullwood, 2016).

In the endometrium, RNA molecules regulate gene expression and many biological functions. In particular, they have been shown to regulate the embryo implantation and the continuity of pregnancy. However, RNAs have been used as biomarkers for the prognosis of endometrial cancer cases in recent studies (Retis-Resendiz et al., 2011).

Endometriosis

Endometriosis is the presence of endometrial tissue in body regions other than the uterus. It is usually seen in the pelvis, including the ovary, fallopian tube, peritoneum, and less commonly in the bowel, ureter, and caesarean section scar. Endometriosis is an estrogen-dependent disease and occurs in approximately 10% of women of reproductive age. Endometriosis related tumors develop in approximately 1% of patients. These tumors almost always arise in the ovary (Lokuhetty et al., 2020).

Hypotheses about the pathophysiology of endometriosis have been described as due to metaplasia and developed from müllerian remnants. However, the widely believed hypothesis is that retrograde transported endometrial tissue. Endometriosis can demonstrate genetic and epigenetic alterations. Mutations of ARID1A, PTEN, K-RAS, beta catenin/Wnt, and microsatellite instability can occur in endometirosis. These mutations are also believed to have important roles in the development neoplasms from endometriosis (Kajiyama et al., 2019, Koninckx et al., 2019).

The anormal epigenetic changes can induce the pathophysiological pathways that cause the formation of endometriosis. Moreover, aberrant expression of DNMTs was observed in endometriosis tissue (Wu et al., 2007). Elucidating the genetic and epigenetic mechanisms and pathways in the endometriosis will permit to develop more specific agents for the prevention and treatment of this disease.

Endometrial Cancer

Endometrial cancer, along with ovarian and cervical cancers, is one of the common gynecological malignancies worldwide. In recent years, the incidence of endometrial cancer has increased in women. Endometrial cancer usually occurs in postmenopausal women and is typically present with abnormal bleeding. Advanced cases can present with pelvic and abdominal symptoms. Menopausal status, obesity, diabetes, hypertension, and unopposed estrogen are known certain risk factors of endometrial cancer (Leslie et al., 2012).

Two basic types of endometrial cancer have been recognized: type 1 (estrogen related) and type 2 (estrogen unrelated). Type 1 tumors are usually low grade and endometrioid carcinomas (Bokhman, 1983). These tumors morphologically resemble the normal endometrium and originate from endometrial hyperplasia under unopposed estrogenic stimulation (Figure 2). Type 2 tumors are highly aggressive carcinomas that originate from the atrophic endometrium. Type 2 tumors are not related to estrogen stimulation and show morphological features including serous and clear cell carcinomas (Figure 3). There are overlapping clinical, morphological, and molecular features of type 1 and type 2 tumors. Most type 1 tumors show downregulation or mutation of the PTEN gene that causes enhanced activity of the PIK3/Akt/mTOR signaling pathway. In addition, the expression of mutant tumor protein 53 (TP53) and tumor suppressor protein 16 (P16) has been shown to be highly in type 2 tumors (Vallone et al., 2018). In type 1 endometrioid endometrial carcinomas, the most common genetic changes are microsatellite instability, mutations in PTEN, K-ras, B-raf, FGFR2, PI3K, and beta-catenin.

Four groups of endometrial cancer are identified integrating genomic features by The Cancer Genome Atlas. Group 1 tumors characterize with POLE mutations, and they have a good prognosis. Group 2 tumors that have an intermediate prognosis, including microsatellite instability. Group 3 tumors also have an intermediate prognosis and include low-copy-number alterations; and group 4 tumors have a poor prognosis and include high-copy-number alterations and TP53 mutations (Lokuhetty et al., 2020).

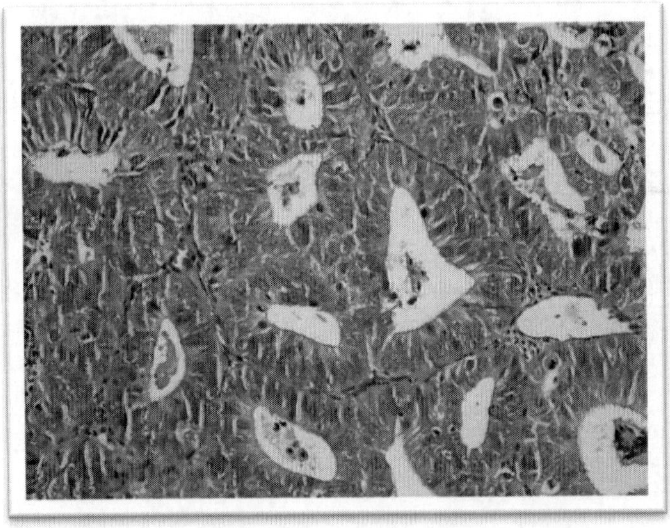

Figure 2. Endometrioid carcinoma, well differentiated: Hyperchromatism, pleomorphism, and mitos are seen in cells of crowded gladular structures.

It is now known that the aberrant DNA methylation can cause the development of endometrial cancer. DNA methylation occurs in cytosines within CpG dinucleotides called CpG islands and is catalyzed by DNA methyltransferase (DNMT). In the human genome, about 80% of all cytosine residues are methylated. The methylation patterns change in different cell types. There are CpG rich and CpG poor sites in the genome.

Promoter hypermethylation is one of the most common epigenetic changes in endometriod endometrial carcinoma. In several methylation studies, hypermethylated tumor suppressor genes and hypomethylated oncogenes have been identified in endometrial cancer. The most known hypermethylated tumor suppressor genes are MLH1, PTEN, p16, APC, MGMT, RASSF1, PR, and CDH1. On the other hand, hypomethylated oncogenes such as BMP, CTCFL, PARP1, and CASP8 are described. Microsatellite instability can present in endometrioid endometrial carcinoma, and it is believed that it provokes changes in many genes associated with DNA repair, apoptosis, and transcriptional regulation during the carcinogenesis process. MLH1 promoter hypermethylation is commonly seen as the mechanism for tumor suppressor gene silencing in endometrial cancers with microsatellite instability. Studies have shown that it is an early change in carcinogenesis.

In endometrioid endometrial carcinoma, PTEN is the most commonly mutated gene, and PTEN promoter methylation may also be associated with advanced stage. Silencing the tumor suppressor genes PTEN and RASSF1A through promoter hypermethylation is related to poor prognosis of the disease. Moreover, MGMT is a silenced DNA repair gene that is present in endometrial cancer and other types of cancer, such as glial tumors.

Recently, HAND2 methylation has been defined in endometrioid endometrial carcinoma. HAND2 is a transcription factor expressed in the endometrial stroma and is found to be hypermethylated in endometrioid endometrial carcinoma and premalignant endometrial lesions (Stampoliou et al., 2016).

Type 2 non-endometrioid carcinoma is more aggressive tumors and mostly invades deeply into the myometrium and spreads extrauterine in the early period. These tumors include different genetic alterations from endometrioid endometrial carcinoma. They are characterized by aberrant p53 mutations. Overexpression of the PI3K/AKT pathway is also observed in these tumors. The PI3K/AKT pathway is a signaling network that regulates the cell cycle and supports cell growth and proliferation.

In addition, non-endometrial carcinoma is associated with Cyclin D1, Cyclin E, and Her2/neu upregulation and reduced E-cadherin gene expression. Loss of progesterone expression is shown in these tumors. Promoter hypermethylation has a less important role in type 2 endometrial carcinoma. DNMT1 and DNMT3B are also downregulated, and this downregulation can cause global hypomethylation in type 2 endometrial carcinoma.

BCOR is an epigenetic regulator gene that regulates cell differentiation. Somatic alterations of BCOR have been described in several types of tumors, such as endometrial stromal sarcoma. Different gene fusions (BCOR-CCNB3, BCOR-MAML3, ZC3H7B-BCOR) and BCOR mutations that cause loss of function can be seen in endometrial stromal sarcoma (Astolfi et al., 2019).

DNA methylation and miRNAs have an important role in the development of endometrial cancer (Banno et al., 2013). There are many methods that have been used to detect DNA methylation such as DNA sequencing, PCR, microarrays, and mass spectrometry. miRNAs can be detected in body fluids of patients with many cancer and can be used as cancer biomarkers to detect the disease.

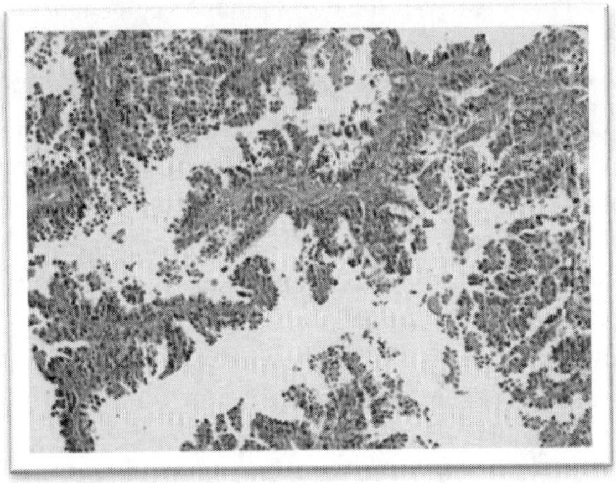

(a)

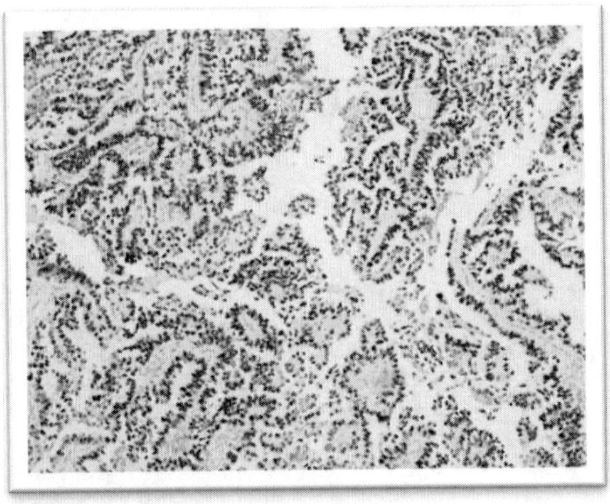

(b)

Figure 3. (a) Serous carcinoma. Papillary structures are seen to consist of cells with high grade nuclei features; (b) There is P53 overexpression in this tumor.

Treatment of the Endometrial Cancer

Endometrial cancer is primarily treated by surgery and is staged. Hysterectomy is usually curative in the early stage endometrial cancers. Advanced endometrial cancers are much more aggressive and fatal. Adjuvant radiotherapy, chemotherapy or hormonal therapy may be applied depending on the risk factors for patients who have undergone appropriate staging and treatment surgery. Chemotherapy is usually chosen for the treatment of metastatic disease (Leslie et al., 2012).

In recent years, studies have focused on increasing numbers of new molecular agents for the treatment of cancer beyond standard chemotherapeutic agents. The new agents that are now in use and in development, blocking important signaling and transcriptional networks in cancer cell. However, it is needed to be more described endometrial carcinogenesis and the molecular pathways which allow malignant cells to escape normal cell cycle. The escape of cancer cells from apoptosis is one of the most important problems in the way of succeeding treatment of patients with endometrial cancer. Aberrant DNA methylation causes the development of apoptosis resistance during endometrial carcinogenesis (Caplakova et al., 2016). It is believed that epigenetic mechanisms can be effective in the development of endometrial cancer, as well as effective in resistance to treatment agents (Balch et al., 2010).

According to further studies using single cell technologies, gene silencing in endometrial cells using CRISPR-Cas9 technology can help to define the specific genes associated with the endometrial pathologies such as endometriosis and endometrial cancer. These studies will provide new data on the endometrial pathologies and new potential therapeutic targets (Hanna and Doench, 2020).

Conclusion

The endometrium is a hormone sensitive functional tissue that undergoes proliferative, secretory and menstrual phases with each menstrual cycle. Genetic and epigenetic alterations play an important role in the regulation of gene expressions and transcriptional networks associated with the cellular processes of the endometrium cycle. Epigenetic changes including DNA methylation, histone modifications, and non-coding RNAs regulate mainly the gene expressions of endometrial epithelial and stromal cells proliferation, angiogenesis, decidualization, and embryo implantation. Moreover, there can be aberrant epigenetic changes in the pathogenesis of endometrial diseases such as endometrial cancer or endometriosis. Abnormal epigenetic changes probably also contribute to implantation failure by preventing the normal menstrual cycle and the formation of a desidualized environment. The definition of epigenetic mechanisms will provide the necessary information to understand the pathogenesis of endometrial diseases and to identify potential therapeutic targets.

References

Astolfi, A., Fiore, M., Melchionda, F., Indio, V., Bertuccio, S. N., Pession, A. (2019). BCOR involvement in cancer. *Epigenomics*, 11(7), 835-855. https://doi.org/10.2217/epi-2018-0195.

Balch, C., Matei, D. E., Huang, T. H., Nephew, K. P. (2010). Role of epigenomics in ovarian and endometrial cancers. *Epigenomics*, 2(3), 419-447. https://doi.org/10.2217/epi.10.19.

Banno, K., Yanokura, M., Kisu, I., Yamagami, W., Susumu, N., Aoki, D. (2013). MicroRNAs in endometrial cancer. *Int. J. Clin. Oncol.*, 18, 186-192. https://doi.org/10.1007/s10147-013-0526-9.

Bokhman, J. V. (1983). Two pathogenetic types of endometrial carcinoma. *Gynecol. Oncol.*, 15(1), 10-17. https://doi.org/10.1016/0090-8258(83)90111-7.

Caplakova, V., Babusikova, E., Blahovcova, E., Balharek, T., Zelieskova, M., Hatok, J. (2016). DNA methylation machinery in the endometrium and endometrial cancer. *Anticancer Res.,* 36(9), 4407-4420. https://doi.org/10.21873/anticanres.10984.

Chi, R. A., Wang, T., Adams, N., Wu, S., Young, S. L., Spencer, T. E., & DeMayo, F. (2020). Human endometrial transcriptome and progesterone receptor cistrome reveal important pathways and epithelial regulators. *J. Clin. Endocrinol. Metab.*, 105(4):e1419-e1439. https://doi.org/10.1210/clinem/dgz117.

Deans, C., Maggert, K. A. (2015). What do you mean, 'epigenetic'?. *Genetics*, 199(4), 887-896. https://doi.org/10.1534/genetics.114.173492.

Egger, G., Liang, G., Aparicio, A., Jones, P. A. (2004). Epigenetics in human disease and prospects for epigenetic therapy. *Nature*, 429, 457-463. https://doi.org/10.1038/nature02625.

Fang, Y., Fullwood, M. J. (2016). Roles, functions and mechanisms of long non-coding RNAs in cancer. *Genomics Proteomics Bioinformatics*, 14(1), 42-54. https://doi.org/10.1016/j.gpb.2015.09.006.

Hanna, R. E., Doench, J. G. (2020). Design and analysis of CRISPR-Cas experiments. *Nat. Biotechnol.*, 38(7), 813-823. https://doi.org/10.1038/s41587-020-0490-7.

Kajiyama, H., Suzuki, S., Yoshihara, M. et al. (2019). Endometriosis and cancer. *Free Radical Biology and Medicine*, 133, 186-192. https://doi.org/10.1016/j.freeradbiomed.2018.12.015.

Koninckx, P. R., Ussia, A., Adamyan, L., Wattiez, A., Gomel, V., Martin, D. C. (2019). Pathogenesis of endometriosis: the genetic/epigenetic theory. *Fertil Steril*, 111(2), 327-340. https://doi.org/10.1016/j.fertnstert.2018.10.013.

Leslie, K. K., Thiel, K. W., Goodheart, M. J., De Geest, K., Jia, Y., Yang, S. (2012). Endometrial cancer. *Obstet. Gynecol. Clin. North Am.*, 39(2), 255-268. https://doi.org/10.1016/j.ogc.2012.04.001.

Lokuhetty, D. White, V. A., Cree, I. A. (Ed.). (2020). *WHO Classification of Tumors: Female Genital Tumors.* Lyon: IARC.

Munro, S. K., Farquhar, C. M., Mitchell, M. D., Ponnampalam A. P. (2010). Epigenetic regulation of endometrium during the menstrual cycle. *Mol. Hum. Reprod.*, 16(5), 297-310. https://doi.org/10.1093/molehr/gaq010.

Retis-Resendiz, A. M., González-García, I. N., León-Juárez, M., Camacho-Arroyo, I., Cerbón, M., Vázquez-Martínez, E. R. (2021). The role epigenetic mechanisms in the regulation of gene expression in the cyclical endometrium. *Clin. Epigenetics*, 13(1), 116. https://doi.org/10.1186/s13148-021-01103-8.

Stampoliou, A., Arapantoni-Dadioti, P., Pavlakis, K. (2016). Epigenetic mechanisms in endometrial cancer. *J. BUON*, 21(2), 301-306.

Taylor, H. S., Arici, A., Olive, D., Igarashi, P. (1998). HOXA10 is expressed in response to sex steroids at the time of implantation in the human endometrium. *J. Clin. Investig.*, 101(7), 1379-1384. https://doi.org/10.1172/JCI1057.

Vallone, C., Rigon, G., Gulia, C., Baffa, A., Votino, R., Morosetti, G., Zaami, S., Briganti, V., Catania, F., Gaffi, M., Nucciotti, R., Costantini, F., Piergentili, R., Putignani, L., & Signore, F. (2018). Non-coding RNAs and endometrial cancer. *Genes*, 9, 187. https://doi.org/10.3390/genes9040187.

Waddington, C. H. (1942). The epigenotype. *Endeavour*, 1, 18-20.

Wu, Y., Strawn, E., Basir, Z., Halverson, G., Guo, S. W. (2007). Aberrant expression of deoxyribonucleic acid methyltransferases DNMT1, DNMT3A and DNMT3B in women with endometriosis. *Fertil. Steril.*, 87, 24-32. https://doi.org/10.1016/j.fertnstert.2006.05.077.

Yamagata, Y., Asada, H., Tamura, I., Lee, L., Maekawa, R., Taniguchi, K., Taketani, T., Matsuoka, A., Tamura, H., & Sugino, N. (2009). DNA methyltransferase expression in the human endometrium: down-regulation by progesterone and estrogen. *Hum. Reprod.*, 24(5), 1126-1132. https://doi.org/10.1093/humrep/dep015.

Zelenko, Z., Aghajanova, L., Irwin, J. C., Giudice, L. C. (2012). Nuclear receptor, coregulator signaling and chromatin remodeling pathways suggest involvement of the epigenome in the steroid hormone response of endometrium and abnormalities in endometriosis. *Reprod. Sci.*, 19(2), 152-162. https://doi.org/10.1177/1933719111415546.

Chapter 24

Epigenetics in PCOS

Sultan Salk*, **MD**
Department of Obstetrics and Gynecology,
Sivas Medicana Hospital, Sivas, Turkey

Abstract

Polycystic ovary syndrome (PCOS) is a common disease in women of reproductive age. Recently, research has shown that the interaction of genomic and environmental factors can modify the clinical condition through epigenetic modifications in the pathophysiology of this disease.

Keywords: epigenetics, polycystic ovary syndrome

Introduction

PCOS affects approximately 5–7% of women of reproductive age. Its clinical features are polycystic ovary's hyperandrogenism, and anovulatory cycle. In these women, insulin resistance, obesity, increase of cardiovascular risk, and atherosclerosis can be found.

Environmental factors influence the clinical condition through epigenetic changes. Genetic and environmental factors acting intrauterine life might determine PCOS develops in life. It is important that epigenetic changes affect gametes, thus affecting future generations.

Epigenetics is molecular events that regulate gene expression without changes in the DNA strain (Chong & Whitelaw, 2004; Jones & Takai, 2001). Epigenetic changes are affected by environmental factors (chemicals, aging, diet, drugs etc.). These changes can occur in the form of DNA methylation, histone modifications, and chromatin changes (Muhonen & Holthofer, 2009; Beisel & Paro, 2011; Shilatifard, 2006; Bonasio et al., 2010). Diseases may occur because of these changes (Bjornsson et al., 2004).

DNA methylation has a role in the development of diseases such as cancer, metabolic diseases, heart diseases, and Polycystic ovary syndrome (PCOS) of fetal origin (Tang & Ho, 2007; Walker & Ho, 2012; Li & Huang, 2008).

The development of PCOS has been studied in animal models such as monkeys, sheep, mice, and rats. It has been shown to occur with prenatal (or perinatal) androgen elevation (Li & Huang, 2008; Dumesic et al., 2007; Xu et al., 2014). PCOS development can be triggered by

---

* Corresponding Author's E-mail: drsultansalk@yahoo.com.

In: Epigenetics: Beyond the Genetics and Medicine
Editors: Sevgi Durna Daştan and Nazan Yurtcu
ISBN: 979-8-88697-228-3

exposure to intrauterine environmental factors and epigenetic mechanisms (Waterland, 2009; Barker, 2004). It is thought that gynecological cancers occur with the effect of intrauterine high estrogen exposure and epigenetic mechanisms with similar mechanisms.

The androgen receptor gene is located on the X chromosome. Studies have been conducted on the role of androgen receptors in the inactivation of the X chromosome in PCOS. In these studies, repeats of the trinucleotide cytosine-adenine-guanine (CAG) were found in the exon 1 part of the androgen receptor. It has been reported that this situation encodes the polyglutamine tract in the transactivation domain and leads to androgen receptor dysfunction (Tut et al., 1997; Beilin et al., 2000; Chamberlain et al., 1994).

Studies have been shown on DNA methylation, which is one of the epigenetic markers in PCOS disease. These studies examined cytosine phosphate guanine (CpG) islands in human promoters. Cytosine methylation is thought to occur in CpG islands. The NIH Roadmap Reference Epigenome Mapping Consortium is developing reference epigenomic maps of human tissues and cells (Saxonov et al., 2006; Maunakea et al., 2010; Lister et al., 2009; Chadwick, 2012).

In women, androgens are produced in the ovaries (Franks & Hardy, 2018), adrenal glands (Burger, 2002), and fat cells (Cadagan et al., 2014). They exhibit their actions through androgen receptors (AR). DNA methylation areas in Androgen receptor (AR), LHCGR (Luteinizing Hormone/Choriogonadotropin Receptor), follicle-stimulating hormone receptor (FSHR) genes were investigated in mice model with PCOS induced by dehydroepiandrosterone (DHEA). It was found that LHCGR methylation in the ovaries of mice was lost (Zhu et al., 2010). This may explain the increased LH level in women with PCOS (Chen et al., 2011).

DNA methylation is increased when the promoter region of the receptor gamma 1 (PPARGC1A) is activated by the peroxisome proliferator. Insulin resistance and high serum androgen levels are associated with decreased PPARGC1A expression in women with PCOS (Zhao et al., 2017). Qu et al., (2021) investigated epigenetic changes peroxisome proliferator-activated receptor gamma 1 (PPARG1), histone deacetylase 3 (HDAC3), and nuclear corepressor 1 (NCOR1) genes of human granulosa cells. They detected hypermethylated CpG regions in PPARG1 genes and hypomethylated CpG regions in NCOR1 genes.

Zhu et al., (2010) reported similar methylation sites in these genes in rats with PCOS. Hyperandrogenism can produce epigenetic changes and lead to ovarian dysfunction.

In another study, methylation levels in the follistatin gene (FST) were measured in women with PCOS and normal women. They reported methylation at only one CpG site. They thought that FST methylation was not associated with PCOS. The limitation in this study was that the body mass index (BMI) of PCOS and normal cases were quite different (Sang et al., 2013).

Recently, microarray techniques have been used for the analysis of differential DNA methylation and gene expression associated with PCOS (Li et al., 2015). Xu et al., (2011) conducted research on visceral adipose tissues in prenatally androgenized (PA) rhesus monkeys. Numerous methylated CpG sites were detected in these tissues. Most of these genes were related to transforming growth factor-β (TGF-β) signaling. The TGF- β signaling lane and the mitogen-activated protein kinase (MAPK) signaling lane have been reported to be involved in PCOS (Cao et al., 2021; Liu et al., 2015). Abnormal levels of the TGF-β family (anti-Müllerian hormone (AMH), inhibin B, activin A, follistatin, and fibrillin 3) have been implicated in PCOS (Jones et al., 2007; Raja-Khan et al., 2010).

It is known that microRNA (miRNA) can lead to the degradation or inhibition of mRNA (Bartel, 2004). Non-coding miRNAs consist of 22 nucleotides. They combine with the RNA-induced silencing complex (RISC) to form double-stranded RNA and generate gene suppression. It has been reported that miRNAs lead to the progression of ovarian tumors by gene expression in human granulosa cells (Toloubeydokhti et al., 2008). It is known that miRNAs have a role in oocyte development and fertility (Hong et al., 2008). Testosterone affects miRNA expression (Delić et al., 2010; Luense et al., 2011). Therefore, it is thought to be PCOS is affected by miRNAs.

Gene instability, DNA damage, and micronucleus formation have been reported in patients with PCOS. These conditions may occur as a result of CpG hypomethylation. In addition, damage to the buccal cells and leukocyte DNA of PCOS patients has been reported (Moran et al., 2008; Nersesyan & Chobanyan, 2010).

There are also studies on histone modifications that play a role in the epigenetic mechanism. Valproate, one of the antiepileptic drugs, stimulates androgen synthesis in theca cells. This occurs through histone acetylation, resulting in increased CYP17 and CYP11A gene expression. This is thought to be similar to the mechanism in women with PCOS who do not use valproate (Nelson-DeGrave et al., 2004).

Hossaini et al., (2019) found that H3K9 di-methylation and DNA methylation and H3K9 acetylation were detected in chromatin of PCOS cumulus cells. HDAC3 is responsible for deacetylations in the lysine 9 (H3-K9) region. Acetylation levels were found in the lysine 9 (H3-K9) region at low levels in the ovaries of the rat PCOS model. Similarly, low levels have been reported in human granulosa cells treated with dihydrotestosterone (Qu et al., 2012). Histone modification is thought to be one of the epigenetic mechanisms in PCOS formation.

In a rat study with S-adenosylmethionine (SAM), the expression levels of several genes associated with ovarian function and insulin release were repaired. (Mimouni et al., 2021).

Conclusion

PCOS is a complex condition confounded by environmental and genetic factors, including miRNA that influence the disease process. There is a role for epigenetics in connecting genotype and phenotype. Epigenetic studies may guide the treatment of PCOS in the future and many studies are needed on this subject.

References

Barker D. J. (2004). The developmental origins of adult disease. *Journal of the American College of Nutrition, 23*(6 Suppl), 588S–595S. https://doi.org/10.1080/07315724.2004.10719428.

Bartel D. P. (2004). MicroRNAs: genomics, biogenesis, mechanism, and function. *Cell, 116*(2), 281–297. https://doi.org/10.1016/s0092-8674(04)00045-5.

Beilin, J., Ball, E. M., Favaloro, J. M., & Zajac, J. D. (2000). Effect of the androgen receptor CAG repeat polymorphism on transcriptional activity: specificity in prostate and non-prostate cell lines. *Journal of Molecular Endocrinology, 25*(1), 85–96. https://doi.org/10.1677/jme.0.0250085.

Beisel, C., & Paro, R. (2011). Silencing chromatin: comparing modes and mechanisms. *Nature Reviews Genetics, 12*(2), 123–135. https://doi.org/10.1038/nrg2932.

Bjornsson, H. T., Fallin, M. D., & Feinberg, A. P. (2004). An integrated epigenetic and genetic approach to common human disease. *Trends in Genetics: TIG, 20*(8), 350–358. https://doi.org/10.1016/j.tig.2004.06.009.

Bonasio, R., Tu, S., & Reinberg, D. (2010). Molecular signals of epigenetic states. *Science (New York, N.Y.), 330*(6004), 612–616. https://doi.org/10.1126/science.1191078.

Burger H. G. (2002). Androgen production in women. Fertility and sterility, *77 Suppl. 4*, S3–S5. https://doi.org/10.1016/s0015-0282(02)02985-0.

Cadagan, D., Khan, R., & Amer, S. (2014). Female adipocyte androgen synthesis and the effects of insulin. *Molecular Genetics and Metabolism Reports, 1*, 254–263. https://doi.org/10.1016/j.ymgmr.2014.05.002.

Cao, P., Yang, W., Wang, P., Li, X., & Nashun, B. (2021). Characterization of DNA Methylation and Screening of Epigenetic Markers in Polycystic Ovary Syndrome. *Frontiers in Cell and Developmental Biology, 9*, 664843. https://doi.org/10.3389/fcell.2021.664843.

Chadwick L. H. (2012). The NIH Roadmap Epigenomics Program data resource. *Epigenomics, 4*(3), 317–324. https://doi.org/10.2217/epi.12.18.

Chamberlain, N. L., Driver, E. D., & Miesfeld, R. L. (1994). The length and location of CAG trinucleotide repeats in the androgen receptor N-terminal domain affect transactivation function. *Nucleic Acids Research, 22*(15), 3181–3186. https://doi.org/10.1093/nar/22.15.3181.

Chen, Z. J., Zhao, H., He, L., Shi, Y., Qin, Y., Shi, Y., Li, Z., You, L., Zhao, J., Liu, J., Liang, X., Zhao, X., Zhao, J., Sun, Y., Zhang, B., Jiang, H., Zhao, D., Bian, Y., Gao, X., Geng, L., Zhao, Y. (2011). Genome-wide association study identifies susceptibility loci for polycystic ovary syndrome on chromosome 2p16.3, 2p21 and 9q33.3. *Nature Genetics, 43*(1), 55–59. https://doi.org/10.1038/ng.732.

Chong, S., & Whitelaw, E. (2004). Epigenetic germline inheritance. *Current Opinion in Genetics & Development, 14*(6), 692–696. https://doi.org/10.1016/j.gde.2004.09.001.

Delić, D., Grosser, C., Dkhil, M., Al-Quraishy, S., & Wunderlich, F. (2010). Testosterone-induced upregulation of miRNAs in the female mouse liver. *Steroids, 75*(12), 998–1004. https://doi.org/10.1016/j.steroids.2010.06.010.

Dumesic, D. A., Abbott, D. H., & Padmanabhan, V. (2007). Polycystic ovary syndrome and its developmental origins. *Reviews in Endocrine & Metabolic Disorders, 8*(2), 127–141. https://doi.org/10.1007/s11154-007-9046-0.

Franks, S., & Hardy, K. (2018). Androgen Action in the Ovary. *Frontiers in Endocrinology, 9*, 452. https://doi.org/10.3389/fendo.2018.00452.

Hong, X., Luense, L. J., McGinnis, L. K., Nothnick, W. B., & Christenson, L. K. (2008). Dicer1 is essential for female fertility and normal development of the female reproductive system. *Endocrinology, 149*(12), 6207–6212. https://doi.org/10.1210/en.2008-0294.

Hosseini, E., Shahhoseini, M., Afsharian, P., Karimian, L., Ashrafi, M., Mehraein, F., & Afatoonian, R. (2019). Role of epigenetic modifications in the aberrant CYP19A1 gene expression in polycystic ovary syndrome. Archives of medical science: *AMS, 15*(4), 887–895. https://doi.org/10.5114/aoms.2019.86060.

Jones, M. R., Wilson, S. G., Mullin, B. H., Mead, R., Watts, G. F., & Stuckey, B. G. (2007). Polymorphism of the follistatin gene in polycystic ovary syndrome. *Molecular Human Reproduction, 13*(4), 237–241. https://doi.org/10.1093/molehr/gal120.

Jones, P. A., & Takai, D. (2001). The role of DNA methylation in mammalian epigenetics. *Science (New York, N.Y.), 293*(5532), 1068–1070. https://doi.org/10.1126/science.1063852.

Li, D., Jiao, J., Zhou, Y. M., & Wang, X. X. (2015). Epigenetic regulation of traf2- and Nck-interacting kinase (TNIK) in polycystic ovary syndrome. *American Journal of Translational Research, 7*(6), 1152–1160.

Li, Z., & Huang, H. (2008). Epigenetic abnormality: a possible mechanism underlying the fetal origin of polycystic ovary syndrome. *Medical Hypotheses, 70*(3), 638–642. https://doi.org/10.1016/j.mehy.2006.09.076.

Lister, R., Pelizzola, M., Dowen, R. H., Hawkins, R. D., Hon, G., Tonti-Filippini, J., Nery, J. R., Lee, L., Ye, Z., Ngo, Q. M., Edsall, L., Antosiewicz-Bourget, J., Stewart, R., Ruotti, V., Millar, A. H., Thomson, J. A., Ren, B., & Ecker, J. R. (2009). Human DNA methylomes at base resolution show widespread epigenomic differences. *Nature, 462*(7271), 315–322. https://doi.org/10.1038/nature08514.

Liu, S., Zhang, X., Shi, C., Lin, J., Chen, G., Wu, B., Wu, L., Shi, H., Yuan, Y., Zhou, W., Sun, Z., Dong, X., & Wang, J. (2015). Altered microRNAs expression profiling in cumulus cells from patients with polycystic ovary syndrome. *Journal of translational Medicine, 13*, 238. https://doi.org/10.1186/s12967-015-0605-y.

Luense, L. J., Veiga-Lopez, A., Padmanabhan, V., & Christenson, L. K. (2011). Developmental programming: gestational testosterone treatment alters fetal ovarian gene expression. *Endocrinology, 152*(12), 4974–4983. https://doi.org/10.1210/en.2011-1182.

Maunakea, A. K., Nagarajan, R. P., Bilenky, M., Ballinger, T. J., D'Souza, C., Fouse, S. D., Johnson, B. E., Hong, C., Nielsen, C., Zhao, Y., Turecki, G., Delaney, A., Varhol, R., Thiessen, N., Shchors, K., Heine, V. M., Rowitch, D. H., Xing, X., Fiore, C., Schillebeeckx, M., Costello, J. F. (2010). Conserved role of intragenic DNA methylation in regulating alternative promoters. *Nature, 466*(7303), 253–257. https://doi.org/10.1038/nature09165.

Mimouni, N., Paiva, I., Barbotin, A. L., Timzoura, F. E., Plassard, D., Le Gras, S., Ternier, G., Pigny, P., Catteau-Jonard, S., Simon, V., Prevot, V., Boutillier, A. L., & Giacobini, P. (2021). Polycystic ovary syndrome is transmitted via a transgenerational epigenetic process. *Cell Metabolism, 33*(3), 513–530.e8. https://doi.org/10.1016/j.cmet.2021.01.004.

Moran, L. J., Noakes, M., Clifton, P. M., Norman, R. J., & Fenech, M. F. (2008). Genome instability is increased in lymphocytes of women with polycystic ovary syndrome and is correlated with insulin resistance. *Mutation Research, 639*(1-2), 55–63. https://doi.org/10.1016/j.mrfmmm.2007.11.007.

Muhonen, P., & Holthofer, H. (2009). Epigenetic and microRNA-mediated regulation in diabetes. *Nephrology, Dialysis, Transplantation, 24*(4), 1088–1096. https://doi.org/10.1093/ndt/gfn728.

Nelson-DeGrave, V. L., Wickenheisser, J. K., Cockrell, J. E., Wood, J. R., Legro, R. S., Strauss, J. F., 3rd, & McAllister, J. M. (2004). Valproate potentiates androgen biosynthesis in human ovarian theca cells. *Endocrinology, 145*(2), 799–808. https://doi.org/10.1210/en.2003-0940.

Nersesyan, A., & Chobanyan, N. (2010). Micronuclei and other nuclear anomalies levels in exfoliated buccal cells and DNA damage in leukocytes of patients with polycystic ovary syndrome. *Journal of B.U.ON. : Official Journal of the Balkan Union of Oncology, 15*(2), 337–339.

Qu, F., Wang, F. F., Yin, R., Ding, G. L., El-Prince, M., Gao, Q., Shi, B. W., Pan, H. H., Huang, Y. T., Jin, M., Leung, P. C., Sheng, J. Z., & Huang, H. F. (2012). A molecular mechanism underlying ovarian dysfunction of polycystic ovary syndrome: hyperandrogenism induces epigenetic alterations in the granulosa cells. *Journal of Molecular Medicine (Berlin, Germany), 90*(8), 911–923. https://doi.org/10.1007/s00109-012-0881-4.

Raja-Khan, N., Kunselman, A. R., Demers, L. M., Ewens, K. G., Spielman, R. S., & Legro, R. S. (2010). A variant in the fibrillin-3 gene is associated with TGF-β and inhibin B levels in women with polycystic ovary syndrome. *Fertility and Sterility, 94*(7), 2916–2919. https://doi.org/10.1016/j.fertnstert.2010.05.047.

Sang, Q., Zhang, S., Zou, S., Wang, H., Feng, R., Li, Q., Jin, L., He, L., Xing, Q., & Wang, L. (2013). Quantitative analysis of follistatin (FST) promoter methylation in peripheral blood of patients with polycystic ovary syndrome. *Reproductive Biomedicine Online, 26*(2), 157–163. https://doi.org/10.1016/j.rbmo.2012.10.011.

Saxonov, S., Berg, P., & Brutlag, D. L. (2006). A genome-wide analysis of CpG dinucleotides in the human genome distinguishes two distinct classes of promoters. *Proceedings of the National Academy of Sciences of the United States of America, 103*(5), 1412–1417. https://doi.org/10.1073/pnas.0510310103.

Shilatifard A. (2006). Chromatin modifications by methylation and ubiquitination: implications in the regulation of gene expression. *Annual Review of Biochemistry, 75*, 243–269. https://doi.org/10.1146/annurev.biochem.75.103004.142422.

Tang, W. Y., & Ho, S. M. (2007). Epigenetic reprogramming and imprinting in origins of disease. *Reviews in Endocrine & Metabolic Disorders, 8*(2), 173–182. https://doi.org/10.1007/s11154-007-9042-4.

Toloubeydokhti, T., Bukulmez, O., & Chegini, N. (2008). Potential regulatory functions of microRNAs in the ovary. *Seminars in Reproductive Medicine, 26*(6), 469–478. https://doi.org/10.1055/s-0028-1096127.

Tut, T. G., Ghadessy, F. J., Trifiro, M. A., Pinsky, L., & Yong, E. L. (1997). Long polyglutamine tracts in the androgen receptor are associated with reduced trans-activation, impaired sperm production, and male infertility. *The Journal of Clinical Endocrinology and Metabolism, 82*(11), 3777–3782. https://doi.org/10.1210/jcem.82.11.4385.

Walker, C. L., & Ho, S. M. (2012). Developmental reprogramming of cancer susceptibility. *Nature Reviews Cancer, 12*(7), 479–486. https://doi.org/10.1038/nrc3220.

Waterland R. A. (2009). Is epigenetics an important link between early life events and adult disease? *Hormone Research, 71,* Suppl 1, 13–16. https://doi.org/10.1159/000178030.

Xu, N., Chua, A. K., Jiang, H., Liu, N. A., & Goodarzi, M. O. (2014). Early embryonic androgen exposure induces transgenerational epigenetic and metabolic changes. *Molecular Endocrinology (Baltimore, MD), 28*(8), 1329–1336. https://doi.org/10.1210/me.2014-1042.

Xu, N., Kwon, S., Abbott, D. H., Geller, D. H., Dumesic, D. A., Azziz, R., Guo, X., & Goodarzi, M. O. (2011). Epigenetic mechanism underlying the development of polycystic ovary syndrome (PCOS)-like phenotypes in prenatally androgenized rhesus monkeys. *PloS One, 6*(11), e27286. https://doi.org/10.1371/journal.pone.0027286.

Zhao, H., Zhao, Y., Ren, Y., Li, M., Li, T., Li, R., Yu, Y., & Qiao, J. (2017). Epigenetic regulation of an adverse metabolic phenotype in polycystic ovary syndrome: the impact of the leukocyte methylation of PPARGC1A promoter. *Fertility and Sterility, 107*(2), 467–474.e5. https://doi.org/10.1016/j.fertnstert.2016.10.039.

Zhu, J. Q., Zhu, L., Liang, X. W., Xing, F. Q., Schatten, H., & Sun, Q. Y. (2010). Demethylation of LHR in dehydroepiandrosterone-induced mouse model of polycystic ovary syndrome. *Molecular Human Reproduction, 16*(4), 260–266. https://doi.org/10.1093/molehr/gap089.

Chapter 25

Epigenetics and Preeclampsia

Aslihan Yurtkal* **and Mujde Canday**
Kafkas University, Faculty of Medicine,
Department of Gynecology and Obstetrics, Kars, Turkey

Abstract

Preeclampsia (PE) is a disease that affects pregnant women at rates ranging from 2% to 10%, causing perinatal and maternal morbidity as well as maternal and perinatal mortality. PE is typically characterized by the onset of new hypertension with proteinuria at and after the 20th week of pregnancy; It may be associated with various causes such as inflammatory cytokines and poor trophoblast invasion. Several epigenetic changes can be associated with PE, such as histone modifications, environmental factors, microRNAs (miRNAs), and DNA methylation. In this perspective, the most important epigenetic factor associated with PE; is abnormal DNA methylation during placentation. In addition, acetylation-like histone modifications and low regulation of miRNAs or the effect of ovarian regulation and long non-coding RNAs in various signaling pathways may be involved in the etiology of PE and its epigenetics. PE is associated with low birth weight (LBW) and intrauterine growth restriction (IUGR). When children born as a result of pregnancies with a diagnosis of PE were followed, it was determined that these children were at risk of cardiovascular disease. The cause of PE, which carries serious risks for the mother and the child, is unfortunately not known precisely, and there is no effective treatment to cope with the acute and chronic consequences of the disease. Although it is an obvious fact that the placenta is essential for fetal development, it is known that epigenetic factors have a role in placental processes such as spiral artery remodeling and trophoblast invasion.

Epigenetic mechanisms leading to changes in placental gene expression in PE mediate processes that contribute to the development of placental malfunction, impaired fetal growth, and IUGR, a critical mission in the onset of PE. Lightening the epigenetic processes that conduce to routine placental growth and the triggering incidents in the etiopathogenesis of PE may contribute to the clear etiology of the disease and may lead to the discovery of new treatments.

This review aims to shed light on the epigenetic relationship with PE in light of these perspectives.

Keywords: preeclampsia, epigenetics, DNA methylation, histone modification, miRNA

---

* Corresponding Author's E-mail: aslihan_md@yahoo.com.

In: Epigenetics: Beyond the Genetics and Medicine
Editors: Sevgi Durna Daştan and Nazan Yurtcu
ISBN: 979-8-88697-228-3

Introduction

Vicissitudes in gene expression without heritable changes in the DNA sequence are the common definitions of epigenetics (Stotz & Griffiths, 2016). Influencing how the cell nucleus interprets genes, it includes diversities that occur with the removal and addition of specific molecules from DNA (B. Huang et al., 2014).

Epigenetic alterations may be de novo processes in response to environmental factors besides normal cellular stages such as survival, transcription, signal transduction, progression, metabolism, migration, replication, and damage repair, which profoundly affect numerous organisms (Chao & D'Amore, 2008).

PE is a disease that increases maternal and fetal morbidity and mortality as a cause of severe obstetric complications. (Ananth et al., 2013).

According to United States data, PE affects pregnant women between 5% and 7% and causes approximately 70,000 maternal deaths and 50,000 fetal losses globally. (*WHO Recommendations for Prevention and Treatment of Pre-eclampsia and Eclampsia*, n.d.).

PE is characterized by hypertension with proteinuria and edema at and after 20 weeks of gestation (Ananth et al., 2013).

PE, especially in developed countries, placental pathogenesis is one of the actual reasons for neonatal, fetal, and maternal death (Kleinrouweler et al., 2012).

With the current literature, it is not a routinely used biomarker for PE, and there is no effective treatment method for preeclampsia. Expulsion of the placenta and baby birth is the only treatment option existing in serious cases, as the pathological placenta is believed to be the organ that causes the development of preeclampsia (Leavey et al., 2018).

Although endocrine, genetic, environmental, and immunological factors are thought to be effective in the development of the disease, unfortunately the molecular mechanism, and exact pathogenesis have not been revealed (Espinoza, 2012).

It has been revealed that endothelial dysfunction is the foremost determinant causing PE-related edema, high blood pressure, and proteinuria. PE progression: Many changes in coagulation pathways, such as tissue factor inhibitor and tissue factor, have been reported to contribute significantly to thrombosis (Mastrolia et al., 2015).

The abnormal reason for PE is inaccurate; superficial extravillous trophoblast invasion was concluded in insufficiently reshaped spiral arteries and impaired blood flow to the placenta. (Burton et al., 2009).

Consequently, this process generates stress on trophoblasts and impairs maternal and fetal endothelial function by releasing extracellular vesicles, cell fragments, and micro-particles into the maternal circulation (C. Escudero et al., 2014; J. M. Roberts & Escudero, 2012; Tannetta et al., 2013).

In the light of the available data on the etiopathogenesis of PE, factors such as inflammatory cytokines, weak trophoblast cell invasion, oxidative stress, genetic factors, diet, endothelial dysfunction, and imbalances between antiangiogenic and proangiogenic factors can be counted (Bartha et al., 2002; Granger et al., 2001; Noris et al., 2004; Saftlas et al., 2005).

It is crucial to identify variations in various epigenetic processes associated with PE. Considering that mighty epigenetic alteration may be returned, elucidating epigenetic factors will enable different therapeutic strategies to be suggested. This review aims to reveal epigenetic variations in patients with PE and to create a perspective for studies aiming to create treatment options against these epigenetic factors.

Epigenetic Alterations

The methylation of DNA, post-translational histone modification, and small RNAs are considered epigenetic signals (Bonasio et al., 2010).

DNA Methylation

It is the most widely acknowledged epigenetic process. DNA methylation occurs by adding methyl groups to cytosine in CpG-rich areas of the genome. (Ahmadi et al., 2017). Methylation in DNA has a vital role in the development of advanced organisms. In the methylation procedure, the methyl groups are attached at the position of the 5-cytosine pyrimidine ring or the 6-nitrogen purine adenine ring. Methylation times may show hereditary features with cell division processes. Methylation of DNA is associated with many vital processes, including suppression of transposable elements, inactivation, X-chromosome, carcinogenesis, genomic imprinting, and aging.

Histone Modification

Protein structures called histones are found in eukaryotic living cell nuclei and have a mission in the chromosomes' formation (Kornberg, 1974). Nucleosomes are formed by wrapping DNA strands on histones.

Modifications of histone comprise deamination, ubiquitination, the addition of adenosine diphosphate (ADP)-ribosylation at the tails of histones, phosphorylation, methylation, acetylation, and sumoylation (Kouzarides, 2007).

Through enzymes, stimulating or inhibiting the expression of a gene in mammals is a histone alteration or a combined ADP-dependent chromatin-modification.

Histone deacetylases (HDACs) and sirtuins are enzymes involved in the deacetylation of histones (Im & Choi, 2013).

Arginine and lysine methyl groups in the histone structure are transferred by the histone-modifying enzyme called histone methyltransferase (Lomniczi & Ojeda, 2016).

Non-Coding RNAs

Short non-coding RNAs, long non-coding RNAs (lncRNAs), small RNAs, and messenger RNAs (mRNAs) can be counted as RNA molecules that make up the heterochromatin form (Holoch & Moazed, 2015).

lncRNAs do not code for proteins. lncRNAs with RNA larger than 200 nucleotides are involved in epigenetic changes. They also involve cellular activities such as post-transcriptional changes and gene expressions. They are also involved in X-chromosome inactivation and imprinting processes (Ransohoff et al., 2018). While each lncRNA can undertake multiple tasks with different functions, their role in placental processes has not fully appeared yet. However, lncRNAs have roles in some essential trophoblast functions, which can be expressed as migration and invasion of trophoblasts. The oldest known lncRNA, H19 (Brannan et al., 1990), inhibits apoptosis in trophoblasts by downregulation while inhibiting proliferation (L. Yu et al., 2009). Its presence in the placenta is controlled by PLAGL1. PLAGL1 is the zinc finger transcription factor. H19 is found in a wide imprinted area on the 11th chromosome (Iglesias-Platas et al., 2014).

TUG1, MEG3, MALAT1, and SPRY4-IT1 can be counted among the IncRNAs that have been shown to have a role in placental processes by studies on the expression of IncRNAs in choriocarcinoma cells in vitro. MIR503HG and RPAIN can be added to these IncRNAs along with lincRNA, LINC00629.

While the role of siRNAs in different functions in the cell is the issue, similarly, the intracellular functions of miRNAs vary according to their location. These structures target mRNAs in the cytoplasmic structure and are interrelated in the post-transcriptional silence of genes; in the cell nucleus, they can mediate histone modification and DNA methylation while simultaneously forming an integral component of chromatin (L. C. Li, 2014).

PrimiRNA is transubstantiated to mature miRNA through enzymes called Drosha and Dicer within the nucleus with the cytoplasm. miRNAs; aim at particular mRNAs by conjunctive to its 30 untranslated regions (UTR) (Hammond, 2015).

Depending on their location in the cell, lncRNAs such as miRNA and siRNA own various functions within the cytoplasm and play a role in the control of miRNA action, gene regulation, siRNA formation, protein, and mRNA stability (Khorkova et al., 2015).

PE and Epigenetic Changes

Considering the epigenetic factors in the etiopathogenesis of PE, the most frequently revealed studies are the methylation patterns that occur during the growth of the placenta (Huppertz, 2018; Jankovic-Karasoulos et al., 2018; Kamrani et al., 2019).

DNA hypomethylation and hypermethylation patterns have been studied in the differentiation and regulation processes of trophoblastic cells used in the present studies. (Gamage et al., 2018). By revealing epigenetic factors, the DNA methylation process determined the methylation patterns of the HSD11B2, RUNX3, and LINE-1 genes. (Majchrzak-Celińska et al., 2017).

Apart from methylation, deacetylation or acetylation mechanisms are also involved in histone modifications and epigenetic processes.

HDAC inhibition resulting from H3 acetylation detected in the JEG-3 cell line results in up-regulation of pregnancy-associated glycoproteins (Abell et al., 2011; Camolotto et al., 2013).

The acetylation of H2A and H2B is also an example of the acetylation model.

It occurs in murine trophoblast stem cells named MAP3K4. Deacetylation processes are functional epigenetic determinants when HDAC effects are taken into account.

Non-coding RNAs are one of the widespread epigenetic promoters. These are the untranslated region (UTRs) components. Studies on epigenetic processes in the literature are often associated with lncRNAs and miRNAs. Considering the adverse processes related to the placental development process in the etiopathogenesis of PE, the presence of lncRNA has been revealed. Many lncRNAs possess the ability to regulate the migration and invasion of trophoblastic cells during placental development.

PE and DNA Methylation

Evidence from studies shows that it is often emphasized that DNA methylation has a vital role in placental processes and the function of the placenta. Based on this point, it can be suggested that DNA methylation is associated with pregnancy complications such as preeclampsia and IUGR. (Jankovic-Karasoulos et al., 2018).

In the diagnosis of preeclampsia, which has an important place among the hypertensive diseases of pregnancy, PE-related DNA methylation is the most important factor among epigenetic changes. Abnormal DNA methylation during placentation is involved in the etiopathogenesis of PE. Changing global DNA patterns in preeclamptic placentas are correlated with maternal blood pressure (Gao et al., 2011; Julian et al., 2015; Kulkarni et al., 2011).

Xuan et al. formed 12 PE patients, and the same number of control groups confronted DNA methylation alterations and determined different amounts of methylation in patients with PE according to the number of promoters containing high, medium, and low CpG (Xuan et al., 2016).

Studies have suggested that differentially methylated regions (DMRs) in the placenta of patients with PE are correlated with the expression of genes associated with endothelial dysfunctions, inflammation, apoptosis, and trophoblastic adhesion, differentiation, and invasion disorders, which are effective in the etiopathogenesis of the disease (Bellido et al., 2010; Chu et al., 2014; Sundrani et al., 2013; Yeung et al., 2016).

Considering the methylation levels in the DMR regions, a difference was made between preterm preeclampsia and term preeclampsia, and more DMR related to altered cell adhesion was demonstrated, especially in preterm preeclampsia (Anton et al., 2014). Anomalous DMR-related methylation in suppressor genes has been demonstrated in the etiopathogenesis of PE. (Rahat et al., 2017). Animal studies on DNA methylation in the placenta revealed remarkable alterations in fetal sex-specific differences in female fetus placentas. (Chu et al., 2014).

11 beta-hydroxysteroid dehydrogenase type 2 is found in the placenta and testis-like tissues and has an essential role in blood pressure regulation by inhibiting mineralocorticoid receptor activation through the HSD11B2 gene that encodes it (Friso et al., 2015).

Majchrzak-Celinska et al. studies have evaluated the relationship between HSD11B2, RUNX3, and LINE-1 genes and PE disease (Majchrzak-Celińska et al., 2017). Majchrzak-Celinska et al. reported hypomethylation templates in HSD11B2, LINE-1, and RUNX3 genes in their study; however, the results were not meaningful when these genes were compared with the control group; however, a positive correlation was demonstrated with LINE-1, RUNX3 and HSD11B2, methylation in patients with PE, with gestational age, delivery of children and birth weight (Majchrzak-Celińska et al., 2017).

Angiotensinogen (AGT) is released in leukocytes, the liver, and the placenta (Gomez et al., 1993). A special form of high molecular weight angiotensin is elevated in the serum of pregnant women (Tewksbury, 1996). Hypomethylation of AGT in patients with PE resulted in increased AGT transcription and blood pressure. Some studies observed hypomethylation patterns in angiotensinogen (Anton & Brosnihan, 2008).

Mammary serine protease inhibitor (MASPIN) hypomethylation has been detected in extravillous trophoblasts, which has been shown to play an essential role in the invasion and migration process in trophoblastic cells; researchers correlated hypoxic states in PE with up-regulation of MASPIN (Shi et al., 2015).

In the study by Wong et al., the adenomatous polyposis coli (APC) gene hypermethylation in placental choriocarcinoma cells was detected; there is an association with the amount of invasion of trophoblasts via the Wnt/beta-catenin (WNT2) pathway. In the same study, it was emphasized that the down-regulation of the APC gene has a role in tumorigenesis and the importance of tumor suppressor genes silencing in pluripotent stem cells for the growth of the placenta. (Wong et al., 2008).

It has been found that sFRP4, a glycol protein that induces the WNT2 route, is down-regulated in the etiopathogenesis of PE (Z. Zhang et al., 2013). WNT2 expression is essential in placental development in reducing the invasion of spiral arteries. WNT2 expression is decreased in patients with PE (Z. Zhang et al., 2013).

WNT2 attaches to the receptors named as Frizzled family, activating the Wnt/β-catenin route. Within studies conducted on rats, WNT2 deficiency; has been revealed that placental defects such as fetal loss, decreased vascularization, and spiral artery invasion is detected (Monkley et al., 1996).

Yeung et al. revealed that DNA methylation increased in the WNT2 promoter area in placentas diagnosed with PE. (Yeung et al., 2016).

Bisphenol A (BPA) is a monomer in the structure of polycarbonate and epoxy resins. Epoxy resins and polycarbonates; are found in plastics. It is an endocrine-distorting chemical.

It imitates the hormone system in the body and disrupts body development.; It can be detected in placental tissues, urine, and serum of pregnant women (Dodson et al., 2012; Peretz et al., 2014).

In a publication on mice, it has been suggested that BPA subjugation during pregnancy affects placental morphology and angiogenesis (Tait et al., 2015).

Studies show a positive correlation between maternal BPA exposure and PE-like findings such as hypertension or circulatory disorders, and studies reveal changes in global DNA methylation levels in mouse placenta exposure to BPA (Nahar et al., 2015; Ye et al., 2017).

Ye et al. showed that if the pregnant woman has come into contact with BPA during her pregnancy, it prevents remodeling of spiral artery and invasion of trophoblast in placental development. Also reported that it caused placentation changes and PE in pregnant mice (Ye et al., 2019).

Fetal endothelial colony-forming cells (ECFC) are the proliferative endothelial progenitor cells. The low activity of ECFC in the etiopathogenesis of PE; has been associated with aberrant fetal ECFC methylation, which causes atypical cellular communication and the Wnt pathway. (Brodowski et al., 2019).

The Homeobox gene family regulates placental growth and is important in placental differentiation and development (Novakovic et al., 2017). Typically, homeoboxes up-regulation is substantial in placental development. In the publication, HOX genes hypermethylation and down-regulation are expressed as distal-less homeobox 5, T-cell leukemia homeobox 1, and HOXA10 found in the human placenta (Novakovic et al., 2017). Considering this study, down-regulation of homeobox appears to be important during late pregnancy.

RASSF1A gene initiator hypermethylation has been derivable in the placenta and has been suggested to possess an act in PE because of its effects on cytotrophoblast growth (Abraham et al., 2018; Chiu et al., 2007).

Matrix metalloproteinases (MMPs) adenosine up-regulation, which act as endopeptidase receptors within nitrogen dioxide, was demonstrated in an association study in the field of epigenetics (Abraham et al., 2018). Curiously, placental growth in the etiopathogenesis of PE is highly likely associated with atmospheric pollution of hypoxic conditions. An enzyme with an essential factor in the regulation of trophoblasts migration (via demethylation of the promoter MMP-9) is TET2 (Rahat, Thakur, et al., 2016). MMPs, which involve in trophoblasts and perform extracellular matrix regulation with endopeptidase activity, are required to invade trophoblast cells.

TET2 enzyme; The promoter region has a fundamental act in the arrangement invading trophoblasts by organizing matrix metalloproteinase-9 (MMP-9) initiator demethylation in the -712 CpG and -233 CpG domains (Rahat, Thakur, et al., 2016).

Li et al., in the PE group in their studies, showed more methylation of the MMP-9 initiator within the -233 bp domain (X. Li et al., 2018).

The Thromboxane A synthase 1 (TBXAS1) gene has been related to epigenetic mechanisms involved in the etiopathogenesis of PE.

Signs of prostacyclin reduction and upregulation of thromboxane have been associated with hypomethylation in the initiator site of TBXAS1. (Saha et al., 2017).

According to Musa et al., their study detected decreased methylation in the initiator region of TBXAS1 located in the neutrophil-like cell line (HL-60 cells) of the thromboxane encoding gene in the etiopathogenesis of PE. In the same study, the authors claimed that tumor necrosis factor-α secretion and increased thromboxane synthase production might also be associated with PE etiopathogenesis (Mousa et al., 2012).

By evaluating the GWAS data, the levels of 5mCs and 5hmCs were measured, and RNA binding protein tyrosine phosphatase receptor type N2 (PTPRN2), fox-1 homolog 1, chloride intracellular channel 6, protocadherin 9, proteinase 3 (ACPA), GATA4, and the coiled-coil domain containing 149 genes were detected to be hypermethylated. The role of PTPRN2 in the epigenetic pathogenesis of PE is intriguing. (Gao et al., 2012).

In the pathogenesis of PE, hypoxia develops at the implantation site due to insufficient perfusion; it damages trophoblasts by increasing (ROS) production, inflammation, and apoptosis (Bosco Becerra et al., 2016; Harmon et al., 2016). It has been demonstrated that DNA methylation changes in the etiopathogenesis of PE effectively affect the expression of genes that regulate processes in the preeclamptic placenta (Yeung et al., 2016). NADPH oxidase 5 are enzymes that control reactive oxygen generation in tumors and the placenta. There are studies in which hypermethylation templates at NADPH oxidase 5 (NOX5) were also revealed within PE. Yeung et al. reported NOX5 CpG domain hypermethylation in the group diagnosed with PE in the same study (Yeung et al., 2016). NOX5 belongs to the NADPH oxidase family and is a fount of reactive oxygen species. Downregulation of NOX5 causes a decrease in proliferation and differentiation, as well as loss of apoptotic potential.

ROS has functions in different processes such as transformation, differentiation, apoptosis, proliferation, and NOX5 gene hypermethylation is related to gravidity pathologies. Yeung et al. reported NOX5 CpG domain hypermethylation in the group diagnosed with PE in the same study (Yeung et al., 2016).

Chelbi and Vaiman suggested in their study that the serine protease inhibitor (SERPIN) gene group members are SERPING1, SERPINE1, and SERPINE2 induced by hypoxia (oxygen deficiency) and are altered for expression in placentas of preeclampsia pregnancies (Abraham et al., 2018). Chelbi et al. found that the initiator of the SERPINA3 was hypomethylated within preeclamptic placenta compared to the normal placentas (Nardozza et al., 2017).

Numerous genome-wide studies have associated abnormal methylation with preeclampsia. Several epigenetic mechanisms separate late-onset and early-onset preeclampsia (E-PE) (Gao et al., 2011). While high expression of DNMT1 resulting in more LINE1 methylation is associated with the pathogenesis of early-onset preeclampsia, similar abnormal methylation patterns are not expected in late-onset preeclampsia. Alike, Yuen et al. declared 34 loci in early-onset preeclampsia against four loci within less methylation in late-onset preeclampsia compared with control pregnancies.

Ma et al. In their study, the authors showed that IGF-1 was considerably attenuated in hypoxic trophoblasts on the preeclamptic placenta, and the pyrophosphate sequence of the IGF-1 initiator was hypermethylated in preeclamptic placentas through DNMT-1. (HTR8) also revealed that IGF-1 expression increased significantly (Ma et al., 2018).

Ruebner et al. showed that the quantity of methylated CpGs initiator of ERVW-1 is associated within decreased gene expression of syncytin-1 in their study and also showed that DNMTs are overexpressed in pathological placentas as in PE disease, and hypermethylation occurs in CpGs located in the ERVW-1 promoter (Ruebner et al., 2013). Zhu et al. evaluated the quantity of 5-methyl cytosine (5mc) and 5-hydroxymethyl cytosine (5hmc) in late-onset preeclamptic women and the control group in their study. They revealed differences in the levels of 5mc and 5hmc in seven genes, including PCDH9, CLIC6, CCDC149, RBFOX1, GATA4, ACAP2, and PTPRN2, when PE disease was compared to the control group (L. Zhu et al., 2015).

Some oncogenes and tumor suppressor genes are involved in the invasion process in trophoblastic cells. Abnormal expressions in these regulatory genes are associated with aberrant initiator methylation, contributing to the pathogenesis of preeclampsia. (Rahat et al., 2014).

NDRG1 (N-myc downstream-regulated gene 1) limits the placental reply to hypoxia by restricting invasion of trophoblast by decreasing the expression of matrix metalloproteinases (MMP-2 and MMP-9) (Fu Y, et al.). Augmented NDRG1 expression decreases the invasion of trophoblast invasion by the ERK/MMP-9 route in preeclampsia.

Impairment of invasion and differentiation in trophoblast cells is a feature of preeclampsia (Rui Zhe Jia et al., 2012). CDX1 (Caudal-associated homeobox transcription factor 1) and CDH11 NDRG1 are modulators of trophoblast differentiation/invasion found to be altered and correlated with DMRs in preeclamptic placentas (Anton et al., 2014). The hypomethylated NDRG1 promoter may describe its overexpression in the placenta with preeclampsia. CDX1 arranges differentiation, proliferation, and invasion of trophoblastic cells by inducing specific signaling pathways such as PI3K, Ras, and Rho. Jiz et al. declared that CDX1 limits the invasion capacity of HTR-8/SV neotrophoblast cells by preventing MMP-9 expression. (R. Z. Jia et al., 2014). The advanced DNA methylation in the CDX1 promoter region was associated with a lower level of mRNA expression in the PE placenta compared to the control group. (Rui Zhe Jia et al., 2012). CDH11 has been shown to have the greatest change (18.3%) in DNA methylation in preterm PE placentas (Maccalman et al., 1996). CDH11 conduces to extravillous trophoblast (EVT) migration and differentiation of trophoblasts; thence, hypermethylation of CDH11 consequences in under-expression of CDH11 mRNA is related to reduced invasion capacity of preeclamptic placental trophoblast

It has been found that overexpression of proteins such as Leptin, Inhibin, sFLT1, and PAPPA in the preeclamptic placenta in the last trimester of pregnancy (Kleinrouweler et al., 2012). In a study, a potent correlation was found among hypomethylation of DNA and expressions of PAPPA-like factors, FLT1, LEP, and INHBA, in the preeclamptic placenta, and it was suggested that the DNA methylation mechanisms might be helpful to as a non-invasive prenatal diagnosis of high-risk pregnancies (Blair et al., 2013; Louwen et al., 2012).

Activation of A2B adenosine receptors (ADORA2B), which has a role in PE disease, has two CpGs that correlate significantly with atmospheric pollutants with methylation levels (Abraham et al., 2018; Iriyama et al., 2015). Huang et al. suggested increased hypermethylation of DNA, which is placental intracellular adenosine-mediated and alters PE-associated placental gene expression. In the study, which revealed that placental adenosine increased in patients with PE; It has been reported that this increase may cause the pathogenesis of PE in two ways, namely ADORA2B and pathogenic autoantibodies produced, and it was determined that the expression of the ADORA2B gene, which encodes the Adenosine receptor, is increased in patients with PE.

Down-regulation of The von Hipper Lindau (VHL) tumor suppressor gene in patients with PE is substantial for intact placental growth (Alahari, Garcia, et al., 2018).

In their study, Alahari et al. drew attention to increasing methylation in a CpG-rich area of the VHL gene in E-PE.

Anderson et al. declared alterations in the methylation of white blood cell genes owned by maternal peripheric blood in the diagnosis of PE in their study (Anderson et al., 2014). They also reported that 64% of the genes examined were related to a considerable methylation income and that 36% of the differentially methylated regions of methylated DNA-binding protein (M-PB) concerned severe methylation reduction.

In their study, Iriyama et al. stated that syncytin-1 is obligatory for villous cytotrophoblastic cell fusion to the multinucleated syncytial trophoblastic cells in the placenta (Iriyama et al., 2015). Studies have shown that syncytin-1 expression is reduced in IUGR, increases liver enzymes, and decreases platelet and the etiopathogenesis of PE (Ruebner et al., 2010).

Hypermethylation has been demonstrated in patients with PE's SPESP1 promoter CpG region. SPESP1 is required for accomplished fertilization by startling fusion of the egg plasma membrane (Fujihara et al., 2010; Wolkowicz et al., 2003).

Yeung et al. found that ALCAM (Activated leukocyte cell adhesion molecule), which is expressed in various structures such as endothelial, hematopoietic, and epithelial cells, was down-regulated in the preeclamptic placenta, and they found ALCAM hypermethylation is higher in the PE group comparing to the control (Yeung et al., 2016).

Ligand Gated Ion Channel 4 (P2RX4; P2X4) and Purinergic Receptor P2X, belonging to the Purinergic receptor family, control cytotrophoblastic apoptosis and differentiation in the placenta by organizing intracellular ion (Kþ/Ca2þ) flux.

Chu. T et al. suggested a correlation between CpG hypomethylation in the P2RX4 initiator and altered transcription of the elevated gene into the trophoblast cell cycle and increased apoptosis in the preeclamptic placenta (V. H. J. Roberts et al., 2006).

The calcitonin-related polypeptide (CALCA) is associated with adaptation of vasodilatation, pain and nerve conduction, Ca++ balance, and angiogenesis in pregnancy; It is produced in the leukocytes, placenta, and vessels (Chu et al., 2014).

Maternal serum G protein-coupled receptor (CGRP) levels decrease after birth. However, CGRP levels increase in pregnant women with untreated PE (Ariza et al., 2009; Yallampalli et al., 2002).

Dimethylarginine dimethylaminohydrolase 1 (DDAH1) contributes to nitric oxide formation by asymmetric dimethylarginine metabolism, and its level will change in PE, with a change in DDAH1 methylation hypothesized to alter gene expression in PE (Savvidou et al., 2003).

Hypermethylation of IG-DMR, up-regulation of DLK1, and down-regulation of MEG3 in umbilical vein epithelial cells have been detected in cases of preeclampsia. According to the control, another study found that protein levels and the transcription grade of Phlda2 were prominently increased in the PE patient's placenta.

Proopiomelanocortin (POMC) produces a hormone premise that gives rise to different proteins, such as a β-endorphin, adrenocorticotropic hormone (ACTH), and α-melanocyte-stimulating hormone. When the pregnant and non-pregnant groups were compared, serum ACTH and β-endorphin levels were higher in the pregnancy group. POMC can be found in the serum in the first trimester of pregnancy but disappears days after delivery (Jin et al., 2015; Y. C. Yu et al., 2019).

White et al. showed various methylation in the CpG regions of the CALCA, POMC, DDAH1, and AGT genes in the PE patients according to the normal.

In summary, in the early diagnosis of PE, the mentioned disorders in the methylation of different genes may cause irregularities of varied gene methylation may cause PE due to assorted reasons such as oxygen homeostasis or hypoxia in E-PE, trophoblast invasion, neutrophils, and hypoxic trophoblast, leaking from maternal systemic blood vessels. (White et al., 2016).

PE and Histone Modification

There are also many publications on different epigenetic modifications, such as histone acetylation, mainly histone H3, associated with increased transcriptional activation of related genes (Gebremedhin & Rademacher, 2016).

Like many diseases, PE is associated with histone acetylation changes (Tsaprouni et al., 2011).

The effects of hypoxic-chronic ischemia processes on universal epigenetic modifications, especially histone modification, are investigated using BeWo placental trophoblast cells in vitro and rodent placenta in vivo (Eddy et al., 2019). In their study, Eddy et al. showed that the global H3 methylation levels, which increased in response to chronic ischemia of the placenta, were considerably reduced in K18, K56, K27, H3K9, and K14 in the diagnosis of PE when BeWo placental trophoblast cells were exposed to acute hypoxia, they were observed in K56, K9, K27, and K9 in the diagnosis of PE. They also revealed that histone acetylation was increased (Eddy et al., 2019).

The expression of the angiotensin 2 - producing enzyme chymase is found in maternal vascular endothelial cells and is elevated in PE. In the vascular endothelium in patients with PE, chymase increases angiotensin 2 yields by alterations in the modification of histone. Prevention of histone deacetylase increases angiotensin 2 production and initiates the activation of chymase (Togher et al., 2017).

HDAC significantly affects the arrangement of gene expression and chromosomal composition. Research shows that HDAC has an essential role in balancing the placenta's function and maintaining healthy gravidity (Seto & Yoshida, 2014; Togher et al., 2017).

Chromatin changes have an essential role in the gene transcription process, with the mechanisms of stimulation or suppression. HDACs organize histone deacetylation and have gained popularity as they play a direct role in remodeling nucleosome composition and transcription factor binding sites to suppress gene transcription. Deacetylation mechanisms are a beneficial epigenetic sign for understanding the effects and functionalizing HDACs. Down-regulation of HDAC9 in PE is another crucial point. Among TIMP metallopeptidase inhibitor 3 (TIMP3) regulators, HDAC9 is located. The dysarranegement of HDAC9 in the PE patient's placenta has been detected to be associated with changes in the expression of TIMP3, an important regulator of trophoblast migration and invasion, and TIMP3 has a vital role in regulating cellular processes such as apoptosis and invasion in trophoblastic cells by antagonizing MMPs and protecting the extracellular matrix from destruction. (Xie et al., 2019; Yuen et al., 2010). In another study, it was reported that HDAC6 expression was remarkably decreased and was associated with less expression of the angiogenic factors such as PLGF and VEGF through the regulation of miRNA-199a-5p in the preeclamptic placenta (Mei et al., 2019).

Trimethylated histone H3K9/27me3 affects regulating MMP 9 and 2. MMP 9 and 2 disrupt collagen 4 between other structures in the uterine wall and are required for implantation with this effect (Rahat, Sharma, et al., 2016). These are found with elevated templates of trimethylation in H3K9/27me3, resulting in reduced amounts of MMPs. Epigenetic regulation of H3K9/27me3 in cytotrophoblasts was detected among GWAS recordings (Ellery et al., 2009; Fogarty et al., 2015). With another GWAS data, one of the histone methylation patterns, H3K4Me2 and H4K20me3, was found to be regulators of RNA polymerase II in syncytiotrophoblast nuclei.

TIMP3 is an MMP antagonist that prevents the degradation of the extracellular matrix by regulating MMPs and regulates cell missions such as apoptosis, migration, invasion, and proliferation (Cruz-Munoz et al., 2006).

In studies on TIMP3, high expression was detected in PE placentas (Yuen et al., 2010).

In their study, Xie et al. determined that the HDAC promoter plays an important and necessary role in trophoblast migration and invasion by regulating TIMP3 expression by changing histone acetylation (Xie et al., 2019).

Studies have shown deficiencies in placental angiogenesis in mice with VHL deficiency. It has been demonstrated that VHL, a tumor suppressor gene protein, is requisite for the appropriate progression of placental growth (Gnarra et al., 1997). Targeting hypoxia-inducible factor 1a (HIF1a) by VHL; It regulates HIF1a levels in the placenta by forming a ubiquitin ligase complex with elongins C cullin 2 and elongins B for proteasomal degradation and polyubiquitination of the VHL protein and HIF1a (Ietta et al., 2006).

It has been stated about the expression and activity of protein 6 that (JMJD6) contains the Jumonji C (JmjC) domain, an oxygen-dependent histone demethylase, and a ferrous iron (Fe2+), are altered in the preeclamptic placenta (Alahari, Post, et al., 2018). JMJD6 has been demonstrated to arrangement cell migration and proliferation through the demethylation of histone 4 at arginine 3 (H4R3me2a) (Shen et al., 2018). A recent study found a remarkable association between low oxygen tension, decreased JMJD6 demethylase activity, and increased H4R3me2 in the E-PE placenta. This result revealed the complexity of chromatin remodeling regulation in the placenta and its contribution to the pathogenesis of PE (Alahari, Post, et al., 2018).

Protein 6 (JMJD6), containing the Jumonji C (JmjC) domain, is in the family with the JmjC domain and can regulate the HIF1A domain (Alahari et al., 2015). JMJD6 can demethylate histone-arginine dots. Also, histone 3 (H3R2me2s) in the JMJD6 demethylase enzyme arginine

2 and histone 4 (H3R2me2s) in arginine 3. Studies show that it is dimethylated (Aprelikova et al., 2016; Ratovitski et al., 2015).

JMJD6 expression significantly increases in PE (Alahari et al., 2015). apVHL grade and VHL mRNA levels are markedly decreased within the E-PE placenta. Alahari et al. found that histone demethylase of JMJD6 was decreased in both H4R3me2s and H3R2me2s markers and was notably reduced in E-PE compared to Preterm control (PTC) (Alahari, Post, et al., 2018). In their study, the authors found a significant reduction in H3R2me2s and H4R3me2s markers in the PTC group after adding the JMJD6 enzyme, but no difference with the addition of the enzyme in the placental histone of E-PE. Reduced VHL promoter upstream H4R3me2s VHL and H3R2me2s VHL domains compared to PTC (Alahari S, Post M, Rolfo A, Weksberg R, Caniggia I. Compromised JMJD6 histone demethylase activity affects VHL gene repression in preeclampsia. J Clin Endocrinol Metabol. 2018; 103(4):1545–1557.)

Endothelial progenitor cells (EPC) can differentiate from fibroblast-mimic cells and intercede neo-vascularization in vascular damage reparation during embryogenesis. (Bautch, 2011). EPCs express the surface markers CD133 and c-Kit, derived from the hemangioblast (Asahara & Kawamoto, 2004). It has been known that EPC levels decrease in cardiovascular pathologies such as diabetic vasculopathy, atherosclerosis metabolic syndrome, coronary artery disease, etc. (Ebner et al., 2010).

At the same time, there are publications in the literature reporting that EPCs derived from cord blood increase in PE and decrease with aging, respectively (Muñoz-Hernandez et al., 2014).

Directly in utero, EPCs have general differentiation, and action capacity is probably determinative of fetal vascular well-being; in the light of the data, it has been suggested that fetal circulation may be affected by fetal EPCs in the etiopathogenesis of PE. Park et al. found a reduction in the differentiation of CKL− EPCs from human cord blood into outgrowth endothelial cells (OECs) and the amount of OECs in the PE patient group from the healthy group. In addition, the trimethylation levels of the CKL− EPCs histones H3K4 and H3K9 were significantly decreased in PE; however, there were no significant difference in EPCand H3K27me3 levels between the PE groups and the control group. They claimed it could impair their angiogenic capacity (Park et al., 2019).

In some pregnancy pathologies such as PE, cytokine expression changes occur. HDAC inhibition alters protein production and cytokine mRNA expression (Roger et al., 2011).

The arrangement of cytokine instability by HDAC in PE may be a therapeutic target (Munro et al., 2013).

As a result, these changes in histone may result in pathogenic factors released, migration and differentiation of trophoblast cells, changes in iron and oxygen and the proinflammatory response, tissue damage, and hemostasis may belong to PE pathology in the later process.

PE and miRNAs

In current research using microRNAomic as a result of the analysis, attention was drawn to the place of miRs in the etiopathogenesis of PE of preeclampsia (Chen & Wang, 2013). While miRNAs are differentially expressed in the human placenta, they have necessary effects on regulating placental progression (G. Fu et al., 2013).

Pregnancy disorders, such as PE, can occur with abnormal miRNA expression. Considering placental hypoxia in the pathogenesis of PE, insufficient trophoblast invasion and insufficient spiral arterial remodeling draw attention.

The critical roles of miRNAs in placental processes have changed the perspective of placental pathologies such as preeclampsia and IUGR. miRNAs have a vast place in the literature as diagnostic and treatment tools for many diseases, affecting the course of the pathogenesis of diseases with their effects on protein expression.

miRNAs, which have a place in placental development, appear in epigenetic mechanisms in the pathogenesis of PE. The known roles of miRNAs in trophoblastic cell differentiation and proliferation have been demonstrated (Saha et al., 2017). MiR200a-3p and miR-141 bind to the 3'UTR of the transthyretin (TTR), which is involved in the uptake of thyroxine into syncytiotrophoblastic cells and have a regulatory effect. In studies, down-regulation of TTR was determined as a result of the up-regulation of miR-200a-p and miR-141p. It has been suggested that the up-regulation of EDN1, a potent vasoconstrictor peptide, is caused by the up-regulation of miRNAs such as let-7c, 125a, let-7a, 125b, and let-7b detected in the umbilical vein endothelial cells of patients with PE (Caldeira-Dias et al., 2018).

Serpin family A member 3 (SERPINA3) and plasminogen activator inhibitor-1 are involved in trophoblast invasion by up-regulation of miR-34 (Doridot et al., 2014; Umemura et al., 2013). Inhibited by overexpression of miR-34, SERPINA3 is a protease inhibitor among G2-M cell cycle regulators. Hypoxia in the pathogenesis of PE has been associated with the up-regulation of miR-34. Studies have suggested that miR-155 down-regulates extravillous trophoblastic cell division by targeting cyclin D1, which involve in the G1/S phases of cell division, activates cdk4, and regulates DNA synthesis (Dai et al., 2012). Up-regulation of cyclin D1 has been suggested to be associated with increased cell migration, cell adhesion, and growth. Up-regulation of miR-155 results in the down-regulation of cyclin D1 in the pathogenesis of PE, suggesting that it may have an essential link with the absence of migration and invasion of extravillous trophoblastic cells.

Recently, it has been declared that various placental miRNAs originate from chr14 (34 miRNA) and chr19 (54 miRNA) (Morales-Prieto et al., 2012). Changes in the expression patterns of variant miRNAs in the placenta and maternal blood of patients with PE have been reported (Laganà et al., 2018). The majority of miRNA expressed in the placenta of PE patients have been implicated as regulatory genes associated with placental angiogenesis and trophoblast differentiation.

Superficial differentiation of EVT in the PE placenta and remodeling of weak spiral arteries following migration are probably among the notable changes in the PE placenta. Inadequate placental perfusion in PE patients with superficial EVT invasion results in up-regulation of hypoxia-inducible factor-1 (HIF-1), a transcription factor that modulates the cellular response to hypoxia (Caniggia & Winter, 2002). Induction of several miRNA expressions, such as miR-210, miR-517c, miR-218, miR-210, and miR-517a/b, has been observed in the hypoxic placenta.

Modified miR-520g-MMP2, miR-221-3p-IGF2BP1, miR-423-5p-IGF2BP1, miR-137-ESRRA, miR-137-THBS2, and miR-142- Genes with 3p-MMP9 targets have been identified (L. Jiang et al., 2017; Lu et al., 2017).

It has been suggested that patients with PE inhibit trophoblast migration by overexpression of miR-210 in the placenta and serum, causing mitochondria dysfunction, and publications show a strong relationship with the severity and progression of PE.

MiR-210 is a potential PE biomarker as it is traceable in maternal serum (Muralimanoharan et al., 2012; Youssef & Marei, 2019).

A relationship between placental neovascularization disorder and downregulation of vascular endothelial growth factor (VEGF) has been reported in the pathogenesis of PE.

Many microRNAs targeting placental VEGF, such as miR-126, miR-199a-5p, miRNA-518b, and miR-203, are involved in the pathogenesis of PE (Mei et al., 2019).

Mei et al. suggested in their study that there is a relationship between the overexpression of miR-199a-5p and the decreased protein histone deacetylase 6 (HDAC6) in the PE placenta.

Another critical factor in the pathogenesis of PE is the increased production of the placental antiangiogenic protein soluble FMS-like tyrosine kinase-1 (sFlt-1). It has been suggested that increased sFLT1 expression in the PE placenta is associated with miR-517c and miR-517a/b overexpression (Takizawa et al., 2012).

Has-miR-210 is the significant marker of hypoxic responses in endothelial and trophoblast cells, including Has-miR-210 (Biró et al., 2019; Chan and Loscalzo, 2010). Biro et al. revealed that placental has-miR-210, Ago-bound plasma, and exosome levels were significantly increased compared to the control group in the pathogenesis of PE. Has-miR-517c, expressed in the placenta, is a primate-specific C19MC miRNA family member. Has-miR-16, which is among the abundant miRNAs in blood, is generally represented by red blood cells (Pritchard et al., 2012).

In their study, Brio et al. found that the placenta has-miR-517c level was up-regulated in the PE group. Still, they could not detect a significant difference between the PE and normal groups in the has-miR-517c level in exosome and Ago-bound plasma. The level of has-miR-16 in plasma that binds to the placenta, exosome, and Ago did not differ statistically between the two groups. At the same time, researchers claimed in their studies that considering the data obtained about exosomal has-miR-210, it had been suggested that it may be involved in the pathogenesis of PE and may affect intracellular communication. In addition, it has been suggested that the release of has-miR-210 due to Ago may be associated with PE complications and cell death-related products (Biró et al., 2019).

Brio et al. MiRNA concentrations in exosome samples were six times higher in severe PE and three times higher in moderate PE compared to the normotensive group. In addition, although the expression of exosomal has-miR-210-3p was higher in the severe PE group than in the moderate group, they were higher in both groups (Biró et al., 2017).

Endothelin-1 (ET-1), frequently the subject of research on the pathogenesis of PE, is an effective vasoconstrictor peptide (Aydin et al., 2004). miRNAs affect the ET-1 gene (EDN1) via post-transcriptional arrangement (Jacobs et al., 2013).

Dias et al. detected high levels of Let-7c miRNA 125b, Let-7a, miRNA 125a, Let-7b, and human umbilical vein endothelial cell (HUVEC) derivated from serum in patients with PE in HUVEC supernatants after transfection of miRNA mimic Let-7b. It showed that the ET-1 level was significantly reduced (approximately 25%) (Caldeira-Dias et al., 2018).

The MIR218-2 and MIR218-1 genes may be conducted by the miR-218-5p MIR218-2 and MIR218-1 genes located in the SLIT3 and SLIT2 gene introns. (Small et al., 2010).

Xu et al. showed that their studies showed that the miR-218-5p level decreased in the PE placenta (P. Xu et al., 2014).

Transforming growth factor -β (TGF-β) signaling possesses diverse roles within the placenta, such as regulating trophoblastic invasion, survival, and trophoblast proliferation.

Research has shown that TGF-β is up-regulated within women with PE (G. Fu, Ye et al., 2013; Nadeem et al., 2011).

Brkic et al. suggest that miR-218-5p is essential for intact placental growth as it enhances differentiation, invasion, and migration of EVT by down-regulation of miR-218-5p is partly caused by inhibition of TGF-β2 signaling that may cause pathogenesis (Brkić et al., 2018).

miR-34a-5p can regulate cancer cell migration and invasion by targeting Smad family member 4 (Smad4) (G. Huang et al., 2018).

Xue et al. In their study, miR-34a-5p was prominently reduced in patients with PE according to the healthy group. They also reported that miR-34a-upregulation targeting 5p, Smad4, and transfected miR-34a-5p inhibitor markedly prevented the migration of the trophoblasts (HTR8/SVnevo) and increased the invasion of HTR8/Svnevo (Xue et al., 2019).

The Rho E protein (RND3) is crucial in the progress of prostate cancer, melanoma, and gastric cancer (Nadiminty et al., 2010).

In the studies by Fang et al., miRNA-182-5p expression was elevated within the patients with PE, and it was suggested that high expression of miR-182-5p could prevent the migration and invasion of HTR8/SVnevo cells. It has been claimed that miR-182-5p can attach to the 30-UTR of RND3 and create down-regulation of RND3 in patients with PE (Fang et al., 2018).

The MMP-2 gene, a member of the MMP family, plays a role in the migration of different cells such as endometriosis cells and trophoblast cells, and the pathogenesis of cervical cancer with similar cell migration (Ahn et al., 2015).

In the studies by Fu et al., the miR-517-5p expression level was higher in patients with PE. It was revealed that this causes proliferative and invasive inhibition of JAR cells in the preeclamptic placenta. 2 showed decreased mRNA levels (J. Y. Fu et al., 2018).

miR-26a acts as a VEGF regulator on the endothelial cell through the Nago-B receptor and has a role in endothelial cell functions such as angiogenesis and apoptosis. (Icli et al., 2016).

Studies draw attention to an imbalance between vasodilator and vasoconstrictor mechanisms in the formation of endothelial dysfunction in the pathogenesis of PE.

VEGF/VEGFR imbalance can be detected as a manifestation of endothelial dysfunction in preeclamptic women and their children (C. A. Escudero et al., 2016).

Pathologies of various angiogenic genes such as sFlt-1, EGFR, kinase splice domain, and VEGF that affect placental methylation have been associated with the pathogenesis of preeclampsia (Sundrani et al., 2013).

Eskandari et al. stated that the PrimiRNA-26a1 rs7372209 polymorphism might be a preserver for PE, and this polymorphism may be related to less risk of severe and mild preeclampsia (Eskandari et al., 2019).

Phosphatidylinositol 3-kinase (PI3K)/protein kinase B (AKT)/mammalian target of rapamycin (mTOR) signaling is a critical pathway in cell proliferation, apoptosis, growth, and metabolism (F. Wang et al., 2015).

AKT activation can regulate PI3K and AKT by targeting mTOR, initiating biological information transmission (Y. Zhu et al., 2013).

In the study by Xu et al., evidence was presented that the expression of taurine up-regulated 1 (TUG1), which is the lncRNA that leads to the up-regulation of the Rnd3 protein, a member of the GTPase family, is decreased in the pathogenesis of PE. In normal placental growth, TUG1 interacts with the enhancer of the zeste 2 polycomb repressor complex with two subunits (EZH2), silencing the transcription of a protein named Rho family GTPase 3 (RND3) (Y. Xu et al., 2017). EZH2 is a repressor of RNA transcription through histone modification included in cell maturation and proliferation (Y. Xu et al., 2017). Separate lncRNA, the RPA-interacting protein (RPAIN), is up-regulated in PE pathogenesis. More expression of RPAIN prevents trophoblast implantation and proliferation adequacy. High RPAIN concentrations are related to preventing complement protein 1 (C1q) expression. Regularly, overexpression of C1q arranges invasion of trophoblastic cells; thus, a reduction in C1q will cut the adequacy of the trophoblast to meet implantation (Song et al., 2017). The lncRNA named Metastasis-associated adenocarcinoma transcript 1 (MALAT-1), included in migration and proliferation processes and cell cycle regulation, is down-regulated in the pathogenesis of PE. This lncRNA down-regulation has inhibited migration, invasion, proliferation, and even cell cycle arrest at G0/G1 in trophoblastic cells (Rahat et al., 2014).

Maternally expressed gene 3 (MEG3), which contributes to increased migration in placental development among incRNAs and functions as a tumor suppressor, is down-regulated in the pathogenesis of PE. Down-regulated MEG3 levels, which were detected lower in placental development, were associated with reduced invasion and migration adequacy in the pathogenesis of PE. (Y. Zhang et al., 2015).

Han et al. suggested that up-regulation of miR-145 may improve and support the PI3K/AKT/mTOR signaling pathway, inhibit p53 expression, and subsequently inhibit PE disease. They suggested that EVCT increased cell proliferation (Han et al., 2017).

In the studies by Khaliq et al., miR-181a and miR-29a were significantly elevated in patients with PE; on the other hand, miR-222 was reduced in patients with PE, and these miRNAs additionally affected the PI3K/AKT pathways in the placenta (Khaliq et al., 2018).

MiR-19a expression has been shown to protect endothelial cells from lipopolysaccharide-induced apoptosis (W. L. Jiang et al., 2015). The expression of miR-19a-3p has been shown to increase cell invasion with the expression of MMP-9, increase proliferation with the expression of Ki67, and reduce apoptosis (indicated by the expression of caspase-3). It has been suggested that miR-19a-3p expression is less in the preeclamptic placenta, and higher expression of miR-19a-3p may cause elevated migration and invasion of cells underneath hypoxia (N. Wang et al., 2019). IL1RAP, the mRNA, and PSG10p, the IncRNA, can activate IL1RAP by regulating IL-1, which is involved in varying immune-inflammatory responses (Jensen et al., 2000). IL1RAP is associated with decreased MMP-9 and increased caspase three activity and significantly affects the apoptotic process. Wang et al. claimed that the expressions of PSG10p and IL1RAP were more in the preeclamptic placenta than in the control group and showed that it promoted the growth and migration of trophoblast cells. Furthermore, transfection of miR-19a-3p mimics in HTR-8/SVnevo, PSG10p expression was subsequently decreased; thus, these consequences powerfully suggest that disorders of the lncRNA-PSG10p/miR19a-3P/IL1RAP systems can lead to the pathogenesis of PE.

25-Hydroxy vitamin D (25-OH-VD) is necessary to influence the level of vitamin D reserve in the body (Wei et al., 2013). The level of serum 25-OH-VD is visibly lower in the patients with PE according to healthy pregnant women. In addition, Baker et al. explained that expression of miRNA-376c is less in patients with PE. Together with disease advancement, it has been found that miRNA expression is elevated (G. Fu, Ye et al., 2013).

These data suggested that 25-OH-VD mRNA and miRNA-376c dysregulation are significantly related to blood pressure and urinary protein in pregnant women and that miRNA-376c and 25-OH-VD impact with each other and complicate pregnancy like PE. The authors examined placental samples in their study and suggested that miR-145-5p, miR-194, miR-149, miR-260-5p, miR-16-5p, miR-, miR-103a-3p expressions have a role in the progression and formation of hypertensive disorder. (Chiofalo et al., 2017). The presence of miR-221-3p and 100-5p downregulation in the pathogenesis of PE has been demonstrated. In some publications, up-regulation of miR-449a-5p, miR-204, miR-520a, miR-92b, miR520-h, miR-516-5p, and miR-191 in the pathogenesis of PE have been revealed in examinations of placental specimens. (Chiofalo et al., 2017; Laganà et al., 2018). Consequently, these irregularities of miRNAs may affect the development of PE. A large number of non-coding genes indicates the range of genome arrangement and diversity and compels us to admit that our work is still at the very beginning of this issue.

Maternal Blood Epigenetic Marks in Preeclampsia

In White et al. study with patients diagnosed with PE, were able to reveal hypermethylation in white blood maternal cells by using methylation-27k sequences obtained through Illumina in 2013 (White et al., 2013). This study found that BEX1, PCDHB7, GABRA1, and GRIN2b were methylated by enrichment via the neuropeptide signaling pathway. When the methylation levels of the genes revealed in the leukocytes circulating in the serum of mothers with PE were reanalyzed; When CpG methylation in PE-related genes DDAH1, POMC, CALCA, and AGT was compared with the moderately methylated control, different (<6%) methylation levels were revealed in these patients. It is known that four genes that attract this attention change the immunomodulation and inflammatory response. In the light of this information, it is assumed that preeclamptic placental changes have epigenomic effects on cells in the maternal circulation (White et al., 2016).

During pregnancy, between 3% and 6% of cell-free DNA in maternal plasma is derived from the placenta. In a study, oxidative stress was detected in the pathogenesis of PE, the release of SCT microparticles, and increased trophoblast apoptosis. It was claimed that there was a 5 to 10-fold increase in fetal DNA circulating in the bloodstream of preeclamptic maternal preeclampsia compared to the control group (Levine et al., 2004; Taglauer et al., 2014). Detection of free-floating fetal molecules and their methylation status and levels have been discussed as a non-invasive biomarker in diagnosing fetal and placental pathologies before the onset of symptoms.

Conclusion

Preeclampsia is a kind of hypertensive pregnancy complication characterized by systemic endothelial cell injury, the cause of which has not been fully elucidated and may cause maternal and fetal mortality. Many factors, including maternal metabolic conditions, genetics, and inflammatory processes, can be associated with PE pathology. It has been shown that many factors contribute to maternal endothelial dysfunction and poor placentation in etiopathogenesis. Severe E-PE occurs at 20 weeks of pregnancy and usually needs pre-mature delivery (before 34 weeks of gestation). Pre-mature birth has a serious risk to the immediate and long-term well-being of the newborn and is related to neonatal intensive care expenses (Toal et al., 2007). In addition, maternal and fetal mortality are severe enough to focus attention on the disease.

Recent publications have revealed possible links between epigenetic mechanisms and the pathophysiology of PE (Agius et al., 2018; Perucci et al., 2017). More studies are needed to learn more about the potential role of epigenetic modifications in the development and progression of PE disease.

In recent years, more research has emerged focusing on the effect of epigenetics on the arrangement of placental growth and its probable impact on placental dysfunctions. We have not had conclusive data on how these epigenetic modifications relate to gene expression so far. Incredibly, we have restricted information on how Histone modifications or DNA methylation modifications affect gene expression in intact and abnormal placental growth. Moreover, our information on the mechanisms of adjustment and the characteristics of the formation of varied epigenetic signs throughout the story is still insufficient. On the other hand, current publications have begun to uncover how epigenetics plays a role in regulating essential processes in placental development, such as EVT migration and invasion, cell fate determination, or syncytialization. The new technologies that allow the study of transcriptomic and epigenetic mechanisms of different cell varieties of the placenta will undoubtedly contribute significantly to improving our understanding of epigenetics in the placenta.

Furthermore, studies analyzing epigenetic modifications in the context of PE have centered on the placenta. However, cytotoxic factors and antiangiogenic derived from the PE placenta have the eventual stimulation of epigenetic changes in maternal tissues. Overall, understanding epigenetic regulation in preeclampsia, both at the level of the placenta and other related organs, may provide new biomarkers and therapeutic targets to improve the management of this disease. Currently, data from epigenetic studies have not been successfully applied as a diagnosis or prognosis of preeclampsia.

The technological inconsistency of removing circulating RNAs from plasma results in inconsistent results among various laboratories, leading to a lack of consensus on the definition of a diagnostic miRNA panel, resulting in data that are not reflected in routine practice. These problems may develop with new data in the future and may significantly use these markers in complex diseases, including preeclampsia. It may be a suggestion for future studies to reveal the fundamental epigenetic changes in the etiopathogenesis of PE, intervene in these changes, and open therapeutic approaches to research.

References

Abell, A. N., Jordan, N. V., Huang, W., Prat, A., Midland, A. A., Johnson, N. L., Granger, D. A., Mieczkowski, P. A., Perou, C. M., Gomez, S. M., Li, L., & Johnson, G. L. (2011). MAP3K4/CBP-regulated H2B acetylation controls epithelial-mesenchymal transition in trophoblast stem cells. *Cell Stem Cell*, *8*(5), 525–537. https://doi.org/10.1016/J.STEM.2011.03.008.

Abraham, E., Rousseaux, S., Agier, L., Giorgis-Allemand, L., Tost, J., Galineau, J., Hulin, A., Siroux, V., Vaiman, D., Charles, M. A., Heude, B., Forhan, A., Schwartz, J., Chuffart, F., Bourova-Flin, E., Khochbin, S., Slama, R., & Lepeule, J. (2018). Pregnancy exposure to atmospheric pollution and meteorological conditions and placental DNA methylation. *Environment International*, *118*, 334–347. https://doi.org/10.1016/J.ENVINT.2018.05.007.

Agius, A., Sultana, R., Camenzuli, C., Calleja-Agius, J., & Balzan, R. (2018). An update on the genetics of pre-eclampsia. *Minerva Ginecologica*, *70*(4), 465–479. https://doi.org/10.23736/S0026-4784.17.04150-8.

Ahmadi, M., Gharibi, T., Dolati, S., Rostamzadeh, D., Aslani, S., Baradaran, B., Younesi, V., & Yousefi, M. (2017). Epigenetic modifications and epigenetic based medication implementations of autoimmune diseases. *Biomedicine & Pharmacotherapy = Biomedecine & Pharmacotherapie*, *87*, 596–608. https://doi.org/10.1016/J.BIOPHA.2016.12.072.

Ahn, J. H., Choi, Y. S., & Choi, J. H. (2015). Leptin promotes human endometriotic cell migration and invasion by up-regulating MMP-2 through the JAK2/STAT3 signaling pathway. *Molecular Human Reproduction*, *21*(10), 792–802. https://doi.org/10.1093/MOLEHR/GAV039.

Alahari, S., Garcia, J., Post, M., & Caniggia, I. (2018). The von Hippel Lindau tumour suppressor gene is a novel target of E2F4-mediated transcriptional repression in preeclampsia. *Biochimica et Biophysica Acta. Molecular Basis of Disease*, *1864*(10), 3298–3308. https://doi.org/10.1016/J.BBADIS.2018.07.016.

Alahari, S., Post, M., & Caniggia, I. (2015). Jumonji Domain Containing Protein 6: A Novel Oxygen Sensor in the Human Placenta. *Endocrinology*, *156*(8), 3012–3025. https://doi.org/10.1210/EN.2015-1262.

Alahari, S., Post, M., Rolfo, A., Weksberg, R., & Caniggia, I. (2018). Compromised JMJD6 Histone Demethylase Activity Affects VHL Gene Repression in Preeclampsia. *The Journal of Clinical Endocrinology and Metabolism*, *103*(4), 1545–1557. https://doi.org/10.1210/JC.2017-02197.

Ananth, C. V., Keyes, K. M., & Wapner, R. J. (2013). Pre-eclampsia rates in the United States, 1980-2010: age-period-cohort analysis. *BMJ*, *347*. https://doi.org/10.1136/BMJ.F6564.

Anderson, C. M., Ralph, J. L., Wright, M. L., Linggi, B., & Ohm, J. E. (2014). DNA methylation as a biomarker for preeclampsia. *Biological Research for Nursing*, *16*(4), 409–420. https://doi.org/10.1177/1099800413508645.

Anton, L., & Brosnihan, K. B. (2008). Systemic and uteroplacental renin–angiotensin system in normal and pre-eclamptic pregnancies. *Therapeutic Advances in Cardiovascular Disease*, *2*(5), 349. https://doi.org/10.1177/1753944708094529.

Anton, L., Brown, A. G., Bartolomei, M. S., & Elovitz, M. A. (2014). Differential Methylation of Genes Associated with Cell Adhesion in Preeclamptic Placentas. *PLOS One*, *9*(6), e100148. https://doi.org/10.1371/JOURNAL.PONE.0100148.

Aprelikova, O., Chen, K., El Touny, L. H., Brignatz-Guittard, C., Han, J., Qiu, T., Yang, H. H., Lee, M. P., Zhu, M., & Green, J. E. (2016). The epigenetic modifier JMJD6 is amplified in mammary tumors and cooperates with c-Myc to enhance cellular transformation, tumor progression, and metastasis. *Clinical Epigenetics*, *8*(1). https://doi.org/10.1186/S13148-016-0205-6.

Ariza, A. C., Bobadilla, N., Díaz, L., Avila, E., Larrea, F., & Halhali, A. (2009). Placental gene expression of calcitonin gene-related peptide and nitric oxide synthases in preeclampsia: effects of magnesium sulfate. *Magnesium Research*, *22*(1), 44–49. https://doi.org/10.1684/MRH.2009.0154.

Asahara, T., & Kawamoto, A. (2004). Endothelial progenitor cells for postnatal vasculogenesis. *American Journal of Physiology, Cell Physiology*, *287*(3). https://doi.org/10.1152/AJPCELL.00330.2003.

Aydin, S., Benian, A., Madazli, R., Uludağ, S., Uzun, H., & Kaya, S. (2004). Plasma malondialdehyde, superoxide dismutase, sE-selectin, fibronectin, endothelin-1 and nitric oxide levels in women with preeclampsia. *European Journal of Obstetrics, Gynecology, and Reproductive Biology*, *113*(1), 21–25. https://doi.org/10.1016/S0301-2115(03)00368-3.

Bartha, J. L., Romero-Carmona, R., Torrejon-Cardoso, R., & Comino-Delgado, R. (2002). Insulin, insulin-like growth factor-1, and insulin resistance in women with pregnancy-induced hypertension. *American Journal of Obstetrics and Gynecology*, *187*(3), 735–740. https://doi.org/10.1067/MOB.2002.126283.

Bautch, V. L. (2011). Stem cells and the vasculature. *Nature Medicine 2011 17:11*, *17*(11), 1437–1443. https://doi.org/10.1038/nm.2539.

Bellido, M. L., Radpour, R., Lapaire, O., De Bie, I., Hösli, I., Bitzer, J., Hmadcha, A., Zhong, X. Y., & Holzgreve, W. (2010). MALDI-TOF Mass Array Analysis of RASSF1A and SERPINB5 Methylation Patterns in Human Placenta and Plasma. *Biology of Reproduction*, *82*(4), 745–750. https://doi.org/10.1095/BIOLREPROD.109.082271.

Biró, O., Alasztics, B., Molvarec, A., Joó, J., Nagy, B., & Rigó, J. (2017). Various levels of circulating exosomal total-miRNA and miR-210 hypoxamiR in different forms of pregnancy hypertension. *Pregnancy Hypertension*, *10*, 207–212. https://doi.org/10.1016/J.PREGHY.2017.09.002.

Biró, O., Fóthi, Á., Alasztics, B., Nagy, B., Orbán, T. I., & Rigó, J. (2019). Circulating exosomal and Argonaute-bound microRNAs in preeclampsia. *Gene*, *692*, 138–144. https://doi.org/10.1016/J.GENE.2019.01.012.

Blair, J. D., Yuen, R. K. C., Lim, B. K., McFadden, D. E., von Dadelszen, P., & Robinson, W. P. (2013). Widespread DNA hypomethylation at gene enhancer regions in placentas associated with early-onset pre-eclampsia. *Molecular Human Reproduction*, *19*(10), 697–708. https://doi.org/10.1093/MOLEHR/GAT044.

Bonasio, R., Tu, S., & Reinberg, D. (2010). Molecular Signals of Epigenetic States. *Science (New York, N.Y.)*, *330*(6004), 612. https://doi.org/10.1126/SCIENCE.1191078.

Bosco Becerra, C., Díaz Guerra, E., Gutierrez Rojas, R., González Montero, J., Parra Cordero, M., Ramón Rodrigo Salinas, R., & Barja Yañez, P. (2016). Placental Hypoxia Developed During Preeclampsia Induces Telocytes Apoptosis in Chorionic Villi Affecting The Maternal-Fetus Metabolic Exchange. *Current Stem Cell Research & Therapy*, *11*(5), 420–425. https://doi.org/10.2174/1574888X10666150202144855.

Brannan, C. I., Dees, E. C., Ingram, R. S., & Tilghman, S. M. (1990). The product of the H19 gene may function as an RNA. *Molecular and Cellular Biology*, *10*(1), 28–36. https://doi.org/10.1128/MCB.10.1.28-36.1990.

Brkić, J., Dunk, C., O'Brien, J., Fu, G., Nadeem, L., Wang, Y. ling, Rosman, D., Salem, M., Shynlova, O., Yougbaré, I., Ni, H., Lye, S. J., & Peng, C. (2018). MicroRNA-218-5p Promotes Endovascular Trophoblast Differentiation and Spiral Artery Remodeling. *Molecular Therapy*, *26*(9), 2189–2205. https://doi.org/10.1016/J.YMTHE.2018.07.009/ATTACHMENT/5C56F506-C674-47DB-93B1-52AF36025D30/MMC1.PDF.

Brodowski, L., Zindler, T., von Hardenberg, S., Schröder-Heurich, B., von Kaisenberg, C. S., Frieling, H., Hubel, C. A., Dörk, T., & von Versen-Höynck, F. (2019). Preeclampsia-associated alteration of DNA methylation in fetal endothelial progenitor cells. *Frontiers in Cell and Developmental Biology*, *7*(MAR). https://doi.org/10.3389/FCELL.2019.00032/FULL.

Burton, G. J., Charnock-Jones, D. S., & Jauniaux, E. (2009). Regulation of vascular growth and function in the human placenta. *Reproduction (Cambridge, England)*, *138*(6), 895–902. https://doi.org/10.1530/REP-09-0092.

Caldeira-Dias, M., Luizon, M. R., Deffune, E., Tanus-Santos, J. E., Freire, P. P., Carvalho, R. F., Bettiol, H., Cardoso, V. C., Antonio Barbieri, M., Cavalli, R. C., & Sandrim, V. C. (2018). Preeclamptic plasma stimulates the expression of miRNAs, leading to a decrease in endothelin-1 production in endothelial cells. *Pregnancy Hypertension*, *12*, 75–81. https://doi.org/10.1016/J.PREGHY.2018.03.001.

Camolotto, S. A., Racca, A. C., Ridano, M. E., Genti-Raimondi, S., & Panzetta-Dutari, G. M. (2013). PSG Gene Expression Is Up-Regulated by Lysine Acetylation Involving Histone and Nonhistone Proteins. *PLOS One*, *8*(2), e55992. https://doi.org/10.1371/JOURNAL.PONE.0055992.

Caniggia, I., & Winter, J. L. (2002). Adriana and Luisa Castellucci Award lecture 2001. Hypoxia inducible factor-1: oxygen regulation of trophoblast differentiation in normal and pre-eclamptic pregnancies--a review. *Placenta*, *23 Suppl A*(SUPPL. 1). https://doi.org/10.1053/PLAC.2002.0815.

Chan, S. Y., & Loscalzo, J. (2010). MicroRNA-210: a unique and pleiotropic hypoxamir. *Cell Cycle (Georgetown, Tex.)*, *9*(6), 1072–1083. https://doi.org/10.4161/CC.9.6.11006.

Chao, W., & D'Amore, P. A. (2008). IGF2: Epigenetic regulation and role in development and disease. *Cytokine & Growth Factor Reviews*, *19*(2), 111–120. https://doi.org/10.1016/J.CYTOGFR.2008.01.005.

Chen, D., & Wang, W. (2013). Human placental microRNAs and preeclampsia. *Biology of Reproduction*, *88*(5). https://doi.org/10.1095/BIOLREPROD.113.107805.

Chiofalo, B., Laganà, A. S., Vaiarelli, A., La Rosa, V. L., Rossetti, D., Palmara, V., Valenti, G., Rapisarda, A. M. C., Granese, R., Sapia, F., Triolo, O., & Vitale, S. G. (2017). Do miRNAs Play a Role in Fetal Growth Restriction? A Fresh Look to a Busy Corner. *BioMed Research International*, *2017*. https://doi.org/10.1155/2017/6073167.

Chiu, R. W. K., Chim, S. S. C., Wong, I. H. N., Wong, C. S. C., Lee, W. S., To, K. F., Tong, J. H. M., Yuen, R. K. C., Shum, A. S. W., Chan, J. K. C., Chan, L. Y. S., Yuen, J. W. F., Tong, Y. K., Weier, J. F., Ferlatte, C., Leung, T. N., Lau, T. K., Lo, K. W., & Lo, Y. M. D. (2007). Hypermethylation of RASSF1A in human and rhesus placentas. *The American Journal of Pathology*, *170*(3), 941–950. https://doi.org/10.2353/AJPATH.2007.060641.

Chu, T., Bunce, K., Shaw, P., Shridhar, V., Althouse, A., Hubel, C., & Peters, D. (2014). Comprehensive Analysis of Preeclampsia-Associated DNA Methylation in the Placenta. *PLOS One*, *9*(9), e107318. https://doi.org/10.1371/JOURNAL.PONE.0107318.

Cruz-Munoz, W., Sanchez, O. H., Di Grappa, M., English, J. L., Hill, R. P., & Khokha, R. (2006). Enhanced metastatic dissemination to multiple organs by melanoma and lymphoma cells in timp-3−/− mice. *Oncogene 2006 25:49*, *25*(49), 6489–6496. https://doi.org/10.1038/sj.onc.1209663.

Dai, Y., Qiu, Z., Diao, Z., Shen, L., Xue, P., Sun, H., & Hu, Y. (2012). MicroRNA-155 inhibits proliferation and migration of human extravillous trophoblast derived HTR-8/SVneo cells via down-regulating cyclin D1. *Placenta*, *33*(10), 824–829. https://doi.org/10.1016/J.PLACENTA.2012.07.012.

Dodson, R. E., Nishioka, M., Standley, L. J., Perovich, L. J., Brody, J. G., & Rudel, R. A. (2012). Endocrine Disruptors and Asthma-Associated Chemicals in Consumer Products. *Environmental Health Perspectives*, *120*(7), 935. https://doi.org/10.1289/EHP.1104052.

Doridot, L., Houry, D., Gaillard, H., Chelbi, S. T., Barbaux, S., & Vaiman, D. (2014). miR-34a expression, epigenetic regulation, and function in human placental diseases. *Epigenetics*, *9*(1), 142–151. https://doi.org/10.4161/EPI.26196.

Ebner, P., Picard, F., Richter, J., Darrelmann, E., Schneider, M., Strauer, B. E., & Brehm, M. (2010). Accumulation of VEGFR-2+/CD133+ cells and decreased number and impaired functionality of CD34+/VEGFR-2+ cells in patients with SLE. *Rheumatology (Oxford, England)*, *49*(1), 63–72. https://doi.org/10.1093/RHEUMATOLOGY/KEP335.

Eddy, A. C., Chapman, H., & George, E. M. (2019). Acute Hypoxia and Chronic Ischemia Induce Differential Total Changes in Placental Epigenetic Modifications. *Reproductive Sciences*, *26*(6), 766. https://doi.org/10.1177/1933719118799193.

Ellery, P. M., Cindrova-Davies, T., Jauniaux, E., Ferguson-Smith, A. C., & Burton, G. J. (2009). Evidence for Transcriptional Activity in the Syncytiotrophoblast of the Human Placenta. *Placenta*, *30*(4), 329–334. https://doi.org/10.1016/J.PLACENTA.2009.01.002.

Escudero, C., Herlitz, K., Troncoso, F., Acurio, J., Aguayo, C., Roberts, J. M., Truong, G., Duncombe, G., Rice, G., & Salomon, C. (2016). Role of Extracellular Vesicles and microRNAs on Dysfunctional Angiogenesis during Preeclamptic Pregnancies. *Frontiers in Physiology*, *7*(MAR), 98. https://doi.org/10.3389/FPHYS.2016.00098.

Escudero, C., Roberts, J. M., Myatt, L., & Feoktistov, I. (2014). Impaired adenosine-mediated angiogenesis in preeclampsia: potential implications for fetal programming. *Frontiers in Pharmacology*, *5*. https://doi.org/10.3389/FPHAR.2014.00134.

Eskandari, F., Rezaei, M., Mohammadpour-Gharehbagh, A., Teimoori, B., Yaghmaei, M., Narooei-Nejad, M., & Salimi, S. (2019). The association of pri-miRNA- 26a1 rs7372209 polymorphism and Preeclampsia susceptibility. *Clinical and Experimental Hypertension (New York, N.Y.: 1993)*, *41*(3), 268–273. https://doi.org/10.1080/10641963.2018.1469643.

Espinoza, J. (2012). Abnormal Fetal-Maternal Interactions: An Evolutionary Value? *Obstetrics and Gynecology*, *120*(2), 370–374. https://doi.org/10.1097/AOG.0B013E31825CB96D.

Fang, Y. N., Huang, Z. L., Li, H., Tan, W. B., Zhang, Q. G., Wang, L., & Wu, J. L. (2018). Highly expressed miR-182-5p can promote preeclampsia progression by degrading RND3 and inhibiting HTR-8/SVneo cell invasion. *European Review for Medical and Pharmacological Sciences*, *22*(20), 6583–6590. https://doi.org/10.26355/EURREV_201810_16132.

Fogarty, N. M. E., Burton, G. J., & Ferguson-Smith, A. C. (2015). Different epigenetic states define syncytiotrophoblast and cytotrophoblast nuclei in the trophoblast of the human placenta. *Placenta*, *36*(8), 796–802. https://doi.org/10.1016/J.PLACENTA.2015.05.006.

Friso, S., Carvajal, C. A., Fardella, C. E., & Olivieri, O. (2015). Epigenetics and arterial hypertension: the challenge of emerging evidence. *Translational Research: The Journal of Laboratory and Clinical Medicine*, *165*(1), 154–165. https://doi.org/10.1016/J.TRSL.2014.06.007.

Fu, G., Brkić, J., Hayder, H., & Peng, C. (2013). MicroRNAs in Human Placental Development and Pregnancy Complications. *International Journal of Molecular Sciences*, *14*(3), 5519–5544. https://doi.org/10.3390/IJMS14035519.

Fu, G., Ye, G., Nadeem, L., Ji, L., Manchanda, T., Wang, Y., Zhao, Y., Qiao, J., Wang, Y. L., Lye, S., Yang, B. B., & Peng, C. (2013). MicroRNA-376c impairs transforming growth factor-β and nodal signaling to promote trophoblast cell proliferation and invasion. *Hypertension (Dallas, Tex.: 1979)*, *61*(4), 864–872. https://doi.org/10.1161/HYPERTENSIONAHA.111.203489.

Fu, J. Y., Xiao, Y. P., Ren, C. L., Guo, Y. W., Qu, D. H., Zhang, J. H., & Zhu, Y. J. (2018). Up-regulation of miR-517-5p inhibits ERK/MMP-2 pathway: potential role in preeclampsia. *European Review for Medical and Pharmacological Sciences*, *22*(20), 6599–6608. https://doi.org/10.26355/EURREV_201810_16134.

Fujihara, Y., Murakami, M., Inoue, N., Satouh, Y., Kaseda, K., Ikawa, M., & Okabe, M. (2010). Sperm equatorial segment protein 1, SPESP1, is required for fully fertile sperm in mouse. *Journal of Cell Science*, *123*(Pt 9), 1531–1536. https://doi.org/10.1242/JCS.067363.

Gamage, T. K. J. B., Schierding, W., Hurley, D., Tsai, P., Ludgate, J. L., Bhoothpur, C., Chamley, L. W., Weeks, R. J., Macaulay, E. C., & James, J. L. (2018). The role of DNA methylation in human trophoblast differentiation. *Epigenetics*, *13*(12), 1154. https://doi.org/10.1080/15592294.2018.1549462.

Gao, W. L., Li, D., Xiao, Z. X., Liao, Q. P., Yang, H. X., Li, Y. X., Ji, L., & Wang, Y. L. (2011). Detection of global DNA methylation and paternally imprinted H19 gene methylation in preeclamptic placentas. *Hypertension Research 2011 34:5*, *34*(5), 655–661. https://doi.org/10.1038/hr.2011.9.

Gao, W. L., Liu, M., Yang, Y., Yang, H., Liao, Q., Bai, Y., Li, Y. X., Li, D., Peng, C., & Wang, Y. L. (2012). The imprinted H19 gene regulates human placental trophoblast cell proliferation via encoding miR-675 that targets Nodal Modulator 1 (NOMO1). *RNA Biology*, *9*(7), 1002–1010. https://doi.org/10.4161/RNA.20807.

Gebremedhin, K. G., & Rademacher, D. J. (2016). Histone H3 acetylation in the postmortem Parkinson's disease primary motor cortex. *Neuroscience Letters*, *627*, 121–125. https://doi.org/10.1016/J.NEULET.2016.05.060.

Gnarra, J. R., Ward, J. M., Porter, F. D., Wagner, J. R., Devor, D. E., Grinberg, A., Emmert-Buck, M. R., Westphal, H., Klausner, R. D., & Linehan, W. M. (1997). Defective placental vasculogenesis causes embryonic lethality in VHL-deficient mice. *Proceedings of the National Academy of Sciences of the United States of America*, *94*(17), 9102–9107. https://doi.org/10.1073/PNAS.94.17.9102.

Gomez, R. A., Norling, L. L., Wilfong, N., Isakson, P., Lynch, K. R., Hock, R., & Quesenberry, P. (1993). Leukocytes synthesize angiotensinogen. *Hypertension*, *21*(4), 470–475. https://doi.org/10.1161/01.HYP.21.4.470.

Granger, J. P., Alexander, B. T., Llinas, M. T., Bennett, W. A., & Khalil, R. A. (2001). Pathophysiology of hypertension during preeclampsia linking placental ischemia with endothelial dysfunction. *Hypertension (Dallas, Tex. : 1979)*, *38*(3 Pt 2), 718–722. https://doi.org/10.1161/01.HYP.38.3.718.

Hammond, S. M. (2015). An overview of microRNAs. *Advanced Drug Delivery Reviews*, *87*, 3–14. https://doi.org/10.1016/J.ADDR.2015.05.001.

Han, L., Zhao, Y., Luo, Q. Q., Liu, X. X., Lu, S. S., & Zou, L. (2017). The significance of miR-145 in the prediction of preeclampsia. *Bratislava Medical Journal*, *118*(9), 523–528. https://doi.org/10.4149/BLL_2017_101.

Harmon, A. C., Cornelius, D. C., Amaral, L. M., Faulkner, J. L., Cunningham, M. W., Wallace, K., & LaMarca, B. (2016). The role of inflammation in the pathology of preeclampsia. *Clinical Science (London, England : 1979)*, *130*(6), 409. https://doi.org/10.1042/CS20150702.

Holoch, D., & Moazed, D. (2015). RNA-mediated epigenetic regulation of gene expression. *Nature Reviews Genetics 2015 16:2*, *16*(2), 71–84. https://doi.org/10.1038/nrg3863.

Huang, B., Jiang, C., & Zhang, R. (2014). Epigenetics: The language of the cell? *Epigenomics*, *6*(1), 73–88. https://doi.org/10.2217/EPI.13.72.

Huang, G., Du, M. yu, Zhu, H., Zhang, N., Lu, Z. W., Qian, L. X., Zhang, W., Tian, X., He, X., & Yin, L. (2018). MiRNA-34a reversed TGF-β-induced epithelial-mesenchymal transition via suppression of SMAD4 in NPC cells. *Biomedicine & Pharmacotherapy = Biomedecine & Pharmacotherapie*, *106*, 217–224. https://doi.org/10.1016/J.BIOPHA.2018.06.115.

Huppertz, B. (2018). The Critical Role of Abnormal Trophoblast Development in the Etiology of Preeclampsia. *Current Pharmaceutical Biotechnology*, *19*(10), 771–780. https://doi.org/10.2174/1389201019666180427110547.

Icli, B., Nabzdyk, C. S., Lujan-Hernandez, J., Cahill, M., Auster, M. E., Wara, A. K. M., Sun, X., Ozdemir, D., Giatsidis, G., Orgill, D. P., & Feinberg, M. W. (2016). Regulation of impaired angiogenesis in diabetic dermal wound healing by microRNA-26a. *Journal of Molecular and Cellular Cardiology*, *91*, 151–159. https://doi.org/10.1016/J.YJMCC.2016.01.007.

Ietta, F., Wu, Y., Winter, J., Xu, J., Wang, J., Post, M., & Caniggia, I. (2006). Dynamic HIF1A regulation during human placental development. *Biology of Reproduction*, *75*(1), 112–121. https://doi.org/10.1095/BIOLREPROD.106.051557.

Iglesias-Platas, I., Martin-Trujillo, A., Petazzi, P., Guillaumet-Adkins, A., Esteller, M., & Monk, D. (2014). Altered expression of the imprinted transcription factor PLAGL1 deregulates a network of genes in the human IUGR placenta. *Human Molecular Genetics*, *23*(23), 6275–6285. https://doi.org/10.1093/HMG/DDU347.

Im, G. Il, & Choi, Y. J. (2013). Epigenetics in osteoarthritis and its implication for future therapeutics. *Expert Opinion on Biological Therapy*, *13*(5), 713–721. https://doi.org/10.1517/14712598.2013.764410.

Iriyama, T., Sun, K., Parchim, N. F., Li, J., Zhao, C., Song, A., Hart, L. A., Blackwell, S. C., Sibai, B. M., Chan, L. N. L., Chan, T. S., Hicks, M. J., Blackburn, M. R., Kellems, R. E., & Xia, Y. (2015). Elevated placental adenosine signaling contributes to the pathogenesis of preeclampsia. *Circulation*, *131*(8), 730–741. https://doi.org/10.1161/CIRCULATIONAHA.114.013740.

Jacobs, M. E., Wingo, C. S., & Cain, B. D. (2013). An emerging role for microRNA in the regulation of endothelin-1. *Frontiers in Physiology*, *4*. https://doi.org/10.3389/FPHYS.2013.00022.

Jankovic-Karasoulos, T., McAninch, D., McCullough, D., Wilson, R. L., Bianco-Miotto, T., & Roberts, C. T. (2018). Isolation of villous cytotrophoblasts from second trimester human placentas. *Placenta*, *74*, 55–58. https://doi.org/10.1016/J.PLACENTA.2018.11.007.

Jensen, L. E., Muzio, M., Mantovani, A., & Whitehead, A. S. (2000). IL-1 signaling cascade in liver cells and the involvement of a soluble form of the IL-1 receptor accessory protein. *Journal of Immunology (Baltimore, MD : 1950)*, *164*(10), 5277–5286. https://doi.org/10.4049/JIMMUNOL.164.10.5277.

Jia, R. Z., Rui, C., Li, J. Y., Cui, X. W., & Wang, X. (2014). CDX1 restricts the invasion of HTR-8/SVneo trophoblast cells by inhibiting MMP-9 expression. *Placenta*, *35*(7), 450–454. https://doi.org/10.1016/J.PLACENTA.2014.04.011.

Jia, Rui Zhe, Zhang, X., Hu, P., Liu, X. M., Hua, X. D., Wang, X., & Ding, H. J. (2012). Screening for differential methylation status in human placenta in preeclampsia using a CpG island plus promoter microarray. *International Journal of Molecular Medicine*, *30*(1), 133–141. https://doi.org/10.3892/IJMM.2012.983.

Jiang, L., Long, A., Tan, L., Hong, M., Wu, J., Cai, L., & Li, Q. (2017). Elevated microRNA-520g in pre-eclampsia inhibits migration and invasion of trophoblasts. *Placenta*, *51*, 70–75. https://doi.org/10.1016/J.PLACENTA.2017.02.001.

Jiang, W. L., Zhang, Y. F., Xia, Q. Q., Zhu, J., Yu, X., Fan, T., & Wang, F. (2015). MicroRNA-19a regulates lipopolysaccharideinduced endothelial cell apoptosis through modulation of apoptosis signal-regulating kinase 1 expression. *BMC Molecular Biology*, *16*(1), 1–8. https://doi.org/10.1186/S12867-015-0034-8/FIGURES/5.

Jin, F., Qiao, C., Luan, N., & Shang, T. (2015). The expression of the imprinted gene pleckstrin homology-like domain family A member 2 in placental tissues of preeclampsia and its effects on the proliferation, migration and invasion of trophoblast cells JEG-3. *Clinical and Experimental Pharmacology & Physiology*, *42*(11), 1142–1151. https://doi.org/10.1111/1440-1681.12468.

Julian, C. G., Pedersen, B. S., Salmon, C. S., Yang, I. V., Gonzales, M., Vargas, E., Moore, L. G., & Schwartz, D. A. (2015). Unique DNA Methylation Patterns in Offspring of Hypertensive Pregnancy. *Clinical and Translational Science*, *8*(6), 740–745. https://doi.org/10.1111/CTS.12346.

Kamrani, A., Alipourfard, I., Ahmadi-Khiavi, H., Yousefi, M., Rostamzadeh, D., Izadi, M., & Ahmadi, M. (2019). The role of epigenetic changes in preeclampsia. *BioFactors*, *45*(5), 712–724. https://doi.org/10.1002/BIOF.1542.

Khaliq, O. P., Murugesan, S., Moodley, J., & Mackraj, I. (2018). Differential expression of miRNAs are associated with the insulin signaling pathway in preeclampsia and gestational hypertension. *Clinical and Experimental Hypertension (New York, N.Y. : 1993)*, *40*(8), 744–751. https://doi.org/10.1080/10641963.2018.1431257.

Khorkova, O., Hsiao, J., & Wahlestedt, C. (2015). Basic biology and therapeutic implications of lncRNA. *Advanced Drug Delivery Reviews*, *87*, 15–24. https://doi.org/10.1016/J.ADDR.2015.05.012.

Kleinrouweler, C. E., Wiegerinck, M. M. J., Ris-Stalpers, C., Bossuyt, P. M. M., Van Der Post, J. A. M., Von Dadelszen, P., Mol, B. W. J., & Pajkrt, E. (2012). Accuracy of circulating placental growth factor, vascular endothelial growth factor, soluble fms-like tyrosine kinase 1 and soluble endoglin in the prediction of pre-eclampsia: a systematic review and meta-analysis. *BJOG : An International Journal of Obstetrics and Gynaecology*, *119*(7), 778–787. https://doi.org/10.1111/J.1471-0528.2012.03311.X.

Kornberg, R. D. (1974). Chromatin structure: A repeating unit of histones and DNA. *Science*, *184*(4139), 868–871. https://doi.org/10.1126/SCIENCE.184.4139.868/ASSET/F767CB17-9373-448B-A058-D0598FEFAF69/ASSETS/SCIENCE.184.4139.868.FP.PNG.

Kouzarides, T. (2007). Chromatin modifications and their function. *Cell*, *128*(4), 693–705. https://doi.org/10.1016/J.CELL.2007.02.005.

Kulkarni, A., Chavan-Gautam, P., Mehendale, S., Yadav, H., & Joshi, S. (2011). Global DNA methylation patterns in placenta and its association with maternal hypertension in pre-eclampsia. *DNA and Cell Biology*, *30*(2), 79–84. https://doi.org/10.1089/DNA.2010.1084.

Laganà, A. S., Vitale, S. G., Sapia, F., Valenti, G., Corrado, F., Padula, F., Rapisarda, A. M. C., & D'Anna, R. (2018). miRNA expression for early diagnosis of preeclampsia onset: hope or hype? *The Journal of Maternal-Fetal & Neonatal Medicine: The Official Journal of the European Association of Perinatal Medicine, the Federation of Asia and Oceania Perinatal Societies, the International Society of Perinatal Obstetricians*, *31*(6), 817–821. https://doi.org/10.1080/14767058.2017.1296426.

Leavey, K., Wilson, S. L., Bainbridge, S. A., Robinson, W. P., & Cox, B. J. (2018). Epigenetic regulation of placental gene expression in transcriptional subtypes of preeclampsia. *Clinical Epigenetics*, *10*(1). https://doi.org/10.1186/S13148-018-0463-6.

Levine, R. J., Maynard, S. E., Qian, C., Lim, K.-H., England, L. J., Yu, K. F., Schisterman, E. F., Thadhani, R., Sachs, B. P., Epstein, F. H., Sibai, B. M., Sukhatme, V. P., & Karumanchi, S. A. (2004). Circulating angiogenic factors and the risk of preeclampsia. *The New England Journal of Medicine*, *350*(7), 672–683. https://doi.org/10.1056/NEJMOA031884.

Li, L. C. (2014). Chromatin remodeling by the small RNA machinery in mammalian cells. *Epigenetics*, *9*(1), 45–52. https://doi.org/10.4161/EPI.26830.

Li, X., Wu, C., Shen, Y., Wang, K., Tang, L., Zhou, M., Yang, M., Pan, T., Liu, X., & Xu, W. (2018). Ten-eleven translocation 2 demethylates the MMP9 promoter, and its down-regulation in preeclampsia impairs trophoblast migration and invasion. *The Journal of Biological Chemistry*, *293*(26), 10059–10070. https://doi.org/10.1074/JBC.RA117.001265.

Lomniczi, A., & Ojeda, S. R. (2016). The Emerging Role of Epigenetics in the Regulation of Female Puberty. *Endocrine Development*, *29*, 1–16. https://doi.org/10.1159/000438840.

Louwen, F., Muschol-Steinmetz, C., Reinhard, J., Reitter, A., & Yuan, J. (2012). A lesson for cancer research: placental microarray gene analysis in preeclampsia. *Oncotarget*, *3*(8), 759–773. https://doi.org/10.18632/ONCOTARGET.595.

Lu, T. M., Lu, W., & Zhao, L. J. (2017). MicroRNA-137 Affects Proliferation and Migration of Placenta Trophoblast Cells in Preeclampsia by Targeting ERRα. *Reproductive Sciences*, *24*(1), 85–96. https://doi.org/10.1177/1933719116650754.

Ma, M., Zhou, Q. J., Xiong, Y., Li, B., & Li, X. T. (2018). Preeclampsia is associated with hypermethylation of IGF-1 promoter mediated by DNMT1. *American Journal of Translational Research*, *10*(1), 16. /pmc/articles/PMC5801344/.

Maccalman, C. D., Furth, E. E., Omigbodun, A., Bronner, M., Coutifaris, C., & Strauss, J. F. (1996). Regulated Expression of Cadherin-11 in Human Epithelial Cells: A Role for Cadherin-11 in Trophoblast-Endometrium Interactions? *Developmental Dynamics*, *206*, 201–211. https://doi.org/10.1002/(SICI)1097-0177(199606)206:2.

Majchrzak-Celińska, A., Kosicka, K., Paczkowska, J., Główka, F. K., Bręborowicz, G. H., Krzyścin, M., Siemiątkowska, A., Szaumkessel, M., & Baer-Dubowska, W. (2017). HSD11B2, RUNX3, and LINE-1 Methylation in Placental DNA of Hypertensive Disorders of Pregnancy Patients. *Reproductive Sciences (Thousand Oaks, Calif.)*, *24*(11), 1520–1531. https://doi.org/10.1177/1933719117692043.

Mastrolia, S. A., Mazor, M., Holcberg, G., Leron, E., Beharier, O., Loverro, G., & Erez, O. (2015). The physiologic anticoagulant and anti-inflammatory role of heparins and their utility in the prevention of pregnancy complications. *Thrombosis and Haemostasis*, *113*(6), 1236–1246. https://doi.org/10.1160/TH14-10-0848.

Mei, Z., Huang, B., Zhang, Y., Qian, X., Mo, Y., & Deng, N. (2019). Histone deacetylase 6 negatively regulated microRNA-199a-5p induces the occurrence of preeclampsia by targeting VEGFA in vitro. *Biomedicine & Pharmacotherapy = Biomedecine & Pharmacotherapie*, *114*. https://doi.org/10.1016/J.BIOPHA.2019.108805.

Monkley, S. J., Delaney, S. J., Pennisi, D. J., Christiansen, J. H., & Wainwright, B. J. (1996). Targeted disruption of the Wnt2 gene results in placentation defects. *Development (Cambridge, England)*, *122*(11), 3343–3353. https://doi.org/10.1242/DEV.122.11.3343.

Morales-Prieto, D. M., Chaiwangyen, W., Ospina-Prieto, S., Schneider, U., Herrmann, J., Gruhn, B., & Markert, U. R. (2012). MicroRNA expression profiles of trophoblastic cells. *Placenta*, *33*(9), 725–734. https://doi.org/10.1016/J.PLACENTA.2012.05.009.

Mousa, A. A., Strauss, J. F., & Walsh, S. W. (2012). Reduced methylation of the thromboxane synthase gene is correlated with its increased vascular expression in preeclampsia. *Hypertension (Dallas, Tex. : 1979)*, *59*(6), 1249–1255. https://doi.org/10.1161/HYPERTENSIONAHA.111.188730.

Muñoz-Hernandez, R., Miranda, M. L., Stiefel, P., Lin, R. Z., Praena-Fernández, J. M., Dominguez-Simeon, M. J., Villar, J., Moreno-Luna, R., & Melero-Martin, J. M. (2014). Decreased Level of Cord Blood Circulating Endothelial Colony-Forming Cells in Preeclampsia. *Hypertension*, *64*(1), 165. https://doi.org/10.1161/HYPERTENSIONAHA.113.03058.

Munro, S. K., Mitchell, M. D., & Ponnampalam, A. P. (2013). Histone deacetylase inhibition by trichostatin A mitigates LPS induced TNFα and IL-10 production in human placental explants. *Placenta*, *34*(7), 567–573. https://doi.org/10.1016/J.PLACENTA.2013.04.004.

Muralimanoharan, S., Maloyan, A., Mele, J., Guo, C., Myatt, L. G., & Myatt, L. (2012). MIR-210 modulates mitochondrial respiration in placenta with preeclampsia. *Placenta*, *33*(10), 816–823. https://doi.org/10.1016/J.PLACENTA.2012.07.002.

Nadeem, L., Munir, S., Fu, G., Dunk, C., Baczyk, D., Caniggia, I., Lye, S., & Peng, C. (2011). Nodal signals through activin receptor-like kinase 7 to inhibit trophoblast migration and invasion: implication in the pathogenesis of preeclampsia. *The American Journal of Pathology*, *178*(3), 1177–1189. https://doi.org/10.1016/J.AJPATH.2010.11.066.

Nadiminty, N., Dutt, S., Tepper, C., & Gao, A. C. (2010). Microarray analysis reveals potential target genes of NF-kappaB2/p52 in LNCaP prostate cancer cells. *The Prostate*, *70*(3), 276–287. https://doi.org/10.1002/PROS.21062.

Nahar, M. S., Liao, C., Kannan, K., Harris, C., & Dolinoy, D. C. (2015). In utero bisphenol A concentration, metabolism, and global DNA methylation across matched placenta, kidney, and liver in the human fetus. *Chemosphere*, *124*(1), 54–60. https://doi.org/10.1016/J.CHEMOSPHERE.2014.10.071.

Nardozza, L. M. M., Caetano, A. C. R., Zamarian, A. C. P., Mazzola, J. B., Silva, C. P., Marçal, V. M. G., Lobo, T. F., Peixoto, A. B., & Araujo Júnior, E. (2017). Fetal growth restriction: current knowledge. *Archives of Gynecology and Obstetrics*, *295*(5), 1061–1077. https://doi.org/10.1007/S00404-017-4341-9.

Noris, M., Todeschini, M., Cassis, P., Pasta, F., Cappellini, A., Bonazzola, S., Macconi, D., Maucci, R., Porrati, F., Benigni, A., Picciolo, C., & Remuzzi, G. (2004). L-arginine depletion in preeclampsia orients nitric oxide synthase toward oxidant species. *Hypertension (Dallas, Tex.: 1979)*, *43*(3), 614–622. https://doi.org/10.1161/01.HYP.0000116220.39793.C9.

Novakovic, B., Fournier, T., Harris, L. K., James, J., Roberts, C. T., Yong, H. E. J., Kalionis, B., Evain-Brion, D., Ebeling, P. R., Wallace, E. M., Saffery, R., & Murthi, P. (2017). Increased methylation and decreased expression of homeobox genes TLX1, HOXA10 and DLX5 in human placenta are associated with trophoblast differentiation. *Scientific Reports 2017 7:1*, *7*(1), 1–13. https://doi.org/10.1038/s41598-017-04776-5.

Park, Y., Lee, H. J., Jung, Y. J., Kwon, H. Y., Kim, H., Lee, J. H., Kim, Y. H., Kim, H. O., Maeng, Y. S., & Kwon, J. Y. (2019). CD133+/C-kit+Lin - endothelial progenitor cells in fetal circulation demonstrate impaired differentiation potency in severe preeclampsia. *Pregnancy Hypertension*, *15*, 146–153. https://doi.org/10.1016/J.PREGHY.2018.12.005.

Peretz, J., Vrooman, L., Ricke, W. A., Hunt, P. A., Ehrlich, S., Hauser, R., Padmanabhan, V., Taylor, H. S., Swan, S. H., Vandevoort, C. A., & Flaws, J. A. (2014). Bisphenol a and reproductive health: update of experimental and human evidence, 2007-2013. *Environmental Health Perspectives*, *122*(8), 775–786. https://doi.org/10.1289/EHP.1307728.

Perucci, L. O., Corrêa, M. D., Dusse, L. M., Gomes, K. B., & Sousa, L. P. (2017). Resolution of inflammation pathways in preeclampsia-a narrative review. *Immunologic Research*, *65*(4), 774–789. https://doi.org/10.1007/S12026-017-8921-3.

Pritchard, C. C., Kroh, E., Wood, B., Arroyo, J. D., Dougherty, K. J., Miyaji, M. M., Tait, J. F., & Tewari, M. (2012). Blood cell origin of circulating microRNAs: a cautionary note for cancer biomarker studies. *Cancer Prevention Research (Philadelphia, Pa.)*, *5*(3), 492–497. https://doi.org/10.1158/1940-6207.CAPR-11-0370.

Rahat, B., Hamid, A., Najar, R. A., Bagga, R., & Kaur, J. (2014). Epigenetic mechanisms regulate placental c-myc and hTERT in normal and pathological pregnancies; c-myc as a novel fetal DNA epigenetic marker for pre-eclampsia. *Molecular Human Reproduction*, *20*(10), 1026–1040. https://doi.org/10.1093/MOLEHR/GAU053.

Rahat, B., Mahajan, A., Bagga, R., Hamid, A., & Kaur, J. (2017). Epigenetic modifications at DMRs of placental genes are subjected to variations in normal gestation, pathological conditions and folate supplementation. *Scientific Reports*, *7*. https://doi.org/10.1038/SREP40774.

Rahat, B., Sharma, R., Bagga, R., Hamid, A., & Kaur, J. (2016). Imbalance between matrix metalloproteinases and their tissue inhibitors in preeclampsia and gestational trophoblastic diseases. *Reproduction (Cambridge, England)*, *152*(1), 11–22. https://doi.org/10.1530/REP-16-0060.

Rahat, B., Thakur, S., Hamid, A., Bagga, R., & Kaur, J. (2016). Association of aberrant methylation at promoter regions of tumor suppressor genes with placental pathologies. *Http://Dx.Doi.Org/10.2217/Epi.16.7*, *8*(6), 767–787. https://doi.org/10.2217/EPI.16.7.

Ransohoff, J. D., Wei, Y., & Khavari, P. A. (2018). The functions and unique features of long intergenic non-coding RNA. *Nature Reviews. Molecular Cell Biology*, *19*(3), 143. https://doi.org/10.1038/NRM.2017.104.

Ratovitski, T., Arbez, N., Stewart, J. C., Chighladze, E., & Ross, C. A. (2015). PRMT5- mediated symmetric arginine dimethylation is attenuated by mutant huntingtin and is impaired in Huntington's disease (HD). *Cell Cycle (Georgetown, Tex.)*, *14*(11), 1716–1729. https://doi.org/10.1080/15384101.2015.1033595.

Roberts, J. M., & Escudero, C. (2012). The placenta in preeclampsia. *Pregnancy Hypertension*, *2*(2), 72. https://doi.org/10.1016/J.PREGHY.2012.01.001.

Roberts, V. H. J., Greenwood, S. L., Elliott, A. C., Sibley, C. P., & Waters, L. H. (2006). Purinergic receptors in human placenta: evidence for functionally active P2X4, P2X7, P2Y2, and P2Y6. *American Journal of Physiology. Regulatory, Integrative and Comparative Physiology*, *290*(5). https://doi.org/10.1152/AJPREGU.00612.2005.

Roger, T., Lugrin, J., Le Roy, D., Goy, G., Mombelli, M., Koessler, T., Ding, X. C., Chanson, A. L., Reymond, M. K., Miconnet, I., Schrenzel, J., François, P., & Calandra, T. (2011). Histone deacetylase inhibitors impair innate immune responses to Toll-like receptor agonists and to infection. *Blood*, *117*(4), 1205–1217. https://doi.org/10.1182/BLOOD-2010-05-284711.

Ruebner, M., Strissel, P. L., Ekici, A. B., Stiegler, E., Dammer, U., Goecke, T. W., Faschingbauer, F., Fahlbusch, F. B., Beckmann, M. W., & Strick, R. (2013). Reduced syncytin-1 expression levels in placental syndromes correlates with epigenetic hypermethylation of the ERVW-1 promoter region. *PloS One*, *8*(2). https://doi.org/10.1371/JOURNAL.PONE.0056145.

Ruebner, M., Strissel, P. L., Langbein, M., Fahlbusch, F., Wachter, D. L., Faschingbauer, F., Beckmann, M. W., & Strick, R. (2010). Impaired cell fusion and differentiation in placentae from patients with intrauterine growth restriction correlate with reduced levels of HERV envelope genes. *Journal of Molecular Medicine (Berlin, Germany)*, *88*(11), 1143–1156. https://doi.org/10.1007/S00109-010-0656-8.

Saftlas, A. F., Beydoun, H., & Triche, E. (2005). Immunogenetic determinants of preeclampsia and related pregnancy disorders: a systematic review. *Obstetrics and Gynecology*, *106*(1), 162–172. https://doi.org/10.1097/01.AOG.0000167389.97019.37.

Saha, S., Chakraborty, S., Bhattacharya, A., Biswas, A., & Ain, R. (2017). MicroRNA regulation of Transthyretin in trophoblast differentiation and Intra-Uterine Growth Restriction. *Scientific Reports 2017 7:1*, *7*(1), 1–13. https://doi.org/10.1038/s41598-017-16566-0.

Salvianti, F., Inversetti, A., Smid, M., Valsecchi, L., Candiani, M., Pazzagli, M., Cremonesi, L., Ferrari, M., Pinzani, P., & Galbiati, S. (2015). Prospective evaluation of RASSF1A cell-free DNA as a biomarker of pre-eclampsia. *Placenta*, *36*(9), 996–1001. https://doi.org/10.1016/J.PLACENTA.2015.07.003.

Savvidou, M. D., Hingorani, A. D., Tsikas, D., Frölich, J. C., Vallance, P., & Nicolaides, K. H. (2003). Endothelial dysfunction and raised plasma concentrations of asymmetric dimethylarginine in pregnant women who subsequently develop pre-eclampsia. *Lancet (London, England)*, *361*(9368), 1511–1517. https://doi.org/10.1016/S0140-6736(03)13177-7.

Seto, E., & Yoshida, M. (2014). Erasers of histone acetylation: the histone deacetylase enzymes. *Cold Spring Harbor Perspectives in Biology*, *6*(4). https://doi.org/10.1101/CSHPERSPECT.A018713.

Shen, C., Quan, Q., Yang, C., Wen, Y., & Li, H. (2018). Histone demethylase JMJD6 regulates cellular migration and proliferation in adipose-derived mesenchymal stem cells. *Stem Cell Research and Therapy*, *9*(1), 1–13. https://doi.org/10.1186/S13287-018-0949-3/FIGURES/7.

Shi, X., Liu, H., Cao, J., Liu, Q., Tang, G., Liu, W., Liu, H., Deng, D., Qiao, F., & Wu, Y. (2015). Promoter Hypomethylation of Maspin Inhibits Migration and Invasion of Extravillous Trophoblast Cells during Placentation. *PLOS One*, *10*(8), e0135359. https://doi.org/10.1371/JOURNAL.PONE.0135359.

Small, E. M., Sutherland, L. B., Rajagopalan, K. N., Wang, S., & Olson, E. N. (2010). MicroRNA-218 regulates vascular patterning by modulation of Slit-Robo signaling. *Circulation Research*, *107*(11), 1336. https://doi.org/10.1161/CIRCRESAHA.110.227926.

Song, X., Rui, C., Meng, L., Zhang, R., Shen, R., Ding, H., Li, J., Li, J., & Long, W. (2017). Long non-coding RNA RPAIN regulates the invasion and apoptosis of trophoblast cell lines via complement protein C1q. *Oncotarget*, *8*(5), 7637–7646. https://doi.org/10.18632/oncotarget.13826.

Stotz, K., & Griffiths, P. (2016). Epigenetics: ambiguities and implications. *History and Philosophy of the Life Sciences*, *38*(4). https://doi.org/10.1007/S40656-016-0121-2.

Sundrani, D. P., Reddy, U. S., Joshi, A. A., Mehendale, S. S., Chavan-Gautam, P. M., Hardikar, A. A., Chandak, G. R., & Joshi, S. R. (2013). Differential placental methylation and expression of VEGF, FLT-1 and KDR genes in human term and preterm preeclampsia. *Clinical Epigenetics*, *5*(1), 1–11. https://doi.org/10.1186/1868-7083-5-6/TABLES/3.

Taglauer, E. S., Wilkins-Haug, L., & Bianchi, D. W. (2014). Review: cell-free fetal DNA in the maternal circulation as an indication of placental health and disease. *Placenta*, *35 Suppl*(Suppl). https://doi.org/10.1016/J.PLACENTA.2013.11.014.

Tait, S., Tassinari, R., Maranghi, F., & Mantovani, A. (2015). Bisphenol A affects placental layers morphology and angiogenesis during early pregnancy phase in mice. *Journal of Applied Toxicology : JAT*, *35*(11), 1278–1291. https://doi.org/10.1002/JAT.3176.

Takizawa, T., Ishibashi, O., Ohkuchi, A., Moksed Ali, M., Kurashina, R., Luo, S. S., Ishikawa, T., Takizawa, T., Hirashima, C., Takahashi, K., Migita, M., Ishikawa, G., Yoneyama, K., Asakura, H., Izumi, A., Matsubara, S., & Takeshita, T. (2012). Hydroxysteroid (17-β) dehydrogenase 1 is dysregulated by miR-210 and miR-518c that are aberrantly expressed in preeclamptic placentas: a novel marker for predicting preeclampsia. *Hypertension (Dallas, Tex. : 1979)*, *59*(2), 265–273. https://doi.org/10.1161/HYPERTENSIONAHA.111.180232.

Tannetta, D. S., Dragovic, R. A., Gardiner, C., Redman, C. W., & Sargent, I. L. (2013). Characterisation of syncytiotrophoblast vesicles in normal pregnancy and pre-eclampsia: expression of Flt-1 and endoglin. *PloS One*, *8*(2). https://doi.org/10.1371/JOURNAL.PONE.0056754.

Tewksbury, D. A. (1996). Quantitation of five forms of high molecular weight angiotensinogen from human placenta. *American Journal of Hypertension*, *9*(10 Pt 1), 1029–1034. https://doi.org/10.1016/0895-7061(96)00175-6.

Toal, M., Chan, C., Fallah, S., Alkazaleh, F., Chaddha, V., Windrim, R. C., & Kingdom, J. C. P. (2007). Usefulness of a placental profile in high-risk pregnancies. *American Journal of Obstetrics and Gynecology*, *196*(4), 363.e1-363.e7. https://doi.org/10.1016/J.AJOG.2006.10.897.

Togher, K. L., Kenny, L. C., & O'Keeffe, G. W. (2017). Class-Specific Histone Deacetylase Inhibitors Promote 11-Beta Hydroxysteroid Dehydrogenase Type 2 Expression in JEG-3 Cells. *International Journal of Cell Biology*, *2017*. https://doi.org/10.1155/2017/6169310.

Tsaprouni, L. G., Ito, K., Powell, J. J., Adcock, I. M., & Punchard, N. (2011). Differential patterns of histone acetylation in inflammatory bowel diseases. *Journal of Inflammation (London, England)*, *8*(1). https://doi.org/10.1186/1476-9255-8-1.

Tsui, D. W. Y., Chan, K. C. A., Chim, S. S. C., Chan, L. W., Leung, T. Y., Lau, T. K., Lo, Y. M. D., & Chiu, R. W. K. (2007). Quantitative aberrations of hypermethylated RASSF1A gene sequences in maternal plasma in pre-eclampsia. *Prenatal Diagnosis*, *27*(13), 1212–1218. https://doi.org/10.1002/PD.1897.

Umemura, K., Ishioka, S. I., Endo, T., Ezaka, Y., Takahashi, M., & Saito, T. (2013). Roles of microRNA-34a in the pathogenesis of placenta accreta. *The Journal of Obstetrics and Gynaecology Research*, *39*(1), 67–74. https://doi.org/10.1111/J.1447-0756.2012.01898.X.

Wang, F., Li, H., Yan, X. G., Zhou, Z. W., Yi, Z. G., He, Z. X., Pan, S. T., Yang, Y. X., Wang, Z. Z., Zhang, X., Yang, T., Qiu, J. X., & Zhou, S. F. (2015). Alisertib induces cell cycle arrest and autophagy and suppresses epithelial-to-mesenchymal transition involving PI3K/Akt/mTOR and sirtuin 1-mediated signaling pathways in human pancreatic cancer cells. *Drug Design, Development and Therapy*, *9*, 575–601. https://doi.org/10.2147/DDDT.S75221.

Wang, N., Li, R., & Xue, M. (2019). Potential regulatory network in the PSG10P/miR-19a-3p/IL1RAP pathway is possibly involved in preeclampsia pathogenesis. *Journal of Cellular and Molecular Medicine*, *23*(2), 852–864. https://doi.org/10.1111/JCMM.13985.

Wei, S. Q., Qi, H. P., Luo, Z. C., & Fraser, W. D. (2013). Maternal vitamin D status and adverse pregnancy outcomes: a systematic review and meta-analysis. *The Journal of Maternal-Fetal & Neonatal Medicine : The Official Journal of the European Association of Perinatal Medicine, the Federation of Asia and Oceania Perinatal Societies, the International Society of Perinatal Obstetricians*, *26*(9), 889–899. https://doi.org/10.3109/14767058.2013.765849.

White, W. M., Brost, B., Sun, Z., Rose, C., Craici, I., Wagner, S. J., Turner, S. T., & Garovic, V. D. (2013). Genome-wide methylation profiling demonstrates hypermethylation in maternal leukocyte DNA in preeclamptic compared to normotensive pregnancies. *Hypertension in Pregnancy*, *32*(3), 257–269. https://doi.org/10.3109/10641955.2013.796970.

White, W. M., Sun, Z., Borowski, K. S., Brost, B. C., Davies, N. P., Rose, C. H., & Garovic, V. D. (2016). Preeclampsia/Eclampsia candidate genes show altered methylation in maternal leukocytes of preeclamptic women at the time of delivery. *Hypertension in Pregnancy*, *35*(3), 394–404. https://doi.org/10.3109/10641955.2016.1162315.

Wolkowicz, M. J., Shetty, J., Westbrook, A., Klotz, K., Jayes, F., Mandal, A., Flickinger, C. J., & Herr, J. C. (2003). Equatorial Segment Protein Defines a Discrete Acrosomal Subcompartment Persisting Throughout Acrosomal Biogenesis. *Biology of Reproduction*, *69*(3), 735–745. https://doi.org/10.1095/BIOLREPROD.103.016675.

Wong, N. C., Novakovic, B., Weinrich, B., Dewi, C., Andronikos, R., Sibson, M., Macrae, F., Morley, R., Pertile, M. D., Craig, J. M., & Saffery, R. (2008). Methylation of the adenomatous polyposis coli (APC) gene in human placenta and hypermethylation in choriocarcinoma cells. *Cancer Letters*, *268*(1), 56–62. https://doi.org/10.1016/J.CANLET.2008.03.033.

World Health Organization. (2011). *WHO recommendations for prevention and treatment of pre-eclampsia and eclampsia*. Retrieved May 11, 2022, from https://www.who.int/publications/i/item/97892415 48335.

Xie, D., Zhu, J., Liu, Q., Li, J., Song, M., Wang, K., Zhou, Q., Jia, Y., & Li, T. (2019). Dysregulation of HDAC9 Represses Trophoblast Cell Migration and Invasion Through TIMP3 Activation in Preeclampsia. *American Journal of Hypertension*, *32*(5), 515–523. https://doi.org/10.1093/AJH/HPZ006.

Xu, P., Zhao, Y., Liu, M., Wang, Y., Wang, H., Li, Y. X., Zhu, X., Yao, Y., Wang, H., Qiao, J., Ji, L., & Wang, Y. L. (2014). Variations of microRNAs in human placentas and plasma from preeclamptic pregnancy. *Hypertension (Dallas, Tex. : 1979)*, *63*(6), 1276–1284. https://doi.org/10.1161/HYPERTENSIONAHA.113.02647.

Xu, Y., Ge, Z., Zhang, E., Zuo, Q., Huang, S., Yang, N., Wu, D., Zhang, Y., Chen, Y., Xu, H., Huang, H., Jiang, Z., & Sun, L. (2017). The lncRNA TUG1 modulates proliferation in trophoblast cells via epigenetic suppression of RND3. *Cell Death & Disease*, *8*(10). https://doi.org/10.1038/CDDIS.2017.503.

Xuan, J., Jing, Z., Yuanfang, Z., Xiaoju, H., Pei, L., Guiyin, J., & Yu, Z. (2016). Comprehensive analysis of DNA methylation and gene expression of placental tissue in preeclampsia patients. *Hypertension in Pregnancy*, *35*(1), 129–138. https://doi.org/10.3109/10641955.2015.1117099.

Xue, F., Yang, J., Li, Q., & Zhou, H. (2019). Down-regulation of microRNA-34a-5p promotes trophoblast cell migration and invasion via targetting Smad4. *Bioscience Reports*, *39*(2). https://doi.org/10.1042/BSR20181631.

Yallampalli, C., Chauhan, M., Thota, C. S., Kondapaka, S., & Wimalawansa, S. J. (2002). Calcitonin gene-related peptide in pregnancy and its emerging receptor heterogeneity. *Trends in Endocrinology and Metabolism: TEM*, *13*(6), 263–269. https://doi.org/10.1016/S1043-2760(02)00563-5.

Ye, Y., Tang, Y., Xiong, Y., Feng, L., & Li, X. (2019). Bisphenol A exposure alters placentation and causes preeclampsia-like features in pregnant mice involved in reprogramming of DNA methylation of WNT2. *FASEB Journal: Official Publication of the Federation of American Societies for Experimental Biology*, *33*(2), 2732–2742. https://doi.org/10.1096/FJ.201800934RRR.

Ye, Y., Zhou, Q., Feng, L., Wu, J., Xiong, Y., & Li, X. (2017). Maternal serum bisphenol A levels and risk of pre-eclampsia: a nested case-control study. *European Journal of Public Health*, *27*(6), 1102–1107. https://doi.org/10.1093/EURPUB/CKX148.

Yeung, K. R., Chiu, C. L., Pidsley, R., Makris, A., Hennessy, A., & Lind, J. M. (2016). DNA methylation profiles in preeclampsia and healthy control placentas. *American Journal of Physiology. Heart and Circulatory Physiology*, *310*(10), H1295–H1303. https://doi.org/10.1152/AJPHEART.00958.2015.

Youssef, H. M. G., & Marei, E. S. (2019). Association of MicroRNA-210 and MicroRNA-155 with severity of preeclampsia. *Pregnancy Hypertension*, *17*, 49–53. https://doi.org/10.1016/J.PREGHY.2019.05.010.

Yu, L., Chen, M., Zhao, D., Yi, P., Lu, L., Han, J., Zheng, X., Zhou, Y., & Li, L. (2009). The H19 gene imprinting in normal pregnancy and pre-eclampsia. *Placenta*, *30*(5), 443–447. https://doi.org/10.1016/J.PLACENTA.2009.02.011.

Yu, Y. C., Jiang, Y., Yang, M. M., He, S. N., Xi, X., Xu, Y. T., Hu, W. S., & Luo, Q. (2019). Hypermethylation of delta-like homolog1/maternally expressed gene 3 loci in human umbilical veins: Insights into offspring vascular dysfunction born after preeclampsia. *Journal of Hypertension*, *37*(3), 581–589. https://doi.org/10.1097/HJH.0000000000001942.

Yuen, R. K. C., Pẽaherrera, M. S., Von Dadelszen, P., McFadden, D. E., & Robinson, W. P. (2010). DNA methylation profiling of human placentas reveals promoter hypomethylation of multiple genes in early-onset preeclampsia. *European Journal of Human Genetics 2010 18:9*, *18*(9), 1006–1012. https://doi.org/10.1038/ejhg.2010.63.

Zhang, Y., Zou, Y., Wang, W., Zuo, Q., Jiang, Z., Sun, M., De, W., & Sun, L. (2015). Down-regulated long non-coding RNA MEG3 and its effect on promoting apoptosis and suppressing migration of trophoblast cells. *Journal of Cellular Biochemistry*, *116*(4), 542–550. https://doi.org/10.1002/JCB.25004.

Zhang, Z., Zhang, L., Zhang, L., Jia, L., Wang, P., & Gao, Y. (2013). Association of Wnt2 and sFRP4 Expression in the Third Trimester Placenta in Women With Severe Preeclampsia. *Reproductive Sciences*, *20*(8), 981. https://doi.org/10.1177/1933719112472740.

Zhu, L., Lv, R., Kong, L., Cheng, H., Lan, F., & Li, X. (2015). Genome-Wide Mapping of 5mC and 5hmC Identified Differentially Modified Genomic Regions in Late-Onset Severe Preeclampsia: A Pilot Study. *PloS One*, *10*(7). https://doi.org/10.1371/JOURNAL.PONE.0134119.

Zhu, Y., Pereira, R. O., O'Neill, B. T., Riehle, C., Ilkun, O., Wende, A. R., Rawlings, T. A., Zhang, Y. C., Zhang, Q., Klip, A., Shiojima, I., Walsh, K., & Dale Abel, E. (2013). Cardiac PI3K-Akt impairs insulin-stimulated glucose uptake independent of mTORC1 and GLUT4 translocation. *Molecular Endocrinology (Baltimore, Md.)*, *27*(1), 172–184. https://doi.org/10.1210/ME.2012-1210.

Chapter 26

Epigenetics and Pain

Emel Guler*, MD

Department of Physical Medicine and Rehabilitation,
Division of Pain Management Section,
Sivas Cumhuriyet University, Sivas, Turkey

Abstract

Pain and its chronicity in the following process are the main subjects of numerous studies nowadays with the adverse impacts of pain on quality of life, loss of workforce it causes, and still not completely explained pathophysiological mechanisms. The difficulties in treating symptoms that accompany pain and individual differences in response to applied treatment methods have accelerated genetic and epigenetic research. Epigenetics, which we have heard frequently in recent years, is the formation of different genetic variations under the influence of various factors and is now accepted as a significant mechanism in the unknown etiology of numerous diseases. Different epigenetic modifications have been described in the formation, typing, and treatment of pain, and new information is obtained with ongoing studies. The difficulties experienced in treatment due to changes at the molecular level caused by the chronic pain process and the activation of sensitization mechanisms have brought about epigenetic mechanisms both in etiopathogenesis studies and in the development of novel treatment approaches.

Keywords: pain, epigenetic mechanism, pain type

Introduction

The International Association for the Study of Pain (IASP) defines pain as "the existing or potential tissue damage or an unpleasant emotional and sensory experience associated with this damage" (Aydede, 2017). However, debates are still ongoing about the inadequacy of this definition to fully express the sensation of pain (Treede, 2018).

The complex structure of pain, difficulties experienced in treatment, and the fact that the treatment response differs from person to person reveal the necessity of a multi-faceted approach to painful patients. Pain perception is an experience that differs among individuals due to genetic, psychosocial, and demographic variables. Chapman and Jones stated the following: "A striking variation in the intensity of pain experienced in diseases with similar

---

* Corresponding Author's E-mail: dremelguler@gmail.com.

In: Epigenetics: Beyond the Genetics and Medicine
Editors: Sevgi Durna Daştan and Nazan Yurtcu
ISBN: 979-8-88697-228-3

lesions is a common observation" (Chapman and Jones, 1944). Pain was classically classified according to its duration, pathophysiology, and localization, and the treatment plan was shaped in line with these characteristics. In the definition of the duration used in pain typing, pain complaints lasting 3 months and more are defined as chronic (Haefeli and Elfering, 2006). Nociceptive, neuropathic, and nociplastic pain definitions were made with the activation of pathophysiological mechanisms in pain. It is possible to define nociceptive pain transmission as the perception and transmission of painful stimuli. Pain emerges when peripheral nociceptors are stimulated by mechanical, chemical, or thermal injuries. Following injury, inflammatory mediators are released from the damaged tissue, nociceptors are stimulated, and sensation is transmitted first to the spinal centers through peripheral Aδ and C fibers and then to the supraspinal centers through the afferent pathways of pain transmission. This is defined as nociceptive pain (Polomano et al., 2008). Although different definitions have been utilized over the years, the latest and the most common definition of neuropathic pain is pain caused by a lesion or disease of the somatosensory system. It originates from a lesion or disease of the somatosensory system, including peripheral fibers (Aβ, Aδ, and C fibers) and central neurons, and occurs in 7-10% of the general population (Colloca et al., 2017). What is nociplastic pain that we have frequently encountered in the literature in recent years? It is described as an increase in pain perception and sensitivity due to changes in sensory conduction pathways with a role in pain transmission in the peripheral and central nervous systems (Fitzcharles et al., 2021). It is found in individuals with nociceptive or neuropathic chronic pain, in isolation or in the form of comorbidity (Woolf, 2011). In 2021, four criteria were stated for the definition of nociplastic pain:

1. Existence for at least 3 months
2. Showing not regional but different pain distribution
3. Pain that cannot be explained by nociceptive or neuropathic mechanisms
4. The presence of clinical signs of pain hypersensitivity at least in the pain region (e.g., hot or cold allodynia, static or dynamic mechanical allodynia) (Nijs et al., 2021).

Epigenetic Mechanisms

So when and where do epigenetic mechanisms come into play in pain? First, to talk about epigenetic mechanisms briefly, they were described for the first time by Conrad Waddington in 1942 (Waddington, 2016). They are defined as phenotypic inherited gene expression as a result of DNA methylation, histone modification, and changes in the structure of chromatin without any changes in the DNA sequence (Choi and Friso, 2010). Epigenetic mechanisms are now blamed for many diseases, whose etiopathogenesis has not been fully explained (Portela and Esteller, 2010), and are assessed under three main headings.

DNA Methylation; DNA methylation has a role in the diversification of genome function at the stage of embryogenesis and during cellular differentiation. DNA methylation patterns were believed to remain fixed throughout life after their formation during embryogenesis. Nevertheless, it has been demonstrated that environmental signals can impact DNA methylation patterns other than embryogenesis and cellular differentiation, especially in the early stages of development, occurring after birth (Szyf and Bick, 2013). Methylation is the conversion of the cytosine base to 5-methylcytosine by methylation at particular sites on DNA during epigenetic regulation. The 5-methylcytosine (5-mC) modification, also named the fifth base, is located in DNA regions, also called CpG islands, where 5'-cytosine-phosphate-guanosine-3' dinucleotides are frequently found. DNA methylation is also possible in other regions of the genome. DNA methyltransferase (DNMT) enzymes, comprising three isoforms, DNMT1, DNMT3a, and DNMT3b, ensure the addition of methyl groups to regions on DNA. Whereas DNMT1 copies the methylation profile to newly formed cells during mitotic cell division, DNMT3a and 3b act as de-novo methylase enzymes (Eser et al., 2016; Jones, 2012; Zhang et al., 2020).

Histone modification: The histone complex facilitates the condensation of genomic DNA and impacts post-transcriptional modification. Varied changes, e.g., acetylation, methylation, and phosphorylation, take place on conserved lysine in histone tails. Histone acetylation and deacetylation modifications during cell proliferation are necessary for gene regulation and are in the close relationship with DNA replication-coupled nucleosome assembly (Surgun, 2019). The mentioned assembly is important for inheriting epigenetic information during DNA replication and repair. The nucleosome is comprised of 147 base pairs of DNA wrapped around an octamer of quaternary histone proteins (H2A, H2B, H3, and H4) (Zhu and Wani, 2010). Acetylation usually indicates active transcription, whereas deacetylation indicates inactive transcription. Histone acetylation and deacetylation are related to inflammatory or neuropathic pain. Many studies indicate that histone deacetylation induces chronic pain (Khangura et al., 2017). Histon methylation, seen as mono, di, and trimetilation, with different effects of each, may indicate active and inactive transcription. The enzyme that performs this metilation is histon methyltransferase (HMTs). Histone modification in H3 is the most studied and characterized (Nakayama et al., 2001). Any mutation of histone-related enzymes can make a contribution to the development of diseases such as cancers, neurologic diseases, and psychological disorders (Yuen and Knoepfler, 2013).

MicroRNA; miRNAs are a class of small non-coding RNAs, approximately 20-30 nucleotides in length. MicroRNAs are complementary to a single or a set of messenger RNAs (mRNAs). They are not translated into protein; however, their main function is known to be regulating the expression of up to 30% of human genes and at least 60% of protein-coding genes (Tufarelli et al., 2003). Emerging evidence shows that miRNAs take essential parts in cell division, differentiation, and development, as well as in controlling DNA methylation and histone modification. Abnormalities in miRNA are related to various human diseases, such as cancer, neurodegenerative, and heart diseases (Calin et al., 2002).

Epigenetic Mechanisms in Chronic Pain

Chronic pain impacts approximately a quarter of the population (Goldberg and McGee, 2011). Many factors are blamed for the chronicity of pain, and the mentioned process is attempted to be explained, particularly by genetic mechanisms and gene expressions (Bai, Ren, and Dubner, 2015). Continuous nociceptive hypersensitivity leads to functional and structural changes (changes called plasticity and occurring at the molecular level) in both the peripheral and central nervous systems. It has been revealed that epigenetic mechanisms are involved in many physiological and pathological processes, such as neuronal plasticity and cancer, including environmental factors (Musselman et al., 2012). A study carried out on twins demonstrated the impact of environmental factors on pain sensitivity and opioid analgesic response (Angst et al., 2012). In another study conducted on the chronicity of pain, environmental factors, rather than genetic factors, gained importance in neck pain research in monozygotic twins after a particular age (Fejer et al., 2006). A study conducted on individuals using drugs and smoking observed that pain became chronic due to epigenetic changes in the nervous system and emphasized the relationship of chronic pain with numerous diseases, such as cancer and diabetes, caused by epigenetic mechanisms (Suter et al., 2012; Villeneuve and Natarajan, 2010).

Qui et al. mentioned hydrogen sulfide, an endogenous gas molecule synthesized by cystathionine-β-synthase (CBS), which is necessary for the excitability of neurons in the dorsal root ganglia (DRG), mechanical pain hypersensitivity, and demonstrated the demethylation of the cystathionine-β-synthase (CBS) gene in DRG after the induced peripheral inflammation (Qi et al., 2013). Whereas no change was observed in the expression and activity of DNMT in DRG in peripheral inflammation, it could not be explained how demethylation occurred in DRG in chronic pain (Rahn et al., 2013). In the study by Aroke et al., involving 50 nonspecific low back pain cases and 48 healthy volunteers, hyper and hypomethylated areas were found in the CpG regions, the difference in methylation was revealed to be statistically significant, and methylation was detected in 50% of the CpG regions and 48% of the promoter regions. Different gene-related methylation sites were observed in regions previously found to take part in immune signal transduction, G-protein coupled transduction, and enchondral ossification. These data revealed the significance of epigenetic mechanisms in pathophysiological changes in nonspecific low back pain (Aroke et al., 2020). Recent research has demonstrated the relationship of DNA methylation modification in GABAergic neurons in chronic pain. It has been emphasized that the decreased methylation level in the spinal dorsal horn and, accordingly, the inhibition of DNA methylation in GABAergic neurons in the dorsal horn can enhance the functions of the mentioned neurons and provide analgesic impacts (Xu et al., 2021). DNMT3a and DNMT3b, among DNA methyltransferases, represent proteins most commonly involved in the change of DNA methylation models in relation to chronic pain. DNMT3a takes part in the hypermethylation of gene loci regulating the addition of Ca ion channel to nociceptors in DRG following peripheral nerve injury (Lipscombe and Lopez-Soto, 2021).

Histone modification, another mechanism, acts in a different way. Histone acetylation is catalyzed by histone acetyltransferase (HAT) and provides gene transcriptional activity, whereas histone deacetylation suppresses transcriptional activity by histone deacetylase (HDAC) activity. HDAC inhibitors have been shown to relieve inflammatory pain. Furthermore, it has been shown that peripheral inflammation induced by complete Freund's adjuvant (CFA) increases class IIa HDAC levels in the spinal dorsal horn, prevents thermal hyperalgesia or alleviates the existing thermal hyperalgesia after intrathecally administered HDAC inhibitors (Liang et al., 2015).

The importance of miRNA in chronic pain is related to epigenetic modification with its impacts on both HDAC and DNMT (Géranton, 2012). The upregulation of the Cav1.2-containing L-type calcium channel (Cav1.2-LTC) in the spinal cord dorsal horn is one of the mechanisms related to chronic pain. Theoretically, miRNAs are capable of regulating multiple mRNAs simultaneously. miR-103, one of the miRNAs, has been demonstrated to regulate the expression of three subunits that constitute Cav1.2-LTC simultaneously, and a study on rats observed an increase in pain following miR-103 degradation (Favereaux et al., 2011). Another study carried out on mice revealed that the dicer enzyme, the dsRNA ribonuclease present in neurons, was deleted and the Nav1.8 channel, a mediator in inflammatory pain, could not be stimulated. Following Dicer deletion, arrangements were observed in the form of upregulation in many mRNA transcripts in DRG but downregulation in nociceptor-associated mRNA transcripts (such as Nav1.8) (Zhao et al., 2010).

Epigenetic Mechanisms in Neuropathic Pain

The International Association for the Study of Pain (IASP) defines neuropathic pain as "pain resulting from a lesion or disease of the peripheral or central somatosensory nervous system" (Russo and Sundaramurthi, 2019). For the first time, in a book chapter in which Mitchell wrote about the sensory effects of nerve injuries in 1872, he defined allodynia as a condition when the sensation that should be perceived only as touch after many injuries could become painful. He also mentioned the loss of sensation in the painful area and signs of neuropathic pain (Mitchell, 1965). Whereas numerous pathophysiological explanations took place in the literature in the following periods, epigenetic mechanisms came into play during the explanation of changes in ion channels while explaining the formation mechanisms of neuropathic pain, and different epigenetic mechanisms were found during pain formation (Luo et al., 2021). DNA methylation or histone deacetylation is functionally effective in the neuropathic pain formation model, as well as in the somatosensory nociceptive pathway (Descalzi et al., 2015). DNA methylation is associated with cortical functions in addition to the brain structure related to pain formation. DNMT1 and DNMT3 have been indicated to regulate the expression of the potassium channel Kcna2 in peripheral neurons following nerve injury and thus contribute to hyperexcitability (Sun et al., 2019). DNMT upregulation is associated with the methylation of μ opioid receptor (MOR) gene promoters in DRG and the spinal cord, which causes the downregulation of opioid receptor expression (Sun et al., 2017). Proteins from the Methyl-CpG-binding domain (MBD) family, such as MBD1-4 and MeCP2, suppress gene transcription by DNA methylation (Turek-Plewa and Jagodzinski, 2005). Oprm1 gene expression, encoding the receptor of MOR and Kcna2 (Kv1.2) from potassium channels, is suppressed by MBD1 and by DNMT3a in DRG neurons. Hypomethylation contributes to an increase in the expression of plasticity occurring in the purinergic receptor P2X ligand-gated ion channel 3 in DRG neurons and contributes to neuropathic pain (H.-H. Zhang, et al., 2015). DNA methylation appears to be one of the potential targets in the management of neuropathic pain.

Histone acetylation has been indicated to increase neuropathic pain-associated gene expression (Liang and Tao, 2018). The oral administration of sodium butyrate, an HDAC inhibitor, following damage to the sciatic nerve caused by chronic compression, reduced both TNF-α increase and pain hypersensitivity (Kukkar et al., 2014). In a study on mice, a change analysis of histone modifications in the dorsal horn was carried out by performing the partial ligation of the sciatic nerve to establish a neuropathic pain model. While no change was observed in DNA methylation in the medulla spinalis, changes in histone methylation were revealed in specific genes. A prominent increase was observed in the expression of monocyte chemotactic protein-3 (MCP-3), a proinflammatory cytokine, in astrocytes in the medulla spinalis two weeks after the nerve ligation (Imai et al., 2011). Brain-derived neurotrophic factor (BDNF) contributes to neuropathic pain by upregulating DRG after peripheral nerve injury. It was revealed that hyperalgesia and allodynia developed following the intrathecal administration of BDNF. Concerning the epigenetic regulation of BDNF gene expression, histone H3 and H4 acetylation and histone acetylation were found to control BDNF exon I expression. This was observed to cause the continuation of neuropathic pain (Uchida et al., 2013). Neuron-restrictive silencer factor (NRSF) is effective in the transcriptional suppression of genes. H4 hyperacetylation was identified in the NRSF promoter II, ensuring an increase in the expression of NRSF in neuropathic pain. As a consequence, MOR and Nav1.8 expressions are adversely impacted (Uchida et al., 2010). It was also observed in the upregulation of Nav1.6 expression in DRG. Acetylation of H3K9ac acetylation in the promoter region of inflammatory mediators and chemokine ligands has been shown to trigger the formation of neuropathic pain (Kiguchi et al., 2014). When Simeoli et al. investigated the role of miRNA21-5p, upregulated after the nerve injury, they observed that it activated macrophages by being released from DRG neurons as a result of nociceptive stimulation. Considering the impact of suppressing miRNA21 expression on immune cells in neuropathic allodynia, decreased hypersensitivity resulting from nerve injury was detected in mice (Simeoli et al., 2017).

Na channels take an essential part in the transmission of hypoesthesia and hypoalgesia. There are 5 isoforms regulating the nociceptive response (Nav1.3, Nav1.6, Nav1.7, Nav1.8, and Nav1.9). While expecting neuropathic pain following nerve injury, hypoesthesia was observed as a result of the epigenetic modification of the Nav1.8 gene with HDAC (Matsushita et al., 2013). The study by Ding et al. showed epigenetic upregulation in the Nav1.6 gene in neuropathic pain induced by a lumbar nerve cut (Ding et al., 2019). Many similar studies demonstrate that epigenetic modifications occur in Na channels, in addition to K channels, in painful conditions.

Conclusion

It is necessary to exhibit a multidisciplinary approach while evaluating pain formation mechanisms and during treatment planning, and biological, psychological, and environmental factors should be addressed as a whole. Numerous studies have discussed epigenetic mechanisms in the pathogenesis of pain, and their impacts on ion channels, receptors, and inflammatory cytokines have been revealed. Additionally, the analgesic effect was provided by the pharmacological regulation of the expression of pain genes, DNA methylation, histone modification, or miRNA expression. However, there is a need for many experimental and clinical studies to see how epigenetic changes will influence germ cells during transmission and what long-term effects the treatment methods developed by targeting epigenetic modulators will have considering the duration and types of pain.

References

Angst MS, Phillips NG, Drover DR, Tingle M, Ray A, Swan GE, Lazzeroni LC and Clark DJ. (2012). Pain sensitivity and opioid analgesia: A pharmacogenomic twin study. *Pain*, 153(7), 1397-1409. https://doi.org/10.1016/j.pain.2012.02.022.

Aroke EN, Overstreet DS, Penn TM, Crossman DK, Jackson P, Tollefsbol TO, Quinn TL, Yi N, and Goodin BR. (2020). Identification of DNA methylation associated enrichment pathways in adults with nonspecific chronic low back pain. *Molecular Pain*, 16, 1744806920972889. https://doi.org/10.1177/1744806920972889

Aydede, M. (2017). Defending the IASP definition of pain. *The Monist,* 100(4), 439-464.

Bai G, Ren K and Dubner R. (2015). Epigenetic regulation of persistent pain. *Translational Research,* 165(1), 177-199.

Calin GA, Dumitru CD, Shimizu M, Bichi R, Zupo S, Noch E, Aldler H, Rattan S, Keating M, Rai K, Rassenti L, Kipps T, Negrini M, Bullrich F and Croce CM. (2002). Frequent deletions and down-regulation of micro-RNA genes miR15 and miR16 at 13q14 in chronic lymphocytic leukemia. *Proceedings of the National Academy of Sciences of the United States of America*, 99(24), 15524-15529. https://doi.org/10.1073/pnas.242606799.

Chapman WP and Jones CM. (1944). Variations in cutaneous and visceral pain sensitivity in normal subjects. *The Journal of Clinical Investigation,* 23(1), 81-91.

Choi S-W and Friso S. (2010). Epigenetics: A new bridge between nutrition and health. *Advances in Nutrition,* 1(1), 8-16.

Colloca L, Ludman T, Bouhassira D, Baron R, Dickenson AH, Yarnitsky D, Freeman R, Truini A, Attal N, Finnerup NB, Eccleston C, Kalso E, Bennett DL, Dworkin RH and Raja SN. (2017). Neuropathic pain. *Nature Reviews. Disease Primers*, 3, 17002. https://doi.org/10.1038/nrdp.2017.2.

Descalzi G, Ikegami D, Ushijima T, Nestler EJ, Zachariou V and Narita M. (2015). Epigenetic mechanisms of chronic pain. *Trends in Neurosciences,* 38(4), 237-246.

Ding HH, Zhang SB, Lv YY, Ma C, Liu M, Zhang KB, Ruan XC, Wei JY, Xin WJ and Wu SL. (2019). TNF-α/STAT3 pathway epigenetically upregulates Nav1.6 expression in DRG and contributes to neuropathic pain induced by L5-VRT. *Journal of Neuroinflammation*, 16(1), 29. https://doi.org/10.1186/s12974-019-1421-8.

Eser BE, Yazgan ÜC, Gürses SA and Aydin M. (2016). Diabetes Mellitus ve Epigenetik Mekanizmalar [*Diabetes Mellitus and Epigenetic Mechanisms*]. *Dicle Tıp Dergisi*, 43(2), 375-382.

Favereaux A, Thoumine O, Bouali-Benazzouz R, Roques V, Papon MA, Salam SA, Drutel G, Léger C, Calas A, Nagy F and Landry M. (2011). Bidirectional integrative regulation of Cav1.2 calcium channel by microRNA miR-103: Role in pain. *The EMBO Journal*, 30(18), 3830-3841. https://doi.org/10.1038/emboj.2011.249.

Fejer R, Hartvigsen J and Kyvik KO. (2006). Heritability of neck pain: a population-based study of 33 794 Danish twins. *Rheumatology,* 45(5), 589-594.

Fitzcharles M-A, Cohen SP, Clauw DJ, Littlejohn G, Usui C and Häuser W. (2021). Nociplastic pain: Towards an understanding of prevalent pain conditions. *The Lancet,* 397(10289), 2098-2110.

Géranton SM. (2012). Targeting epigenetic mechanisms for pain relief. *Current Opinion in Pharmacology,* 12(1), 35-41.

Goldberg DS and McGee SJ. (2011). Pain as a global public health priority. *BMC Public Health,* 11(1), 1-5.

Haefeli M and Elfering A. (2006). Pain assessment. *European Spine Journal,* 15(1), S17-S24.

Imai S, Saeki M, Yanase M, Horiuchi H, Abe M, Narita M, Kuzumaki N, Suzuki T and Narita M. (2011). Change in microRNAs associated with neuronal adaptive responses in the nucleus accumbens under neuropathic pain. *The Journal of Neuroscience: The Official Journal of the Society for Neuroscience*, 31(43), 15294-15299. https://doi.org/10.1523/JNEUROSCI.0921-11.2011.

Jones PA. (2012). Functions of DNA methylation: islands, start sites, gene bodies and beyond. *Nature Reviews Genetics,* 13(7), 484-492.

Khangura RK, Bali A, Jaggi AS, and Singh N. (2017). Histone acetylation and histone deacetylation in neuropathic pain: An unresolved puzzle? *European Journal of Pharmacology,* 795, 36-42.

Kiguchi N, Kobayashi Y, Kadowaki Y, Fukazawa Y, Saika F and Kishioka S. (2014). Vascular endothelial growth factor signaling in injured nerves underlies peripheral sensitization in neuropathic pain. *Journal of Neurochemistry,* 129(1), 169-178.

Kukkar A, Singh N and Jaggi AS. (2014). Attenuation of neuropathic pain by sodium butyrate in an experimental model of chronic constriction injury in rats. *Journal of the Formosan Medical Association,* 113(12), 921-928.

Liang L, Lutz BM, Bekker A and Tao Y-X. (2015). Epigenetic regulation of chronic pain. *Epigenomics,* 7(2), 235-245.

Liang L and Tao Y-X. (2018). Expression of acetyl-histone H3 and acetyl-histone H4 in dorsal root ganglion and spinal dorsal horn in rat chronic pain models. *Life Sciences,* 211, 182-188.

Lipscombe D and Lopez-Soto EJ. (2021). Epigenetic control of ion channel expression and cell-specific splicing in nociceptors: Chronic pain mechanisms and potential therapeutic targets. *Channels,* 15(1), 155-163.

Luo D, Li X, Tang S, Song F, Li W, Xie G, Liang J and Zhou J. (2021). Epigenetic modifications in neuropathic pain. *Molecular Pain*, 17, 17448069211056767. https://doi.org/10.1177/17448069211056767.

Matsushita Y, Araki K, Omotuyi OI, Mukae T and Ueda H. (2013). HDAC inhibitors restore C-fibre sensitivity in experimental neuropathic pain model. *British Journal of Pharmacology,* 170(5), 991-998.

Mitchell SW. (1965). *Injuries of Nerves and their Consequences. (1872).*

Musselman CA, Lalonde M-E, Côté J and Kutateladze TG. (2012). Perceiving the epigenetic landscape through histone readers. *Nature Structural and Molecular Biology*, 19(12), 1218-1227.

Nakayama J-I, Rice JC, Strahl BD, Allis CD and Grewal SI. (2001). Role of histone H3 lysine 9 methylation in epigenetic control of heterochromatin assembly. *Science,* 292(5514), 110-113.

Nijs J, Lahousse A, Kapreli E, Bilika P, Saraçoğlu İ, Malfliet A, Coppieters I, De Baets L, Leysen L, Roose E, Clark J, Voogt L and Huysmans E. (2021). Nociplastic Pain Criteria or Recognition of Central Sensitization? Pain Phenotyping in the Past, Present and Future. *Journal of Clinical Medicine*, 10(15), 3203. https://doi.org/10.3390/jcm10153203.

Polomano RC, Dunwoody CJ, Krenzischek DA and Rathmell JP. (2008). Perspective on pain management in the 21st century. *Pain Management Nursing,* 9(1), 3-10.

Portela A and Esteller M. (2010). Epigenetic modifications and human disease. *Nature Biotechnology,* 28(10), 1057-1068.

Qi F, Zhou Y, Xiao Y, Tao J, Gu J, Jiang X and Xu G-Y. (2013). Promoter demethylation of cystathionine-β-synthetase gene contributes to inflammatory pain in rats. *PAIN®*, 154(1), 34-45.

Rahn EJ, Guzman-Karlsson MC and David Sweatt J. (2013). Cellular, molecular, and epigenetic mechanisms in non-associative conditioning: Implications for pain and memory. *Neurobiol Learn Mem,* 105, 133-150. doi:10.1016/j.nlm.2013.06.008.

Russo MM and Sundaramurthi T. (2019). *An Overview of Cancer Pain: Epidemiology and Pathophysiology.* Paper presented at the Seminars in Oncology Nursing.

Simeoli R, Montague K, Jones HR, Castaldi L, Chambers D, Kelleher JH, Vacca V, Pitcher T, Grist J, Al-Ahdal H, Wong LF, Perretti M, Lai J, Mouritzen P, Heppenstall P and Malcangio M. (2017). Exosomal cargo including microRNA regulates sensory neuron to macrophage communication after nerve trauma. *Nature Communications*, 8(1), 1778. https://doi.org/10.1038/s41467-017-01841-5.

Sun L, Gu X, Pan Z, Guo X, Liu J, Atianjoh FE, Wu S, Mo K, Xu B, Liang L, Bekker A and Tao YX. (2019). Contribution of DNMT1 to Neuropathic Pain Genesis Partially through Epigenetically Repressing *Kcna2* in Primary Afferent Neurons. *The Journal of Neuroscience: The Official Journal of the Society for Neuroscience*, 39(33), 6595-6607. https://doi.org/10.1523/JNEUROSCI.0695-19.2019.

Sun L, Zhao J-Y, Gu X, Liang L, Wu S, Mo K, Bekker A. (2017). Nerve injury-induced epigenetic silencing of opioid receptors controlled by DNMT3a in primary afferent neurons. *Pain,* 158(6), 1153.

Suter MA, Anders AM and Aagaard KM. (2012). Maternal smoking as a model for environmental epigenetic changes affecting birthweight and fetal programming. *MHR: Basic Science of Reproductive Medicine,* 19(1), 1-6.

Szyf M and Bick J. (2013). DNA methylation: A mechanism for embedding early life experiences in the genome. *Child Development,* 84(1), 49-57.

Şurgun E. (2019). Maternal Beslenmenin Epigenetik Mekanizmalar Üzerinden İnfant Sağlığına Etkileri [*The Effects of Maternal Nutrition on Infant Health through Epigenetic Mechanisms*]. *Başkent Üniversitesi Sağlık Bilimleri Fakültesi Dergisi-BÜSBİD,* 4(1).

Treede R-D. (2018). The International Association for the Study of Pain definition of pain: As valid in 2018 as in 1979, but in need of regularly updated footnotes. *Pain Reports,* 3(2).

Tufarelli C, Stanley JAS, Garrick D, Sharpe JA, Ayyub H, Wood WG and Higgs DR. (2003). Transcription of antisense RNA leading to gene silencing and methylation as a novel cause of human genetic disease. *Nature Genetics,* 34(2), 157-165.

Turek-Plewa J and Jagodzinski PP. (2005). The role of mammalian DNA methyltransferases in the regulation of gene expression. *Cellular and Molecular Biology Letters,* 10(4), 631.

Uchida H, Ma L and Ueda H. (2010). Epigenetic gene silencing underlies C-fiber dysfunctions in neuropathic pain. *Journal of Neuroscience,* 30(13), 4806-4814.

Uchida H, Matsushita Y and Ueda H. (2013). Epigenetic regulation of BDNF expression in the primary sensory neurons after peripheral nerve injury: Implications in the development of neuropathic pain. *Neuroscience,* 240, 147-154.

Villeneuve LM and Natarajan R. (2010). The role of epigenetics in the pathology of diabetic complications. *American Journal of Physiology-Renal Physiology,* 299(1), F14-F25.

Waddington CH. (2016). *An Introduction to Modern Genetics*. Routledge.

Woolf CJ. (2011). Central sensitization: implications for the diagnosis and treatment of pain. *Pain,* 152(3), S2-S15.

Xu Q, Bai F and Liu T. (2021). *GABAergic Neuron-Related DNA Methylation Modification and Chronic Pain.* Paper presented at the Fifth International Conference on Biological Information and Biomedical Engineering.

Yuen BT and Knoepfler PS. (2013). Histone H3. 3 mutations: a variant path to cancer. *Cancer Cell,* 24(5), 567-574.

Zhang HH, Hu J, Zhou YL, Qin X, Song ZY, Yang PP, Hu S, Jiang X and Xu GY. (2015). Promoted Interaction of Nuclear Factor-κB with Demethylated Purinergic P2X3 Receptor Gene Contributes to Neuropathic Pain in Rats with Diabetes. *Diabetes*, 64(12), 4272-4284. https://doi.org/10.2337/db15-0138.

Zhang L, Lu Q and Chang C. (2020). Epigenetics in health and disease. *Epigenetics in Allergy and Autoimmunity*, 3-55.

Zhao J, Lee MC, Momin A, Cendan CM, Shepherd ST, Baker MD, Asante C, Bee L, Bethry A, Perkins JR, Nassar MA, Abrahamsen B, Dickenson A, Cobb BS, Merkenschlager M and Wood JN. (2010). Small RNAs control sodium channel expression, nociceptor excitability, and pain thresholds. *The Journal of Neuroscience: The Official Journal of the Society for Neuroscience*, 30(32), 10860-10871. https://doi.org/ 10.1523/ JNEUROSCI.1980-10.2010.

Zhu Q and Wani AA. (2010). Histone modifications: Crucial elements for damage response and chromatin restoration. *Journal of Cellular Physiology,* 223(2), 283-288.

Chapter 27

Epigenetics and Connective Tissue Diseases

Ali Erhan Özdemirel*, MD

Department of Rheumatology, Liv Hospital, Ankara, Turkey

Abstract

Connective tissue diseases (CTDs) are defined as chronic inflammatory diseases that can affect all organs and systems, primarily the joints. The underlying genetic background is very important for the development of these diseases, and environmental factors also contribute to this process. The clinical spectrum can vary considerably from patient to patient in individuals with CTDs, and even responses varying from person to person are observed in treatment responses. The emergence of such different phenotypic characteristics in this group of patients with relatively similar genotypic characteristics has caused the need to investigate them in different models that may contribute to the underlying pathogenetic process.

It has been recently revealed that changes in DNA cannot be explained only by genetics, and the role of epigenetic mechanisms is also quite large. In epigenetics, the DNA sequence does not change. However, since the promoter region of the gene changes, differences occur in gene transcription, in other words, in the end product of the gene. There is no clear factor that induces this change, and epigenetic modifications such as histone modification, DNA methylation, and microRNA (miRNA) that probably occur under the influence of environmental factors have led to the emergence of a new field to explain different phenotypic characteristics in patients.

In this chapter, the characteristics of epigenetic mechanisms in general and the reflections of these modifications on common CTDs, both at the cellular level and clinically, will be discussed.

Keywords: connective tissue diseases, epigenetic, DNA methylation, histone modification

Introduction

Connective tissue diseases (CTDs) represent a group of heterogeneous chronic immune-mediated inflammatory diseases and define a group of diseases that can affect a wide variety of organ systems, particularly connective tissues, and may present with various clinical findings (Mazzone et al., 2019). Systemic lupus erythematosus, Sjogren's syndrome, systemic sclerosis,

---

* Corresponding Author's E-mail: erhanozdemirel@hotmail.com.

In: Epigenetics: Beyond the Genetics and Medicine
Editors: Sevgi Durna Daştan and Nazan Yurtcu
ISBN: 979-8-88697-228-3

rheumatoid arthritis, and inflammatory myopathies are among these diseases. The complex intertwined relationship of genetic and environmental factors has an important role in the occurrence of these diseases, as in many diseases. It has been recently demonstrated that epigenetic modifications induced by environmental factors have an important role in the development of autoimmune diseases in individuals with genetic background, which has revealed the importance of the concept of epigenetics.

In recent years, it has been revealed that changes in DNA cannot be explained only by genetics, and the role of epigenetic mechanisms has also been considerably large. Epigenetic mechanisms are known as mechanisms that do not change the nucleotide sequence, but change the chromatin. In other words, the DNA sequence does not change; however, because the promoter region of the gene changes, quantitative and qualitative changes emerge in gene transcription. The transcription of the relevant gene can be silenced or activated due to transcriptional changes. The mentioned quantitative and qualitative changes are not permanent and can be adjusted in case of need. Additionally, these changes in gene transcription can be transferred to the following generations (Morgan et al., 1999).

Epigenetic Mechanisms

DNA methylation, histone methylation, histone acetylation, histone phosphorylation, histone ubiquitination, histone citrullination, histone ribosylation, non-coding RNAs, and chromatin re-modeling can be mentioned among epigenetic mechanisms (Mazzone et al., 2019). We will examine the most important ones in more detail.

DNA Methylation

Cytosine methylation is known to be the best among epigenetic mechanisms. Typically, a methyl group is transferred from S-adenosine methionine (SAM) to cytosine residues at the C5 position of pyrimidine with the catalyst effect of DNA methyltransferases (DNMTs) (Du et al., 2015). When cytosine is methylated, it transforms into thymine. Thymine pairs with adenine at the next replication, which causes a point mutation. Due to this mutation, transcription is silenced and a number of biological processes, such as chromosomal instability, are impacted. Another critical function of DNA methylation is maintaining T cell regulation (Wadhwa et al., 2016).

Histone Modifications

Histone-modifying enzymes have a very important role in chromatin stability, nucleosomal functioning, and DNA repair (Lawrence et al., 2016). Due to the impact of these enzymes, a helix is formed around the histone complex (H2a, H2b, H3, and H4) and the nucleosome structure is formed. The DNA-histone relationship is impacted and the chromatin structure is changed because of histone methylation, histone acetylation, histone phosphorylation, histone ubiquitination, histone citrullination, and histone ribosylation. When histone is acetylated,

DNA is released and transcription starts. When acetyl groups in histone are removed from the medium, cytosine is methylated and transcription stops. The histone acetyltransferase enzyme is responsible for the binding of the acetyl group, whereas the histone deacetyl transferase enzyme is responsible for its removal (Zwergel et al., 2015). As a result of all these interactions, the functions of T cells, which have a role in the center of immune and inflammatory processes, are impacted (Akimova et al., 2012).

Non-Coding RNAs

Non-coding RNAs (nc-RNA) appear to be the active molecules of RNA. They have many subgroups, including piwi-interacting RNA, small nucleolar RNAs, small interfering RNAs, microRNAs, circular RNAs, antisense RNAs, and long intergenic non-coding RNA. Nevertheless, studies have primarily involved microRNA and long intergenic non-coding RNA (Pea et al., 2021).

Non-coding RNAs may be classified as small or long in accordance with the number of nucleotides they carry. MicroRNAs (miRNAs) are a well-known subgroup of short, non-coding RNAs with a crucial role in regulating host gene expression at the post-transcriptional level. About 2656 mature miRNAs have been identified in humans, which are thought to regulate 60% of gene expression (Kumar et al., 2010). A single miRNA is capable of regulating the expression of dozens of genes by inhibiting protein translation or cleaving mRNA (Garzon et al., 2010). The miRNA expression pattern of each cell type makes a contribution to forming tissue-specific properties and functions. miRNAs can alter gene expression in their genes and act as intercellular communication molecules. Recent research has demonstrated that miRNAs are packaged and released into surrounding tissues or circulation. Based on all this information, miRNAs are considered significant clinical markers in the diagnosis and treatment follow-up (Adams et al., 2017).

The general characteristics of the epigenetic mechanisms are described above, and the epigenetic properties of frequently observed CTDs and their specific reflections on the immune system will be discussed in the following section

Systemic Lupus Erythematosus (SLE)

SLE is a chronic autoimmune disease that affects a lot of organ systems and is characterized by autoantibodies that develop against nuclear antigens. The dysregulation of T lymphocytes is the main pathogenetic process in SLE, and it is the disease in which epigenetic modifications are the most studied among almost all autoimmune diseases, and numerous studies have been recently conducted on this issue.

Many genes present in T lymphocytes, such as CD11a (ITGAL), perforin (PRF1), CD70 (TNFS7), and CD40LG (TNFSF5), have been shown to be hypomethylated in patients with SLE (Richardson, 2007). In these patients, the development of auto-reactivity has been associated with increased CD11a expression, which takes an important part in costimulation and adhesion regulation (Lu et al., 2002).

As is known, SLE usually affects females, and it has been argued that CD40LG methylation may have a role in female predisposition. CD40LG is a costimulatory molecule, and demethylated CD40LG has been indicated to induce T lymphocytes in vitro (Lu et al., 2007). On the other hand, the over-expression of E4BP4, a human transcription factor, has been shown to suppress the autoimmune response in patients with SLE by inhibiting CD40LG expression (Zhao et al., 2013).

CD70 is the ligand of CD27, and it has been demonstrated that a lupus-like disease develops due to the interaction of this binary complex with demethylating agents such as hydralazine and procainamide (Oelke et al., 2004). In a study by Sunahori et al., it increased DNA methylation by inhibiting the catalytic subunit of protein phosphatase 2A, and as a result, a decrease in CD70 gene expression was detected (Sunahori et al., 2013).

PRF1 is a gene with key significance for cytotoxic CD8 lymphocytes, and cytolytic proteins for target surfaces are released with its activation. As a result of increased methylation, the over-expression of PFR1 has been demonstrated in both CD4 and CD8 lymphocytes in SLE patients (Podack et al., 1985).

Among epigenetic changes in patients with SLE, it has been shown that in the context of histone modification, histone acetyltransferases increase the production of autoantibodies, causing tissue damage through STAT3 activation (Hedrich et al., 2014). However, in general, the evidence shows that histone modifications contribute to SLE activation similar to DNA methylation is unclear.

Recent studies have demonstrated that elevated RNA levels contribute to the pathogenesis of SLE. For example, miR-21, miR-148a, and miR-126, regulated by methylation, have been revealed to be correlated with decreased DNMTs expression in CD4 T lymphocytes in SLE patients (Zhao et al., 2011). In another study, miR-155 was overexpressed in regulatory T cells in an MRLlpr mouse model, and accordingly, IL-4 and IL-17A levels were impacted (Xin et al., 2015).

Sjogren's Syndrome (SS)

SS is a chronic autoimmune disease that primarily impacts the exocrine glands and, as a result, is manifested with dry eye and dry mouth symptoms and can also impact other body organs in the advanced stage and is relatively common. Decreased DNA methylation in immune cells is the most researched epigenetic mechanism in SS, as in other autoimmune diseases. A study showed that the hypomethylation of CD70 promoter in SS patients caused the over-expression of CD70, a costimulator for CD4 T lymphocytes (Yin et al., 2010). By contrast, FOXP3 expression was detected to decrease in parallel with DNA hypermethylation in these patients (Yu et al., 2013). It was demonstrated that hypomethylation in the promoter regions of the IF44L and PARP9 loci in patients with SS was associated with increased mRNA expression in B lymphocytes. On the other hand, it was revealed that the RUNX1 gene with a key role in T cell development was hypermethylated, contrary to those mentioned above (Imgenberg Kreuz et al., 2016).

When examined locally, global hypomethylation was detected in the glands of patients with SS. In a study conducted on this issue, it was found that DNA methylation increased in the glands of patients with SS as a result of using rituximab, an anti-CD20 monoclonal antibody (Thabet et al., 2013). Konsta et al. reported that epithelial protein cytokeratin-19 expression increased as a result of decreased DNA methylation in glandular acini of the minor salivary glands (Konsta et al., 2016). Research on histone and mRNA in the context of epigenetic modifications in patients with SS is currently quite inadequate.

Systemic Sclerosis (SSc)

SSc is a chronic inflammatory disease that progresses with fibrosis in organs, primarily the skin. The downregulation of demethylating enzymes such as DNMT1 and MBD3 in SSc results in the hypomethylation of genes that have an important role in SSc genetics, which causes the over-expression of CD40L, CD11a, and CD70, one of the most prominent features of SSc. Especially the over-expression of CD40L has a key role in fibrosis, the most prominent feature of SSc (Fukasawa et al., 2003). Another fibrotic pathway in SSc is the Wnt pathway, and Dickkopf-1, a natural inhibitor of this pathway, is present in a hypomethylated form in dermal fibroblasts. As a result of 5-azacytidine treatment, the Wnt signal decreases and it has been demonstrated that the fibrotic pattern decreases in the mouse model (Dees et al., 2014). Likewise, the inactivated collagen suppressor gene (FLI1) as a result of hyper-fibromethylation causes decreased type-1 collagen production in fibroblasts (Wang et al., 2006).

Similar to SLE, a number of histone modifications were identified in SSc. It has been shown that both H3 and H4 acetylations decrease in fibroblasts, which can be associated with increased fibrosis (Wang et al., 2006).

MicroRNAs have been associated with dysregulated fibrosis in SSc. For instance, miR-29a prevents pulmonary fibrosis; however, as a result of its blocking, the level of pro-fibrotic cytokines such as TGF-beta increases (Xiao et al., 2012). On the contrary, decreased collagen levels were detected as a result of the over-expression of miR-196 (Honda et al., 2012).

Rheumatoid Arthritis (RA)

RA represents a chronic inflammatory disease that leads to joint damage and finally results in destructive arthritis. Epigenetic mechanisms in RA involve various methylation processes, including both T and B lymphocytes and fibroblasts in the target tissue (Smollen et al., 2016). Studies investigating early methylation have determined that T cells in these patients clearly show the global hypomethylation phenotype, just as in SLE (Richardson et al., 1990). It has been demonstrated that methotrexate (MTX), an agent frequently utilized to treat RA, increases protective Treg cells through FOXP3 demethylation and thus may reduce inflammation. Subsequent studies have revealed that MTX reverses the hypomethylation state in mononuclear cells in the peripheral blood (Cribbs et al., 2015).

Less emphasis has been involved in epigenetic studies on histone modification in RA. Dysregulated histone deacetylase (HDAC) activation was detected in these patients. It was even argued that selective HDAC2/3 inhibitors reduced IL-6 release in RA, so they could be utilized as treatment agents in the following period (Gillespie et al., 2012). Another study found that TNF-alpha increased HDAC1 expression in the synovial fibroblasts from patients with RA (Kawabata et al., 2010). One more study showed that IL-6 expression increased in fibroblasts due to the hyperacetylation of histone H3 (Wada et al., 2014).

It was demonstrated that TNF-alpha upregulated miR-146a and downregulated miR-363 and miR-498 in CD4+ cells of patients with RA, but its impact on the pathogenetic and clinical process has not been understood yet (Li et al., 2010). Another study revealed that increased miR-21 expression resulted in increased Treg accumulation in synovial fibroblasts (van der Geest et al., 2015).

Conclusion

CTDs may present with various clinical signs and symptoms. Epigenetic modifications have opened a new era to explain these different clinical spectra that may develop in patients with a similar genetic background. Epigenetic modifications can be characterized as genetic product changes affected by environmental factors in some way, which results in the differentiation of pathogenetic processes from person to person and, therefore, the person-specific development of the clinical spectrum. Although it is emphasized that epigenetic changes develop under the effect of both environmental factors and inflammation in light of the current findings, it is not yet known whether there is a genetic predisposition to epigenetic changes. With an increase in our knowledge of epigenetic modifications, the importance of the contributions of these modifications in terms of individualized treatment approaches, which have been frequently emphasized in recent years, can already be clearly seen.

References

Adams, B. D., Parsons, C., Walker, L., Zhang, W. C. & Slack, F. J (2017). Targeting noncoding RNAs in disease. *J. Clin. Invest*, 127, 761–771.

Akimova, T., Beier, U. H., Liu, Y., Wang, L., Hancock, W. W. (2012). Histone/protein deacetylases and T-cell immune responses. *Blood*, 119(11), 2443–51.

Cribbs, A. P., Kennedy, A., Penn, H., Amjadi, P., Green, P., Read, J. E., Brennan, F., Gregory, B., Williams, R. O. (2015). Methotrexate Restores Regulatory T Cell Function Through Demethylation of the FoxP3 Upstream Enhancer in Patients With Rheumatoid Arthritis. *Arthritis Rheumatol.*, 67(5), 1182-92.

Dees, C., Schlottmann, I., Funke, R., Distler, A., Palumbo-Zerr, K., Zerr, P., Lin, N. Y., Beyer, C., Distler, O., Schett, G., Distler, J. H. (2014). The Wnt antagonists DKK1 and SFRP1 are downregulated by promoter hypermethylation in systemic sclerosis. *Ann. Rheum. Dis.*, 73(6), 1232-9.

Du, J., Johnson, L. M., Jacobsen, S. E., Patel, D. J. (2015). DNA methylation pathways and their crosstalk with histone methylation. *Nat. Rev. Mol. Cell Biol.*, 16(9), 519–32.

Fukasawa, C., Kawaguchi, Y., Harigai, M., Sugiura, T., Takagi, K., Kawamoto, M., Hara, M., Kamatani, N. (2003). Increased CD40 expression in skin fibroblasts from patients with systemic sclerosis (SSc): role of CD40-CD154 in the phenotype of SSc fibroblasts. *Eur. J. Immunol.*, 33(10), 2792-800.

Garzon, R., Marcucci, G. & Croce, C. M. (2010). Targeting microRNAs in cancer: Rationale, strategies and challenges. *Nat. Rev. Drug Discov.*, 9(10), 775–789.

Gillespie, J., Savic, S., Wong, C., Hempshall, A., Inman, M., Emery, P., Grigg, R., McDermott, M. F. (2012). Histone deacetylases are dysregulated in rheumatoid arthritis and a novel histone deacetylase 3-selective inhibitor reduces interleukin-6 production by peripheral blood mononuclear cells from rheumatoid arthritis patients. *Arthritis Rheum.*, 64(2), 418-22.

Hedrich, C. M., Rauen, T., Apostolidis, S. A., Grammatikos, A.P., Rodriguez, R. N., Ioannidis, C., Kyttaris, V. C., Crispin, J. C., Tsokos, G. C. (2014). Stat3 promotes IL-10 expression in lupus T cells through trans-activation and chromatin remodeling. *Proc. Natl. Acad. Sci. USA*, 111(37), 13457-62.

Honda, N., Jinnin, M., Kajihara, I., Makino, T., Makino, K., Masuguchi, S., Fukushima, S., Okamoto, Y., Hasegawa, M., Fujimoto, M., Ihn, H. (2012). TGF-β-mediated downregulation of microRNA-196a contributes to the constitutive upregulated type I collagen expression in scleroderma dermal fibroblasts. *J. Immunol.*, 188(7), 3323-31.

Imgenberg-Kreuz, J., Sandling, J. K., Almlöf, J. C., Nordlund, J., Signér, L., Norheim, K. B., Omdal, R., Rönnblom, L., Eloranta, M. L., Syvänen, A. C., Nordmark, G. (2016). Genome-wide DNA methylation analysis in multiple tissues in primary Sjögren's syndrome reveals regulatory effects at interferon-induced genes. *Ann. Rheum. Dis.*, 75(11), 2029-2036.

Kawabata, T., Nishida, K, Takasugi, K., Ogawa, H., Sada, K., Kadota, Y., Inagaki, J., Hirohata, S., Ninomiya, Y., Makino, H. (2010). Increased activity and expression of histone deacetylase 1 in relation to tumor necrosis factor-alpha in synovial tissue of rheumatoid arthritis. *Arthritis Re.s Ther.*, 12(4), R133.

Konsta, O. D., Le Dantec, C., Charras, A., Cornec, D., Kapsogeorgou, E. K., Tzioufas, A. G., Pers, J. O., Renaudineau, Y. (2016). Defective DNA methylation in salivary gland epithelial acini from patients with Sjögren's syndrome is associated with SSB gene expression, anti-SSB/LA detection, and lymphocyte infiltration. *J. Autoimmun.*, 68,30-8.

Kumar, M., Nath, S., Prasad, H. K., Sharma, G. & Li, Y. (2012). MicroRNAs: A new ray of hope for diabetes mellitus. *Protein Cell*, 3(10), 726–738.

Lawrence, M., Daujat, S., Schneider, R. (2016). Lateral thinking: how histone modifications regulate gene expression. *Trends Genet.*, 32(1), 42–56.

Li, J., Wan, Y., Guo, Q., Zou, L., Zhang, J., Fang, Y., Zhang, J., Fu, X., Liu, H., Lu, L., Wu, Y. (2010). Altered microRNA expression profile with miR-146a upregulation in CD4+ T cells from patients with rheumatoid arthritis. *Arthritis Res. Ther.*, 12(3), R81.

Lu, Q., Kaplan, M., Ray, D., Zacharek, S., Gutsch, D., Richardson, B. (2002). Demethylation of ITGAL (CD11a) regulatory sequences in systemic lupus erythematosus. *Arthritis Rheum.*, 46(5), 1282-91.

Lu, Q., Wu, A., Tesmer, L., Ray, D., Yousif, N., Richardson, B. (2007). Demethylation of CD40LG on the inactive X in T cells from women with lupus. *J. Immunol.*, 179(9), 6352–8.

Mazzone, R., Zwergel, C., Artico, M., Taurone, S., Ralli, M., Greco, A., Mai, A. (2019). The emerging role of epigenetics in human autoimmune disorders. *Clin. Epigenetics*, 11(1), 26-34.

Morgan, H. D., Sutherland, H. G. E. & Martin, D. L. K. (1999). Epigenetic inheritance at the agouti locus in the mouse. *Nat. Genet.*, 23, 314-8.

Oelke, K., Lu, Q., Richardson, D., Wu, A., Deng, C., Hanash, S., Richardson, B. (2004). Overexpression of CD70 and overstimulation of IgG synthesis by lupus T cells and T cells treated with DNA methylation inhibitors. *Arthritis Rheum.*, 50(6), 1850-60.

Pea, A., Jamieson, N. B. & Braconi, C. (2021). Biology and clinical application of regulatory rnas in hepatocellular carcinoma. *Hepatology*, 73(S1):38-48. doi:10.1002/hep.31225.

Podack, E.R., Young, J.D., Cohn, Z.A. (1985). Isolation and biochemical and functional characterization of perforin 1 from cytolytic T-cell granules. *Proc. Natl. Acad. Sci. U S A*, 82(24), 8629–33.

Richardson, B. (2007). Primer: epigenetics of autoimmunity. *Nat. Clin. Pract. Rheumatol.*, 3(9), 521–7.

Richardson, B., Scheinbart, L., Strahler, J., Gross, L., Hanash, S., Johnson, M. (1990). Evidence for impaired T cell DNA methylation in systemic lupus erythematosus and rheumatoid arthritis. *Arthritis Rheum.*, 33(11), 1665–73.

Smolen, J. S., Aletaha, D., McInnes, I. B. (2016). Rheumatoid arthritis. *Lancet*, 388(10055), 2023–38.

Sunahori, K., Nagpal, K., Hedrich, C. M., Mizui, M., Fitzgerald, L. M., Tsokos, G. C. (2013). The catalytic subunit of protein phosphatase 2A (PP2Ac) promotes DNA hypomethylation by suppressing the phosphorylated mitogen-activated protein kinase/extracellular signal-regulated kinase (ERK) kinase (MEK)/ phosphorylated ERK/DNMT1 protein pathway in T-cells from controls and systemic lupus erythematosus patients. *J. Biol. Chem.*, 288(30), 21936–44.

Thabet, Y., Le Dantec, C., Ghedira, I., Devauchelle, V., Cornec, D., Pers, J.O., Renaudineau, Y. (2013). Epigenetic dysregulation in salivary glands from patients with primary Sjögren's syndrome may be ascribed to infiltrating B cells. *J. Autoimmun.*, 41, 175-81.

van der Geest, K. S., Smigielska-Czepiel, K., Park, J. A., Abdulahad, W. H., Kim, H. W., Kroesen, B. J., van den Berg, A., Boots, A. M., Lee, E. B., Brouwer, E. (2015). SF Treg cells transcribing high levels of Bcl-2 and microRNA-21 demonstrate limited apoptosis in RA. *Rheumatology (Oxford)*, 54(5), 950-8.

Wada, T. T., Araki, Y., Sato, K., Aizaki, Y., Yokota, K., Kim, Y. T., Oda, H., Kurokawa, R., Mimura, T. (2014). Aberrant histone acetylation contributes to elevated interleukin-6 production in rheumatoid arthritis synovial fibroblasts. *Biochem. Biophys. Res. Commun.*, 444(4), 682-6.

Wadhwa, E., Nicolaides, T. (2016). Bromodomain inhibitor review: Bromodomain and extra-terminal family protein inhibitors as a potential new therapy in central nervous system tumors. *Cureus,* 8(5), e620.

Wang, Y., Fan, P. S., Kahaleh, B. (2006). Association between enhanced type I collagen expression and epigenetic repression of the FLI1 gene in scleroderma fibroblasts. *Arthritis Rheum.*, 54(7), 2271–9.

Xiao, J., Meng, X. M., Huang, X. R., Chung, A. C., Feng, Y. L., Hui, D. S., Yu, C. M., Sung, J. J., Lan, H. Y. (2012). miR-29 inhibits bleomycin-induced pulmonary fibrosis in mice. *Mol. Ther.*, 20(6), 1251-60.

Xin, Q., Li, J., Dang, J., Bian, X., Shan, S., Yuan, J., Qian, Y., Liu, Z., Liu, G., Yuan, Q., Liu, N., Ma, X., Gao, F., Gong, Y., Liu, Q. (2015). miR-155 Deficiency Ameliorates Autoimmune Inflammation of Systemic Lupus Erythematosus by Targeting S1pr1 in Faslpr/lpr Mice. *J. Immunol.*, 194(11), 5437-45.

Yin, H., Zhao, M., Wu, X., Gao, F., Luo, Y., Ma, L., Liu, S., Zhang, G., Chen, J., Li, F., Zuo, X., Lu, Q. (2010). Hypomethylation and overexpression of CD70 (TNFSF7) in CD4+ T cells of patients with primary Sjögren's syndrome. *J. Dermatol. Sci.*, 59(3), 198-203.

Yu, X., Liang, G., Yin, H., Ngalamika, O., Li, F., Zhao, M., Lu, Q. (2013). DNA hypermethylation leads to lower FOXP3 expression in CD4+ T cells of patients with primary Sjögren's syndrome. *Clin. Immunol.,* 148(2), 254-7.

Zhao, M., Liu, Q., Liang, G., Wang, L., Luo, S., Tang, Q., Zhao, H., Su, Y., Yung, S., Chan, T.M., Lu, Q, (2013). E4BP4 overexpression: a protective mechanism in CD4+ T cells from SLE patients. *J. Autoimmun.,* 41, 152-60.

Zhao, S., Wang, Y., Liang, Y., Zhao, M., Long, H., Ding, S., Yin, H., Lu, Q. (2011). MicroRNA-126 regulates DNA methylation in CD4+ T cells and contributes to systemic lupus erythematosus by targeting DNA methyltransferase 1. *Arthritis Rheum.*, 63(5), 1376-86.

Zwergel, C., Valente, S., Jacob, C., Mai, A. (2015). Emerging approaches for histone deacetylase inhibitor drug discovery. *Expert Opin. Drug Discovery,* 10(6), 599–613.

Chapter 28

Epigenetics and Rheumatoid Arthritis (RA)

Alper Doğancı*, MD

Sivas Cumhuriyet University,
Department of Physical Medicine and Rehabilitation,
Department of Rheumatology, Sivas, Turkey

Abstract

Rheumatoid arthritis (RA) is chronic, autoimmune, erosive inflammatory rheumatism that impacts especially the female population between the ages of 20-50. Its prevalence varies between 0.5-1% worldwide. The etiology of rheumatoid arthritis is multifactorial. The risk factors include genetic, epigenetic, allergic, hormonal, neuroendocrine, reproduction-related factors, comorbid conditions, smoking, air pollution, socioeconomic status, lifestyle, diet, inhalation of dusts such as silica-asbestos-glass powder-textile dyes, microbiota, and infectious agents. After the diagnosis is established with physical examination, laboratory, and imaging methods, an appropriate treatment regimen must be quickly arranged to prevent disability. Pharmacological and non-pharmacological treatments are used to treat RA. There are patient education, psychosocial support, orthoses, exercise program, physical therapy agents, nutritional support and diet, prevention of osteoporosis and other comorbidities among non-pharmacological treatments. Pharmacologically, conventional DMARDs (disease-modifying anti-rheumatic drugs) are initially used (methotrexate, leflunomide, sulfasalazine, and hydroxy-chloroquine). In cases unresponsive to conventional treatments, TNF-a inhibitors (adalimumab, golimumab, infliximab, certolizumab pegol, and etanercept) or non-TNF biologics (rituximab, tocilizumab, anakinra, abatacept, baricitinib, tofacitinib) are utilized. Epigenetics refers to changes in gene expression without any change in DNA sequence. Changes occur in the chromosome, various phenotypes emerge, and the resulting changes can be passed on to the next generations by mitosis or meiosis. Environmental stimuli such as drugs, smoke, and cigarettes can induce epigenetic modifications. Hence, the link between the genome and the environment is ensured by epigenetic mechanisms. Epigenetic mechanisms include DNA methylation, post-translational histone modifications (histone methylation, histone acetylation, histone phosphorylation, histone ubiquitination, histone citrullination, and histone ribosylation), and the expression of non-coding RNAs (ncRNAs) such as microRNA (miRNA). DNA hypomethylation, histone acetylation, histone methylation, micro-RNAs, and long non-coding RNAs are the most accused in the relationship between RA and epigenetics. Nowadays, it is thought that these epigenetic mechanisms detected in RA will be employed as a prognostic factor and will have a role in diagnosis and treatment follow-up and in determining the susceptibility to RA.

---

* Corresponding Author's E-mail: alperdoganci.79@gmail.com.

In: Epigenetics: Beyond the Genetics and Medicine
Editors: Sevgi Durna Daştan and Nazan Yurtcu
ISBN: 979-8-88697-228-3

Keywords: rheumatoid arthritis, epigenetics, DNA methylation, histone modification, miRNAs, lncRNAs

Introduction

Rheumatoid arthritis (RA) is a chronic, immune-mediated multisystem disease of unknown etiology, which causes joint pain, swelling, stiffness, and loss of function. It is the most common among autoimmune diseases and frequently impacts the joints symmetrically and erosively. In general, it occurs 3 times more frequently in females than in males (Gibofsky, 2014). Although it can occur at any age, it is most frequently detected between the ages of 20-50 years. Its prevalence varies between 0.5-1% worldwide (Firestein, 2003).

The risk factors are divided into two subgroups: host-related and environment-related. Genetic, epigenetic, allergic, hormonal (decreased risk during lactation and pregnancy), neuroendocrine, reproduction-related factors, and comorbid conditions are among patient-related factors. Considering environmental factors, smoking (the most accused agent), air pollution, socioeconomic status, lifestyle, diet (the protective role of the Mediterranean diet), inhalation of dusts such as silica-asbestos-glass powder-textile dyes, microbiota (periodontitis), and infectious agents (EBV, CMV, periodontitis, etc.) come to mind (Vasco & Joao, 2021). Hence, the etiology of RA is multifactorial (Fadda et al., 2016). It has been particularly identified in monozygotic twins in which genetics does not have a role alone. The disease is observed in only 9-15% of monozygotic twins (Svendsen et al., 2013). When genetic studies were reviewed, HLA-DRB1 from HLA genes, PAD and PTPN22 polymorphism from non-HLA genes, the presence of the STAT4 variant allele, TRAF1-C5 gene locus, intergenic region between OLIG3 and TNFAIP3 genes, PADI-4 and CTLA4 genes were found to be strongly associated with RA (Araki and Mimura, 2017). There is a strong relationship, especially between ACPA positivity and HLA-DRB1 common epitope and PTPN22 polymorphism.

RA frequently begins with polyarthritis of the hand and foot joints. Cases that start with mono or oligoarthritis are also available. Moreover, constitutional findings may also accompany the clinical picture. Patients describe stiffness, pain, swelling, increased temperature, and loss of function in the affected joints. The disease has an insidious onset in 60% of patients. Extraarticular findings can also be seen in 40% of patients with RA. Advanced age, the presence of HLA-DRB1, early radiological damage, smoking, and seropositivity pose a risk for extraarticular involvement (Turenson & Jacobsson, 2004). Extraarticular system involvements include hematological, renal, gastrointestinal system, eye, neurological, pulmonary, cardiovascular system, rheumatoid vasculitis, osteoporosis, and muscle involvement.

In addition to physical examination, laboratory findings and imaging methods are also utilized to diagnose RA. RF (rheumatoid factor) and ACPA (anti-citrulline protein antibody) antibody positivities are valuable in diagnosis (Whiting et al., 2010). Furthermore, acute phase markers such as erythrocyte sedimentation rate (ESR) or c-reactive protein (CRP) may be elevated in the blood.

It is possible to detect the joint damage caused by RA by conventional radiography, ultrasonography, magnetic resonance imaging, scintigraphy, and computed tomography. It should not be forgotten that the said imaging modalities may be normal in early RA. Furthermore, a synovial fluid analysis can be used in diagnosing inflammatory arthritis.

The classification criteria recommended by the ACR (American College of Rheumatology)/EULAR (The European League Against Rheumatism) are employed in early RA (Figure 1). For the patient to be definitely diagnosed with RA, the total score to be acquired from the categories in Figure 1 must be ≥ 6.

Classification criteria for RA (Score-based algorithm: add score of categories A-D) A score of ≥ 6/10 is needed for a definite classification of a patient with RA.	
Joint involvement[A]	
1 large[B] joint	0
2-10 large joints	1
1-3 small[C] joints (with or without involvement of large joints)	2
4-10 small joints (with or without involvement of large joints)	3
>10 joints[D] (at least one small joint)	5
Serology[E] (at least one test result is needed for classification)	
Negative RF **and** negative ACPA	0
Low positive RF **or** low positive ACPA	2
High positive RF **or** high positive ACPA	3
ACUTE PHASE REACTANTS[F] (at least one test result is needed for classification)	
Normal CRP **and** normal ESR	0
Abnormal CRP **or** abnormal ESR	1
Duration of symptoms[G]	
< 6 weeks	0
≥ 6 weeks	1

[A]Joint involvement refers to any swollen or tender joint on examination, which may be confirmed by imaging evidence of synovitis. Distal interphalangeal joints (DIPs), 1st carpo-metacarpal (CMC) joint, and 1st metatarso-phalangeal (MTP) joint are *excluded from assessment*. Categories of joint distribution are classified according to the location and number of the involved joints, with placement into the highest category possible based on the pattern of joint involvement.

[B]Large joints refer to shoulders, elbows, hips, knees and ankles.

[C]Small joints refer to the wrists, metacarpo-phalangeal (MCP) joints, proximal interphalangeal (PIP) joints, thumb interphalangeal (IP) joints and metatarsophalangeal (MTP).

[D]In this category, at least 1 of the involved joints must be a small joint ; the other joints can include any combination of large and additional small joints, as well as other joints not specifically listed elsewhere (e.g. temperomandibular, acromioclavicular and sternoclavicular joints).

ENegative refers to international unit (IU) values that are £ upper limit of normal ULN for the lab and assay. Low titre refers to IU values that are > ULN but £ 3X ULN for lab and assay. High titre positive: > 3X ULN for lab and assay. Where RF is only available as positive or negative, a positive results should be scored as 'low positive' for RF.

FNormal /abnormal is determined by local laboratory standards (*Other causes for elevated acute phase reactants should be excluded*).

[G]Duration of symptoms refers to patient self-report of the duration of signsor symptoms of synovitis (e.g., pain, swelling, tenderness) of joints that are clinically involved at the time of assessment, regardless of treatment status.

RF = rheumatoid factor; ACPA = anti-citrullinated protein/ peptide antibodies; ULN = upper limit of normal; ESR = erythrocyte sedimentation rate; CRP = C-reactive protein.

Figure 1. RA 2010 ACR/EULAR classification criteria (Aletaha et al., 2010).

Pharmacological and non-pharmacological treatments are utilized to treat RA. Patient education, psychosocial support, orthoses, exercise program, physical therapy agents, nutritional support, and diet, prevention of osteoporosis and other comorbidities are among non-pharmacological treatments. In pharmacological treatments, conventional DMARDs (disease-modifying anti-rheumatic drugs) are used initially (methotrexate, leflunomide, sulfasalazine, and hydroxychloroquine). In cases unresponsive to conventional treatments, TNF-a inhibitors (adalimumab, golimumab, infliximab, certolizumab pegol, and etanercept) or non-TNF biologics (rituximab, tocilizumab, anakinra, abatacept, baricitinib, and tofacitinib) are utilized.

Epigenetic Mechanisms

Epigenetics refers to changes in gene expression without any change in DNA sequence. Changes occur in the chromosome, various phenotypes emerge, and the resulting changes can be passed on to the next generations by mitosis or meiosis (Berger et al., 2009).

Environmental stimuli such as drugs, smoke, and cigarettes can induce epigenetic modifications. Hence, the link between the genome and the environment is ensured by epigenetic mechanisms (Costenbader et al., 2012). DNA methylation, post-translational histone modifications, and the expression of non-coding RNAs (ncRNAs) such as microRNAs (miRNAs) take place among epigenetic mechanisms.

DNA methylation occurs when a methyl group is attached to the carbon at position 5 of the cytosine base in a region rich in cytosine and guanine bases, named the CpG island. S-adenosyl methionine (SAM) is a methyl donor, and the reaction is catalyzed by the enzyme DNA methyltransferase (DNMT). As a result of this reaction, transcription factors cannot bind to DNA, and transcription is silenced. Additionally, DNA methylation suppresses the expression of potentially harmful transposons and viral elements in the genome (Araki & Mimura, 2016).

Nucleosomes represent one of the main targets of epigenetic modifications. A nucleosome consists of the histone octamer formed by H2A, H2B, H3, and H4 and 146 bp DNA wrapped around the histone in the form of a double helix. Acetylation, methylation, ubiquitination, phosphorylation, sumoylation, citrullination, ADP ribosylation, and proline isomerization are listed among histone modifications. Studies have mostly been done on histone acetylation and methylation. Due to these modifications, transcription factors cannot bind to DNA, and gene expression is silenced (Zhao et al., 2015).

Non-coding RNAs (nc-RNAs) are actually an umbrella term. The sub-groups involve piwi-interacting RNA, small nucleolar RNAs, small interfering RNAs, microRNAs, circular RNAs, antisense RNAs, and long intergenic non-coding RNAs (lncRNAs). Nevertheless, studies have included especially microRNA and long intergenic non-coding RNAs (Pea et al., 2021).

MicroRNAs are comprised of approximately 22 nucleotides, whereas long non-coding RNAs consist of over 200 nucleotides. Especially miRNAs have a role in post-transcriptional control pathways in numerous biological functions. They bind to one or more mRNAs, take part in the degradation of mRNAs, or inhibit mRNA translation. Thus, gene expression is silenced (Hausser & Zavolan, 2014).

RA and Epigenetics

DNA methylation, post-translational histone modifications, and non-coding RNAs take place among epigenetic mechanisms contributing to the formation of RA. These epigenetic changes lead to synovial inflammation by increasing the expression of particularly metalloproteinases and inflammatory cytokines in RA. As a result, the severity and course of RA are impacted.

Hypo- or hypermethylation of specific promoter regions causes an increase or decrease in pro- and anti-inflammatory genes (Rhead et al., 2017).

Varied joint involvement patterns in patients with RA have been associated with different methylation models in key genes having a role in the pathogenesis of RA (Frank Bertonceli et al., 2017).

Especially global DNA hypomethylation has been identified in RA patients in comparison with healthy controls. Moreover, DNA hypomethylation has been detected in fibroblast-like synoviocytes and synovial tissue/fluid in RA.

Studies performed on RA synovial fibroblasts and peripheral blood mononuclear cells detected abnormalities in the methylation profile in single gene promoters, such as IL-6, IL-10, IL1-R2, DR3, and CXCL12 (Picascia et al., 2015).

CD40L is an X chromosome gene. As a result of the demethylation of this gene, the gene escapes X-chromosome inactivation. The mentioned gene is overexpressed, particularly in female RA patients, which also explains the predominance of RA disease in females (Liao et al., 2012).

A study conducted in 2014 determined a significant decrease in the DNA methylation of the FOXP3 promoter in RA T regulatory cells in comparison with healthy controls (Kennedy et al., 2014).

It is interesting that methotrexate treatment has been demonstrated to reverse global hypomethylation in T cells, B cells, and monocytes. Additionally, T regulatory cell function was also restored through the demethylation of the FOXP3 locus with methotrexate treatment (Cribbs et al., 2015).

The PIBF1 promoter was revealed to be hypermethylated in RA. AZU1, LTBR, CCR6, CMTM5, IL10RA, IL21R, IL32, and RTEL1 promoters were found to be significantly hypomethylated (Wang et al., 2018).

Less is known about the role of histone modifications in RA. Especially acetylation, methylation, phosphorylation, citrullination, and others, among histone modifications, lead to changes in the structure of chromatin and thus gene transcription.

Most studies have concentrated on measuring the expression of histone-modifying enzymes, histone deacetylases (HDACs) and histone acetyltransferases, in blood and synovial tissue in patients with RA (Kawabata et al., 2010). In particular, it is thought to be more important to measure histone deacetylases rather than histone acetyltransferases. Furthermore, various studies have shown the impacts of HDAC inhibitors in suppressing inflammation [especially IL-6 and type-I interferon (IFN)], angiogenesis, and the function and survival of fibroblast-like synoviocytes and macrophages (Angiolli et al., 2017).

Both HDAC activity and expression in the synovial tissues of RA patients were observed to be significantly decreased compared to healthy individuals. Histone acetylase/HDAC balance shifted toward the hyperacetylation of histones in patients with RA (Picascia et al., 2015).

Importantly, smoking, a significant environmental risk factor for RA, has recently been demonstrated to increase two key HDAC levels [sirtuin (SIRT1) 1 and (SIRT6)]. This shows the significance of the impact of environmental factors on epigenetics (Engler et al., 2016).

It was revealed that histone phosphorylation levels increased in mice with arthritis.

Comprehensive studies have been done on both microRNAs and long non-coding RNAs, among non-coding RNAs, in the suspicion, severity, and treatment of RA (Li et al., 2018).

miRNAs are non-coding RNAs that bind to mRNA, cause its degradation, or inhibit its translation. miRNA-155 and miRNA-146a are the most studied among them. They have been detected in many cells and tissues from patients with RA. Whereas both induce the inflammatory response, they suppress joint destruction (Kmiolek&Paradowska-Gorycka, 2022).

The levels of miR-16, miR-103a, miR-145, miR-146a, miR-155, miR-221, miR-22, and miR-301a increased, while the level of let7a, miR-21, miR-125b, and miR-548a decreased in peripheral blood mononuclear cells of patients with RA (Lin et al., 2020).

It was determined that let-7a, miR-26, miR-146a, miR-146b, miR-150, and miR-155 have a role in the pathogenesis of RA by causing IL-17 increase.

miR-132 levels were lower in RA patients than in healthy controls (Tsai et al., 2021).

It was demonstrated that miRNA-223 increased and miRNA-124a decreased in RA synovial tissue, fibroblast-like synoviocytes, and blood cells, and they contributed directly to the regulation of osteoclastogenesis, fibroblast-like synoviocyte proliferation, and T cell and macrophage-mediated inflammation.

It was argued that an increase in miR-203 expression might indicate the active phenotype of RA disease.

The results of plasma studies on patients with RA showed that an increase in the plasma concentrations of miR-24 and miR-125a-5p could be a diagnostic biomarker for RA.

A study performed by Liu et al., in 2017 determined that the miR-29a level was very high in RA synovial fibroblasts, and this elevation inhibited proliferation and suppressed the expression of inflammatory cytokines (Liu et al., 2017).

Moreover, miRNA levels differ according to the developmental stage of RA. Serum miR-16, miR-146a, miR-155, and miR-223 levels are lower in early-stage RA than in advanced-stage RA (Lennert & Fardo, 2017). Lower miR-16 and miR-223 levels were detected in early-stage RA than healthy controls. Therefore, these markers can be utilized as biomarkers to distinguish patients with early RA from healthy controls.

Nowadays, the view that miRNAs detected in RA will be utilized as a prognostic factor, will have a role in diagnosis and treatment follow-up and determining susceptibility to RA has started to dominate.

Long non-coding RNAs (lncRNAs) have recently started to be researched due to their functions as nuclear and cytoplasmic regulators of gene transcription and mRNA translation in RA. The most characteristic lncRNA is HOTAIR (HOX antisense intergenic RNA), which suppresses the expression of matrix metalloproteinases MMP-2 and MMP-13. It has been revealed to be increased in peripheral blood mononuclear cells, fibroblast-like synoviocytes in the lower or upper extremity joints of RA patients. It is considered that HOTAIR is another mechanism involved in the RA joint involvement pattern (Elhai et al., 2019).

Conclusion

Rheumatoid arthritis (RA) is a chronic, immune-mediated, multisystem disease of unknown etiology, which causes joint pain, swelling, stiffness, and loss of function. It is the most common among autoimmune diseases. There is a female predominance in RA. It may present with both articular and extraarticular manifestations. Although numerous factors such as genetics, environmental factors, viruses, hormones, and diet are blamed for the etiology of RA, the role of epigenetics has recently been emphasized. Epigenetics represents a collection of mechanisms that do not change the DNA base sequence but change chromatin. Quantitative and qualitative changes emerge in gene transcription as a result of changes in chromatin. Hence, the transcription of the relevant gene is silenced or activated. The said changes in gene transcription can also be transferred to the next generations. DNA hypomethylation, histone acetylation, histone methylation, micro-RNAs, and long non-coding RNAs take place among the most accused in the RA-epigenetics relationship.

References

Aletaha D, Neogi T, Silman A J, Funovits J, Felson D T, Bingham C O, Birnbaum N S, Burmester G R, Bykerk V P, Cohen M D, Combe B, Costenbader K H, Dougados M, Emergey P, Ferraccioli G, Hazes J M W, Hobbs K, Huizinga T W J, Kayanaugh A, Hawker G (2010). Rheumatoid Arthritis Classification Criteria An American College of Rheumatology/European League Against Rheumatism Collaborative Initiative. *Arthritis & Rheumatism*, 62(9): 2569-2581.

Angiolli C, Kabala P A, Grabiec A M, Baarsen I M V, Ferguson B S, Garcia S, Fernandez B M, McKinsey T A, Tak P P, Fossati G, Mascagni P, Baeten D L & Reedquist K A (2017). Histone deacetylase 3 regulates the inflammatory gene expression programme of rheumatoid arthritis fibroblast-like synoviocytes. *Ann. Rheum. Dis.,* 76: 277–85. doi: 10.1136/annrheumdis-2015- 209064.

Araki Y, Mimura T (2016). The mechanisms underlying chronic inflammation in rheumatoid arthritis from the perspective of the epigenetic landscape. *Journal of Immunology Research*, 1-11.

Araki Y & Mimura T (2017). The histone modification code in the pathogenesis of autoimmune diseases. *Mediators of Inflammation*, 1-13.

Berger S L, Kouzarides T, Shiekhattar R & Shilatifard A (2009). An operational definition of epigenetics. *Genes & Development*, 23(7): 781-783.

Costenbader K H, Gay S, Alarcón-Riquelme M E, Iaccarino L &Doria A (2012). Genes, epigenetic regulation and environmental factors: which is the most relevant in developing autoimmune diseases? *Autoimmun. Rev.*, 11:604–9. http://doi: 10.1016/j.autrev.2011.10.022.

Cribbs A P, Kennedy A, Penn H, Amjadi P, Green P, Read J E, Brennan F, Gregory B & Williams R O (2015). Methotrexate restores regulatory T cell function through demethylation of the FoxP3 upstream enhancer in patients with rheumatoid arthritis. *Arthritis Rheumatol*, 67:1182–92 doi: 10.1002/art.39031.

Elhai M, Frank-Bertoncelj M, Klein K, Distler O & Ospelt C (2019). HOTAIR is involved in joint patterning by regulating FGFR2, BMP2 and WNT pathways. *Ann. Rheum. Dis.*, 78(Suppl. 2): 226–7. doi: 10.1136/annrheumdis-2019-eular.4370.

Engler A, Tange C, Frank-Bertoncelj M, Gay R E, Gay S & Ospelt C (2016). Regulation and function of SIRT1 in rheumatoid arthritis synovial fibroblasts. *J. Mol. Med.*, 94: 173–82. http://doi: 10.1007/s00109-015-133 2-9.

Fadda S, Abolkheir E, Afifi R & Gamal M (2016). Serum matrix metalloproteinase-3 in rheumatoid arthritis patients: Correlation with disease activity and joint destruction. *The Egyptian Rheumatologist*, 38(3): 153-159.

Firestein, G S (2003). Evolving concepts of rheumatoid arthritis. *Nature*, 423, 356–361.

Kolling, C, Armaka, M, Filer, A, Michel, B A, Gay, R E, Buckley, C D, Kollias, G, Gay, S, & Ospelt, C (2017). Epigenetically-driven anatomical diversity of synovial fibroblasts guides joint-specific fibroblast functions. *Nature communications*, *8*, 14852.

Gibofsky A (2014). Epidemiology, pathophysiology, and diagnosis of rheumatoid arthritis: A Synopsis. *The American Journal of Managed Care*, 20 (7 Suppl): 128-35.

Hausser J &Zavolan M (2014). Identification and consequences of miRNA–target interactions beyond repression of gene expression. *Nature Reviews Genetics*, 15(9): 59.

Kawabata T, Nishida K, Takasugi K, Ogawa H, Sada K, Kadota Y, Inagaki J, Hirohata S, Ninomiya Y & Makino H (2010). Increased activity and expression of histone deacetylase 1 in relation to tumor necrosis factor-alpha in synovial tissue of rheumatoid arthritis. *Arthritis Res. Ther.*, 12:R133. http://doi.10.11 86/ar3071.

Kennedy, A, Schmidt, E M, Cribbs, A P, Penn, H, Amjadi, P, Syed, K, Read, J E, Green, P, Gregory, B, & Brennan, F M (2014). A novel upstream enhancer of FOXP3, sensitive to methylation-induced silencing, exhibits dysregulated methylation in rheumatoid arthritis Treg cells. *European Journal of Immunology*, *44*(10): 2968–2978. https://doi.org/10.1002/eji.201444453.

Kmiolek T & Paradowska-Gorycka A (2022). miRNAs as Biomarkers and Possible Therapeutic Strategies in Rheumatoid Arthritis. *Cells*, 11: 452. https://doi.org/10.3390/cells11030452.

Lennert, A & Fardo, D W (2017). Detecting novel micro RNAs in rheumatoid arthritis with gene-based association testing. *Clin. Exp. Rheum.*, 35: 586–592.

Li Z, Li X, Jiang C, Qian W, Tse G, Chan M T V & Wu W K K (2018). Long non-coding RNAs in rheumatoid arthritis. *Cell Prolif.*, 51:e12404. doi: 10.1111/cpr.12404.

Liao, J, Liang, G, Xie, S, Zhao, H, Zuo, X, Li, F, Chen, J, Zhao, M, Chan, T M, & Lu, Q (2012). CD40L demethylation in CD4(+) T cells from women with rheumatoid arthritis. *Clinical Immunology 145*(1): 13–18. https://doi.org/10.1016/j.clim.2012.07.006.

Lin, S, Wang, S, Zhang, Z, Lu, Y, Yang, M, Chen, P, Chen, L & Wang, M (2020). MiRNA-6089 inhibits rheumatoid arthritis fibroblast-like synoviocytes proliferation and induces apoptosis by targeting CCR4. *Arch. Physiol. Biochem*, 17: 1–8.

Liu J, Fei D, Xing J & Du J (2017). MicroRNA-29a inhibits proliferation and induces apoptosis in rheumatoid arthritis fibroblast-like synoviocytes by repressing STAT3. *Biomedicine & Pharmacotherapy*, 96: 173-181.

McInnes I B, Schett G (2011). The pathogenesis of rheumatoid arthritis. *New England Journal of Medicine*, 365(23): 2205-2219.

Nemtsova M V, Zaletaev D V, Bure I V, Mikhaylenko D S, Kuznetsova E B, Alekseeva E A, Beloukhova M I, Deviatkin A A, Lukashev A N & Zamyatnin A A (2019). Epigenetic changes in the pathogenesis of rheumatoid arthritis. *Front Genet*, 10:570. doi: 10.3389/fgene.2019.00570.

Pea A, Jamieson N B & Braconi C (2021). Biology and clinical application of regulatory RNAs in hepatocellular carcinoma. *Hepatology*, 73(S1):38-48. doi:10.1002/hep.31225.

Picascia A, Grimaldi V, Pignalosa O, De Pascale M R, Schiano C & Napoli C (2015). Epigenetic control of autoimmune diseases: from bench to bedside. *Clinical Immunology*, 157(1): 1-15.

Rhead B, Holingue C, Cole M, Shao X, Quach H L, Quach D, Shah K, Sinclair E, Graf J, Link T, Harrison R, Rahmani E, Halperin E, Wang W, Frestein G S, Barcellos L F & Criswell L A. Rheumatoid arthritis naive T cells share hypermethylation sites with synoviocytes (2017). *Arthritis Rheumatol.*, 69: 550–9. doi: 10.1002/art. 39952.

Svendsen A J, Kyvik K O, Houen G, Junker P, Christensen K & Christiansen L (2013). On the origin of rheumatoid arthritis: the impact of environment and genes—a population based twin study. *PLoS ONE*. 8:e57304. doi: 10.1371/journal.pone.00 57304.

Tsai C H, Hsieh S C, Liu C W, Lu C H, Liao H T, Chen M H, Li K J, Wu C H, Shen C Y, Kuo Y M & Yu C L (2021). The Expression of Non-Coding RNAs and Their Target Molecules in Rheumatoid Arthritis: A Molecular Basis for Rheumatoid Pathogenesis and Its Potential Clinical Applications. *Int. J. Mol. Sci*, 22: 5689. https://doi.org/ 10.3390/ijms22115689.

Turenson C & Jacobsson L T (2004). Epidemiology of extraarticular manifestations in rheumatoid arthtritis. *Scand. J. Rheumatol.*, 33 (2): 65-72.

Vasco C R & João E F (2021). Etiology and Risk Factors for Rheumatoid Arthritis: A State-of-the-Art Review. *Frontiers in Medicine*. volume 8. doi: 10.3389/fmed.2021.689698.

Wang, X, Lei, D, Ding, J, Liu, S, Tao, L, Zhang, F, Peng, J, & Xu, J (2018). A DNA-Methylated Sight on Autoimmune Inflammation Network across RA, pSS, and SLE. *Journal of Immunology Research*, 4390789. https://doi.org/10.1155/2018/4390789.

Whiting P F, Smidt N & Sterna J A (2010). Systematic review: accuracy of anti-citrullinated peptide antibpdies for diagnosing rheumatoid arthritis. *Ann. Intern. Med.*, 152: 456-64.

Zhao M, Wang Z, Yung S & Lu Q (2015). Epigenetic dynamics in immunity and autoimmunity. *The International Journal of Biochemistry & Cell Biology*, 67: 65-74.

Chapter 29

Inflammatory Bowel Diseases and Epigenetics

İlkay Güler*, MD
Department of General Surgery,
Kayseri City Hospital, Kayseri, Turkey

Abstract

Inflammatory bowel diseases (IBDs) represent a group of diseases, which have a chronic course, cause a decrease in a person's quality of life, and whose etiopathogenesis is still not fully explained. The risk factors include the environment, smoking, diet, genetic factors, a person's immunological status, and the intestinal microbiota. Epigenetic mechanisms have recently begun to take their place in the occurrence mechanism of diseases. The mechanisms described under three main headings, DNA methylation, histone modification, and miRNA, have taken a significant place in the diagnosis and follow-up of many diseases and the treatment protocol. In light of all this information, the association between epigenetics and inflammatory bowel diseases and its place in the future will gain even more importance with new studies.

Keywords: inflammatory bowel diseases, ulcerative colitis, Crohn's disease, epigenetics

Introduction

The pathogenesis of inflammatory bowel diseases (IBDs) still contains many questions for researchers. The mucosal healing, disease remission, and sudden disease activation, which last for years in Crohn's disease, have necessitated clarifying the question of "disease memory" (Rogler et al., 2018). What are the influencing factors here? The environment, smoking, diet, genetics, a person's immunological status, and the intestinal microbiota are the risk factors. However, are they sufficient to explain the pathogenesis? Epigenetic mechanisms come into play here. Studies revealing the role of epigenetic mechanisms in the occurrence of many diseases have recently been carried out. Epigenetics has the potential to be used as a biomarker in the diagnosis, follow-up, and response to disease treatment. In recent years, pharmacoepigenetic studies have gained momentum, and significant advancements have been

* Corresponding Author's E-mail: drilkayguler@gmail.com.

In: Epigenetics: Beyond the Genetics and Medicine
Editors: Sevgi Durna Daştan and Nazan Yurtcu
ISBN: 979-8-88697-228-3

made in epigenetic drug development (Zhang et al., 2020). In line with all these advancements, how can the association between IBDs and epigenetics be explained?

Definition of Epigenetics

The word epigenetics means "the phenotypic change in both prokaryotes and eukaryotes related to the regulation of gene sequence, while there is no change in the DNA sequence, which can be transferred to the next generations" (Jablonka and Lamb, 2015). It shows various gene expressions and activities that occur without changing the DNA sequence or structure. All molecular changes on DNA and in DNA-associated histones are defined as epigenetic modifications, and no change occurs in the nucleotide sequence in this process (Weinhold, 2006). This modification decides which gene to transcribe or whether the gene is switched on or silenced. To define it in another way, just as the DNA of all cells in our body is the same but consists of many functionally differentiated tissues, the epigenetic profile of tissues determines this functional difference in tissues (Talbert and Henikoff, 2006). Hereditary changes are associated with these gene expressions, as well as long-term and stable environmental factors affect these changes. Nevertheless, the mechanism of inheritance has not been fully explained yet. For the purpose of explaining the difference from genetic changes, the phenotypic difference in monozygotic twins with identical DNA sequences is ensured by epigenetic diversity (Coolen et al., 2011; Portela and Esteller, 2010). Various formation mechanisms for epigenetics have been described (İzmirli, 2013).

1- Mechanisms That Control Gene Expression Indirectly (control of gene expression with RNA): Only 3% of protein-coding messenger RNAs (mRNA) are synthesized in the mammalian genome. In the remaining 97%, non-protein-coding RNAs, called non-coding RNA (ncRNA), are synthesized, and some of them are stated to be involved in epigenetic processes (Bora and Yurter, 2007). It is indicated that some ncRNAs can suppress gene expression by breaking down mRNAs in the cytoplasm or by stopping translation, and some ncRNAs by inhibiting the transcription stage in the nucleus (Güzelgül and Aksoy, 2009). Furthermore, it is thought that ncRNAs are the driving force for the initiation of histone modifications and DNA methylation; thus, they keep the DNA quiescent by contributing to the formation of the heterochromatin region (Güngör, 2015).

2-Mechanisms That Control Gene Expression Directly: DNA methylation is the best known and functional form of methylation (Fauque, 2013). In general, DNA methylation occurs with the attachment of a methyl group (-CH3) to cytosine in areas where CpG (C cytosine, p phosphate, G Guanine) dinucleotides (CpG islands) are frequently found in vertebrates (İzmirli, 2013; Orcan, 2006). Although the impacts of methylation have not been fully understood yet, it is considered to have a role in altering gene expression and the emergence of heterochromatin structure. Covalent histone modifications such as acetylation, methylation, phosphorylation, ubiquitination, and sumoylation occur in histone proteins, responsible for packaging DNA, and these modifications cause epigenetic effects since they alter the structure of chromatin (Gürel et al., 2016; Jones and Takai, 2001). Epigenetics, which is attempted to be explained by all these mechanisms, is now associated with many diseases in the field of medicine. Inflammatory bowel diseases are among them (Jenke and Zilbauer, 2012).

Inflammatory Bowel Diseases

Ulcerative colitis (UC) and Crohn's disease (CH) are included under the title of inflammatory bowel diseases (IBDs). They emerge as a chronic inflammatory picture, whose etiopathogenesis has not been fully explained. Although these diseases have different pathological and clinical features, they share many common features. Although both diseases tend to appear in early adulthood, they can also occur at any age from early childhood. Ulcerative colitis is a chronic inflammatory condition characterized by the recurrence and healing of episodes of inflammation limited to the mucosal colon lining. The rectum is frequently involved and the involvement usually continues toward the proximal portion of the colon. Crohn's disease is characterized by transmural inflammation and skipped areas of involvement. The transmural inflammatory nature of Crohn's disease can lead to fibrosis and strictures and obstructive clinical manifestations that are not typically observed in patients with ulcerative colitis. Crohn's disease most commonly impacts the ileum and distal portion of the colon; however, any part of the gastrointestinal tract can be impacted. It presents with diarrhea, abdominal pain, and rectal bleeding in UC (Wehkamp et al., 2016). IBDs are observed more commonly in developed countries and regions with cold climates. They are among the important health problems worldwide, with an incidence of 12.7-24.3 per 100,000people per year in Europe and a prevalence of 0.5-1% (Loddo and Romano, 2015). A study from Turkey detected the incidence of UC in our country as 4.4 per 100,000 and the incidence of CH as 2.2 per 100,000 (Tozun et al., 2009).

Various factors (environmental factors, genetic predisposition, impaired immune response mechanisms, and intestinal microbiota) have been blamed for the etiopathogenesis;

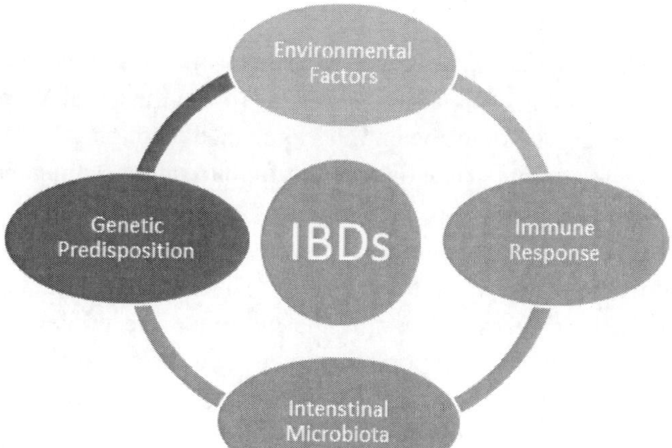

Figure 1. The etiyopathogenesis of IBDs.

Environmental factors: Numerous environmental factors such as smoking, diet, drugs, geography, social stress, and psychological factors have been considered risk factors. While stress definitely has adverse effects, breast milk has a protective role. It has been found that especially smoking increases the risk of CD twice, and passive smoking and exposure at an early age are also effective. Smoking causes inflammatory protein release by increasing CD4 T cells and, accordingly, intestinal inflammation. On the other hand, the protective effects of smoking are mentioned for UC (Corrao et al., 1998; Cosnes et al., 2004; Lakatos et al., 2007). It has been suggested that appendectomy reduces the risk of UC and increases the risk for CD, but the exact mechanism has not been explained (Andersson et al., 2001, 2003). It has been suggested that oral contraceptives among drugs and hormone replacement therapies increase the risk of IBDs by increasing the inflammatory response under the effect of estrogen, isotretinoin causes an increase in the risk of IBDs, although its mechanism of action has not been fully explained, and non-steroidal anti-inflammatory drugs cause an increase in the risk of IBDs by impairing the intestinal epithelial surface and increasing the immune response (Corrao et al., 1998).

Impaired immune response: An association has been revealed between an excessive immune response against microorganisms in the intestinal lumen, abnormal immunoregulation, and increased inflammatory cytokine levels and IBDs (Strober and Fuss, 2011).

Intestinal microbiota: Shigella, Salmonella, Yersinia, Campylobacter, Aeromonas, C. difficile, E. coli, and tuberculosis pathogens have a role in the development of IBDs (Nagalingam and Lynch, 2012; Seyedian et al., 2019). The change in the intestinal microbiota, which has an essential role in developing a person's immune system, is called dysbiosis and is important for the pathogenesis of IBDs (Nishida et al., 2018).

Genetic factors: In monozygotic and dizygotic twins, while the incidences of CH and UC were 36% and 16%, respectively, the incidence of their co-existence was found to be 4%. In 1996, the disease-associated gene was first identified on chromosome 16 (Hugot et al., 1996; Van Limbergen et al., 2007). Different explanations have been remarkable in recent years. A study on twins demonstrated that genetic predisposition had a more significant role in Crohn's disease compared to ulcerative colitis, in contrast to environmental factors (Halfvarson, 2011).

IBDs have complex genetics, and more than 200 loci were identified in genome-wide studies. However, it was attempted to explain this polymorphism located in non-coding regions of the genome through transcriptional regulatory mechanisms, and epigenetic modification was involved in this process (Huang et al., 2017). When the role of the gene-environment interaction in the pathogenesis, which could not be entirely explained through genetic mechanisms, was taken into account, it was attempted to explain the differences in the clinical picture of the onset of IBDs in young and old patients through epigenetic mechanisms. It was highlighted that in addition to genetic and cytogenetic changes, epigenetic changes also had a role in the history of malignancy that occurred afterward (Beaudet, 2008). Furthermore, the genome-environment interaction was revealed by the rapidly increasing incidence and prevalence in IBDs (Kaplan and Ng, 2017). One of the most important known gene regulatory systems is epigenetic modification. In the studies compared with the control group, differences were observed in the expression of specific microRNA (miRNA) in colonic mucosa samples in the group with IBDs. The presence of miRNA in the peripheral blood was recommended as a novel biomarker of the disease (Ventham et al., 2013). miRNAs have a role in the change in the microbiota and the cytokine response to the event, and the dysregulation of miRNA was associated with IBDs, especially in Th17 cells (Chapman and Pekow, 2015).

It is known that diet affects epigenetic changes and gene expression is altered by the disrupted immune system. Recent studies have suggested that gene expression, chromatin modification, and DNA methylation can be modulated by secondary plant metabolites such as polyphenols (Remely et al., 2015). It was demonstrated that DNA methyltransferase activity was inhibited by polyphenols such as epigallocatechin-3-gallate or genistein in green tea or soybeans. Epigenetic effects have also been shown for other dietary components such as curcumin (Reuter et al., 2011). Nutrition supplies the substrates required for DNA methylation and can modulate the activity of enzymes in the one-carbon cycle. Therefore, the pioneers of S-adenosylmethionine, such as methionine, folate, choline, betaine, and vitamins B2, B6, and B12, were enounced to affect DNA methylation patterns (Anderson et al., 2012).

The intestinal microbiota may lead to changes in histone mechanism in the human colon tissue. The end products of fermentation and especially short-chain fatty acids such as acetate, butyrate, and propionate, which are mostly produced by the microbial fermentation of fiber, may be particularly important for the epigenetic regulation of inflammatory reactions (Krautkramer et al., 2016). A diet poor in fiber leads to the suppression of microbiota-derived short-chain fatty acid production and the disruption of chromatin effects (Krautkramer et al., 2016).

Previously mentioned significant results indicating that butyrate-producing bacteria (Faecalibacterium) and SCFA (Short-chain fatty acid)-producing bacteria (Roseburia) decreased in IBDs were obtained (Kostic et al.). Nevertheless, the therapeutic value of pharmabiotic butyrate- bacteria producing in humans was examined because of the difficulty in propagating them in vitro (Eeckhaut et al., 2014).

In the existing studies, it is not certain yet that changes in diet affect epigenetics through the microbiota. Nevertheless, increasing research results have revealed that the metabolites produced by certain microorganisms in the colon impact gene transcription and trigger the potential development of the disease (Aleksandrova et al., 2017; Yi and Kim, 2015).

DNA Methylation in IBDs

The association between the pathogenesis of IBDs and DNA methylation among epigenetic modifications has been revealed. DNA methylation in the cell mostly occurs through the hydroxymethylation of cytosine by the covalent attachment of a methyl group to the cytosine nucleotide in the dinucleotide sequence of cytosine phosphate guanine (CpG), and these epigenetic modifications have been confirmed to have a role in the occurrence and development of diseases (Chen et al., 2017). Issa et al., demonstrated that it was associated with age-related epigenetic modification in the colon, 70% of which was caused by abnormal gene-specific methylation, and it was found that the methylation of the promoter of the tumor suppressor gene ESR1 in the normal colon also increased with age (Issa et al., 1994). The transcriptional activity and expression levels of genes are significantly altered by modifications in the methylation status of genes associated with IBDs. Thus, it shapes the risk and progression of the disease. In addition to the assumption that some DNA profiles are common in CH and UC, it has been demonstrated that some different DNA profiles are specific to CH or UC for both disease classification and treatment. Hypermethylation of the TRAF6 promoter and consequently reduced gene expression in mononuclear cells in peripheral blood were observed in these two diseases (Zhang et al., 2020).

Genome studies found the hypermethylation of the promoters of *AATK, BGN,* and *SERPINA5* in the inflamed mucosa in CD compared to controls (McDermott et al., 2016). A study observed that *FANCC, THRAP2,* and *GBGT1* were hypermethylated in the inflamed mucosa in CD; however, no methylation was detected in these genes in normal mucosal areas and UC (Cooke et al., 2012).

Histone Modification in IBDs

The histone and 147 base pairs of DNA form the nucleosome and are the basic structural units of chromatin. Chromatin plays a role in the gene regulation of histones as the main protein component. There are many modifications in histone, and acetylation and methylation occur most frequently. A study on mice demonstrated higher histone acetylation in the group with colitis compared to normal tissue (De Zoeten et al., 2010; Xu et al., 2022).

Histone acetylation and deacetylation take place through two enzymes (histone acetyltransferases (HATs) and histone deacetylases (HDACs)). These two enzymes have significant roles in cell proliferation and apoptosis. In case of the acetylation of histone, chromatin, which is related to transcriptional activity, is relieved. However, in case of the deacetylation of histone, chromatin is compressed, and transcriptional activity decreases. In their study, Xu et al., demonstrated that it inhibited the proinflammatory response and had a protective role by triggering apoptosis with the HDAC inhibitor in mice with colitis. They also observed higher histone acetylation in intestinal mucosa compared to non-inflamed tissues (Xu et al., 2022).

This histone modification in IBDs may indicate the interaction between intestinal microorganisms and the host. For example, most symbiotic bacteria, such as *Akkermansia muciniphila, Clostridium butyricum*, and *Faecalibacterium prausnitzi*, have an anti-inflammatory effect and a protective effect on the integrity of the epithelial barrier in the host's intestinal tract. However, they are considered HDAC inhibitors, which can inhibit HDAC activity by increasing HAT activity and producing n-butyrate (Chang et al., 2014).

IBDs and microRNA

Among non-coding RNAs, especially miRNAs are short nucleotide sequences that can regulate both transcriptional and post-transcriptional gene expression and thus alter some possible pathways. It was demonstrated that they altered the IL23/Th17 signaling pathways and autophagy mechanisms after the differentiation of T cells in IBDs. The onset and progression of the disease are influenced after this event (Annese, 2020). When many miRNAs, including miR-21, miR-16, and miR-594, were compared to healthy controls, they were found in large amounts in the inflamed mucosa in CD (Soroosh et al., 2018). UC and CH genome studies revealed upregulation in miR-106a, miR23b, and miR-191 and downregulation in miR-629 and miR-19b (Ni et al., 2018).

Another study observed the overexpression of miR-126, miR-9, and miR-130a only in active CH and suggested that these miRNAs might be good markers for treatment due to this situation, which was not encountered in inactive CD and healthy controls, and might contribute to the onset and progression of CH (Moein et al., 2019).

Conclusion

DNA methylation, histone modification, and miRNA are the three principal mechanisms of epigenetics, which are responsible for the arrangement of epigenetic changes and the gene expression profile. They also constitute the cornerstones of a number of cellular processes, including cell differentiation, gene expression, X chromosome inactivation, embryogenesis, and genomic repression. Genetic and environmental factors are known to be risk factors for the occurrence of IBDs. Furthermore, the role of epigenetics in the occurrence of diseases in people has also started to become important in recent years. Epigenetic mechanisms have taken a significant place in the diagnosis, follow-up, and prognosis of diseases and the treatment protocol. The drugs called epidrugs and produced based on these mechanisms were first used in hematological malignancies with the FDA approval. Clinics are also investigating their use as biomarkers. Considering all of these, the importance of an individual approach in evaluating patients has further come to the forefront. Along with the increase in epigenetic studies in the following years, it seems inevitable that we will face concepts such as personalized treatment plans and drug production.

Large-scale studies on epigenetics, which is considered to make significant contributions to humanity today and in the future, are needed. With the advancement of technology, screening, early diagnosis, treatment, and follow-up of diseases will become easier with epigenetics.

References

Aleksandrova, K., Romero-Mosquera, B., & Hernandez, V. (2017). Diet, gut microbiome and epigenetics: emerging links with inflammatory bowel diseases and prospects for management and prevention. *Nutrients, 9*(9), 962.

Anderson, O. S., Sant, K. E., & Dolinoy, D. C. (2012). Nutrition and epigenetics: an interplay of dietary methyl donors, one-carbon metabolism and DNA methylation. *The Journal of Nutritional Biochemistry, 23*(8), 853-859.

Andersson, R. E., Olaison, G., Tysk, C., & Ekbom, A. (2001). Appendectomy and protection against ulcerative colitis. *N. Engl. J. Med., 344*(11), 808-814. doi:10.1056/NEJM200103153441104.

Andersson, R. E., Olaison, G., Tysk, C., & Ekbom, A. (2003). Appendectomy is followed by increased risk of Crohn's disease. *Gastroenterology, 124*(1), 40-46. doi:10.1053/gast.2003.50021

Annese, V. (2020). Genetics and epigenetics of IBD. *Pharmacological Research, 159*, 104892.

Beaudet, A. L. (2008). Epigenetics and complex human disease: is there a role in IBD? *Journal of Pediatric Gastroenterology and Nutrition, 46*, E2.

Bora, G., & Yurter, H. (2007). Epigenetic diseases and treatment approaches. *Hacettepe Medical Journal, 38*, 48-54.

Chang, P. V., Hao, L., Offermanns, S., & Medzhitov, R. (2014). The microbial metabolite butyrate regulates intestinal macrophage function via histone deacetylase inhibition. *Proceedings of the National Academy of Sciences, 111*(6), 2247-2252.

Chapman, C. G., & Pekow, J. (2015). The emerging role of miRNAs in inflammatory bowel disease: a review. *Therapeutic Advances in Gastroenterology, 8*(1), 4-22.

Chen, B., Sun, L., & Zhang, X. (2017). Integration of microbiome and epigenome to decipher the pathogenesis of autoimmune diseases. *Journal of Autoimmunity, 83*, 31-42.

Cooke, J., Zhang, H., Greger, L., Silva, A. L., Massey, D., Dawson, C., Metz, A., Ibrahim, A., & Parkes, M. (2012). Mucosal genome-wide methylation changes in inflammatory bowel disease. *Inflammatory Bowel Diseases, 18*(11), 2128–2137. https://doi.org/10.1002/ibd.22942

Coolen, M. W., Statham, A. L., Qu, W., Campbell, M. J., Henders, A. K., Montgomery, G. W., Martin, N. G., & Clark, S. J. (2011). Impact of the genome on the epigenome is manifested in DNA methylation patterns of imprinted regions in monozygotic and dizygotic twins. *PloS One*, *6*(10), e25590. https://doi.org/10.1371/journal.pone.0025590.

Corrao, G., Tragnone, A., Caprilli, R., Trallori, G., Papi, C., Andreoli, A., Di Paolo, M., Riegler, G., Rigo, G. P., Ferraù, O., Mansi, C., Ingrosso, M., & Valpiani, D. (1998). Risk of inflammatory bowel disease attributable to smoking, oral contraception and breastfeeding in Italy: a nationwide case-control study. Cooperative Investigators of the Italian Group for the Study of the Colon and the Rectum (GISC). *International Journal of Epidemiology*, *27*(3), 397–404. https://doi.org/10.1093/ije/27.3.397.

Cosnes, J., Nion-Larmurier, I., Afchain, P., Beaugerie, L., & Gendre, J. P. (2004). Gender differences in the response of colitis to smoking. *Clin. Gastroenterol. Hepatol.*, *2*(1), 41-48. doi:10.1016/s1542-3565(03) 00290-8.

De Zoeten, E. F., Wang, L., Sai, H., Dillmann, W. H., & Hancock, W. W. (2010). Inhibition of HDAC9 increases T regulatory cell function and prevents colitis in mice. *Gastroenterology, 138*(2), 583-594.

Eeckhaut, V., Ducatelle, R., Sas, B., Vermeire, S., & Van Immerseel, F. (2014). Progress towards butyrate-producing pharmabiotics: Butyricicoccus pullicaecorum capsule and efficacy in TNBS models in comparison with therapeutics. *Gut, 63*(2), 367-367.

Fauque, P. (2013). Ovulation induction and epigenetic anomalies. *Fertility and Sterility, 99*(3), 616-623.

Güngör, Ö. F. (2015). Epigenetik ve genomik baskılanma [*Epigenetic and genomic suppression*]. *Lalahan Hayvancılık Araştırma Enstitüsü Dergisi, 55*(2), 73-81.

Gürel, Ç., Nursal, A., & Yiğit, S. (2016). Epigenetik ve kanser [*Epigenetics and cancer*]. *Turkiye Klinikleri J. Radiat. Oncol-Special Topics, 2*(1), 45-51.

Güzelgül, F., & Aksoy, K. (2009). Kodlanmayan RNA'ların İşlevi ve Tıpda Kullanım Alanları [*Function of Non-Coding RNAs and Their Use in Medicine*]. *Arşiv Kaynak Tarama Dergisi 18*(3), 141-155.

Halfvarson, J. (2011). Genetics in twins with Crohn's disease: less pronounced than previously believed? *Inflamm. Bowel Dis., 17*(1), 6-12. doi:10.1002/ibd.21295.

Huang, H., Fang, M., Jostins, L., Umićević Mirkov, M., Boucher, G., Anderson, C. A., Andersen, V., Cleynen, I., Cortes, A., Crins, F., D'Amato, M., Deffontaine, V., Dmitrieva, J., Docampo, E., Elansary, M., Farh, K. K., Franke, A., Gori, A. S., Goyette, P., Halfvarson, J., … Barrett, J. C. (2017). Fine-mapping inflammatory bowel disease loci to single-variant resolution. *Nature*, *547*(7662), 173–178. https://doi.org/10.1038/nature22969.

Hugot, J. P., Laurent-Puig, P., Gower-Rousseau, C., Olson, J. M., Lee, J. C., Beaugerie, L., Naom, I., Dupas, J. L., Van Gossum, A., Orholm, M., Bonaiti-Pellie, C., Weissenbach, J., Mathew, C. G., Lennard-Jones, J. E., Cortot, A., Colombel, J. F., & Thomas, G. (1996). Mapping of a susceptibility locus for Crohn's disease on chromosome 16. *Nature*, *379*(6568), 821–823. https://doi.org/10.1038/379821a0.

Issa, J.-P. J., Ottaviano, Y. L., Celano, P., Hamilton, S. R., Davidson, N. E., & Baylin, S. B. (1994). Methylation of the oestrogen receptor CpG island links ageing and neoplasia in human colon. *Nature Genetics, 7*(4), 536-540.

İzmirli, M. (2013). Epigenetic Mechanisms and Epigenetic Approaches to Cancer Therapy. *Van Medical Journal, 20*(1), 48-51.

Jablonka, E., & Lamb, M. J. (2015). Commentary: Reflections on: Jablonka E, Lamb MJ. The inheritance of acquired epigenetic variations. *Int. J. Epidemiol., 44*(4), 1103-1105. doi:10.1093/ije/dyv023.

Jenke, A. C., & Zilbauer, M. (2012). Epigenetics in inflammatory bowel disease. *Current Opinion in Gastroenterology, 28*(6), 577-584.

Jones, P. A., & Takai, D. (2001). The role of DNA methylation in mammalian epigenetics. *Science, 293*(5532), 1068-1070.

Kaplan, G. G., & Ng, S. C. (2017). Understanding and preventing the global increase of inflammatory bowel disease. *Gastroenterology, 152*(2), 313-321. e312.

Kostic, A. D., Xavier, R. J., & Gevers, D. (2014). The microbiome in inflammatory bowel disease: current status and the future ahead. *Gastroenterology, 146*(6), 1489-1499.

Krautkramer, K. A., Kreznar, J. H., Romano, K. A., Vivas, E. I., Barrett-Wilt, G. A., Rabaglia, M. E., Keller, M. P., Attie, A. D., Rey, F. E., & Denu, J. M. (2016). Diet-Microbiota Interactions Mediate Global Epigenetic Programming in Multiple Host Tissues. *Molecular Cell*, *64*(5), 982–992. https://doi.org/10.1016/j.molcel.2016.10.025.

Lakatos, P. L., Szamosi, T., & Lakatos, L. (2007). Smoking in inflammatory bowel diseases: good, bad or ugly? *World J. Gastroenterol., 13*(46), 6134-6139. doi:10.3748/wjg.v13.i46.6134.

Loddo, I., & Romano, C. (2015). Inflammatory bowel disease: genetics, epigenetics, and pathogenesis. *Frontiers in Immunology, 6*, 551.

McDermott, E., Ryan, E. J., Tosetto, M., Gibson, D., Burrage, J., Keegan, D., Byrne, K., Crowe, E., Sexton, G., Malone, K., Harris, R. A., Kellermayer, R., Mill, J., Cullen, G., Doherty, G. A., Mulcahy, H., & Murphy, T. M. (2016). DNA Methylation Profiling in Inflammatory Bowel Disease Provides New Insights into Disease Pathogenesis. *Journal of Crohn's & Colitis, 10*(1), 77–86. https://doi.org/10.1093/ecco-jcc/jjv176.

Moein, S., Vaghari-Tabari, M., Qujeq, D., Majidinia, M., Nabavi, S. M., & Yousefi, B. (2019). MiRNAs and inflammatory bowel disease: An interesting new story. *Journal of Cellular Physiology, 234*(4), 3277-3293.

Nagalingam, N. A., & Lynch, S. V. (2012). Role of the microbiota in inflammatory bowel diseases. *Inflamm Bowel Dis, 18*(5), 968-984. doi:10.1002/ibd.21866.

Ni, Y., Song, C., Jin, S., Chen, Z., Ni, M., Han, L., Wu, J., & Jin, Y. (2018). Gene set enrichment analysis: A genome-wide expression profile-based strategy for discovering functional microRNA-disease relationships. *The Journal of International Medical Research*, *46*(2), 596–611. https://doi.org/10.1177/0300060517693719.

Nishida, A., Inoue, R., Inatomi, O., Bamba, S., Naito, Y., & Andoh, A. (2018). Gut microbiota in the pathogenesis of inflammatory bowel disease. *Clinical Journal of Gastroenterology, 11*(1), 1-10.

Orcan, S. (2006). Epigenetics and Epigenomics. *Hacettepe University*.

Portela, A., & Esteller, M. (2010). Epigenetic modifications and human disease. *Nat. Biotechnol., 28*(10), 1057-1068. doi:10.1038/nbt.1685.

Remely, M., Lovrecic, L., de la Garza, A. L., Migliore, L., Peterlin, B., Milagro, F. I., Martinez, A. J., & Haslberger, A. G. (2015). Therapeutic perspectives of epigenetically active nutrients. *British Journal of Pharmacology*, *172*(11), 2756–2768. https://doi.org/10.1111/bph.12854.

Reuter, S., Gupta, S. C., Park, B., Goel, A., & Aggarwal, B. B. (2011). Epigenetic changes induced by curcumin and other natural compounds. *Genes & Nutrition, 6*(2), 93-108.

Rogler, G., Biedermann, L., & Scharl, M. (2018). New insights into the pathophysiology of inflammatory bowel disease: microbiota, epigenetics and common signalling pathways. *Swiss Medical Weekly, 148*, w14599.

Seyedian, S. S., Nokhostin, F., & Malamir, M. D. (2019). A review of the diagnosis, prevention, and treatment methods of inflammatory bowel disease. *J. Med. Life, 12*(2), 113-122. doi:10.25122/jml-2018-0075.

Soroosh, A., Koutsioumpa, M., Pothoulakis, C., & Iliopoulos, D. (2018). Functional role and therapeutic targeting of microRNAs in inflammatory bowel disease. *American Journal of Physiology-Gastrointestinal and Liver Physiology, 314*(2), G256-G262.

Strober, W., & Fuss, I. J. (2011). Proinflammatory cytokines in the pathogenesis of inflammatory bowel diseases. *Gastroenterology, 140*(6), 1756-1767. doi:10.1053/j.gastro.2011.02.016.

Talbert, P. B., & Henikoff, S. (2006). Spreading of silent chromatin: inaction at a distance. *Nat. Rev. Genet., 7*(10), 793-803. doi:10.1038/nrg1920.

Tozun, N., Atug, O., Imeryuz, N., Hamzaoglu, H. O., Tiftikci, A., Parlak, E., Dagli, U., Ulker, A., Hulagu, S., Akpinar, H., Tuncer, C., Suleymanlar, I., Ovunc, O., Hilmioglu, F., Aslan, S., Turkdogan, K., Bahcecioglu, H. I., Yurdaydin, C., & Members of the Turkish IBD Study Group (2009). Clinical characteristics of inflammatory bowel disease in Turkey: a multicenter epidemiologic survey. *Journal of Clinical Gastroenterology*, *43*(1), 51–57. https://doi.org/10.1097/MCG.0b013e3181574636.

Van Limbergen, J., Russell, R. K., Nimmo, E. R., & Satsangi, J. (2007). The genetics of inflammatory bowel disease. *Am. J. Gastroenterol., 102*(12), 2820-2831. doi:10.1111/j.1572-0241.2007.01527.x.

Ventham, N. T., Kennedy, N. A., Nimmo, E. R., & Satsangi, J. (2013). Beyond gene discovery in inflammatory bowel disease: the emerging role of epigenetics. *Gastroenterology, 145*(2), 293-308.

Wehkamp, J., Gotz, M., Herrlinger, K., Steurer, W., & Stange, E. F. (2016). Inflammatory Bowel Disease. *Dtsch. Arztebl. Int., 113*(5), 72-82. doi:10.3238/arztebl.2016.0072.

Weinhold, B. (2006). Epigenetics: the science of change. *Environ. Health Perspect., 114*(3), A160-167. doi:10.1289/ehp.114-a160.

Xu, J., Xu, H. M., Yang, M. F., Liang, Y. J., Peng, Q. Z., Zhang, Y., Tian, C. M., Wang, L. S., Yao, J., Nie, Y. Q., & Li, D. F. (2022). New Insights Into the Epigenetic Regulation of Inflammatory Bowel Disease. *Frontiers in Pharmacology*, *13*, 813659. https://doi.org/10.3389/fphar.2022.813659.

Yi, J. M., & Kim, T. O. (2015). Epigenetic alterations in inflammatory bowel disease and cancer. *Intestinal Research, 13*(2), 112.

Zhang, L., Lu, Q., & Chang, C. (2020). Epigenetics in health and disease. *Epigenetics in Allergy and Autoimmunity*, 3-55.

Chapter 30

Epigenetic Factors and Surgical Approaches in Gastric Cancers

Pınar Koçatakan[*]**, MD**
T. R. Ministry of Health Ankara,
Yenimahalle Training and Research Hospital,
Department of General Surgery,
General Directorate of Public Hospitals,
Department of Health Services, Ankara, Turkey

Abstract

In spite of the decreasing incidence rates of gastric cancer in many industrialized countries, it is still an important cause of death from cancer around the world. Gastric cancer takes the fourth place among causes of death due to cancer worldwide. Gastric cancer incidence in Turkey was detected at 14.2/100,000 among males and 3.4/100,000 among females. Risk factors for gastric cancer involve numerous unmodifiable variables, e.g., sex, age, and race/ethnicity. The remaining risk factors, including smoking, infection with *Helicobacter pylori* (Hp) bacteria, and diets with high nitrate and nitrite contents, are among the controllable causes. Hp represents a Gram-negative microaerophilic bacterium infecting almost half of the population in the world and is considered the main etiologic agent of gastric cancer. Dietary habits and different environmental factors, including Hp infection, and irregularities in genetic and epigenetic mechanisms are involved in forming gastric cancer. While genetic changes lead to loss of function or protein expression in metabolic pathways in different ways, epigenetic alterations cause differentiation in the expressions of tumor suppressor genes and oncogenes.

In gastric cancer surgery, the only curative method in localized gastric cancers is the complete resection of the regional lymph nodes and tumors. Functional surgical methods can be preferred in suitable patients. Pancreas and spleen-preserving D2 dissection is preferred as a standard approach in serosa-positive and/or lymph node-positive cases.

Keywords: gastric cancer, genetic, epigenetic, surgical approaches

Introduction

Despite the decreasing incidence rates of gastric cancer in many industrialized countries, it remains an important cause of death from cancer around the world (Quante and Bornschein,

[*] Corresponding Author's Email: pinar.kocatakan@saglik.gov.tr.

In: Epigenetics: Beyond the Genetics and Medicine
Editors: Sevgi Durna Daştan and Nazan Yurtcu
ISBN: 979-8-88697-228-3

2019). The incidence of cancer increases due to the increased prevalence of established risk factors, e.g., overweight, physical inactivity, smoking, and altered reproductive patterns related to economic development and urbanization, in addition to population growth and aging (Torre et al., 2016). Female breast cancer is the type of cancer diagnosed most frequently, and it has estimated 2.3 million new cases (11.7%), followed by lung (11.4%), colorectal (10.0%), prostate (7.3%), and gastric (5.6%) cancers. Lung cancer continues to be the main cause of death due to cancer, with estimated 1.8 million deaths (18%), followed by colorectal (9.4%), liver (8.3%), gastric (7.7%), and female breast (6.9%) cancers (Sung et al., 2021).

Gastric cancer takes the fourth place among the major causes of death from cancer in the world. Despite the fact that gastric cancer has been frequently detected in industrialized countries before, the recent epidemiological data confirm that more than 70% of new gastric cancer cases occur in developing countries (Quante and Bornschein, 2019). Gastric cancer incidence in Turkey was detected at 14.2/100,000 among males and 3.4/100,000 among females. Considering the distribution of the first ten cancer types in males, gastric cancer makes up 5.5%, while it makes up 3.7% in females (Ministry of Health Statistics Yearbook, 2019).

Risk factors for gastric cancer involve numerous unmodifiable variables, e.g., sex, age, and race/ethnicity. The remaining risk factors, including smoking, infection with *Helicobacter pylori* bacteria, and diets with high nitrate and nitrite contents, constitute the controllable causes. A number of comparatively rare risk factors, including previous gastric surgery, a history of mucosa-associated lymphoid tissue lymphoma, and pernicious anemia, should also not be forgotten. Moreover, the presence of a first-degree family member with gastric cancer constitutes a risk factor. There are a few inherited cancer syndromes known to be related to gastric cancer. It is known that the strongest correlation is revealed in hereditary disseminated gastric cancer (CDH1) syndrome, with the risk of gastric cancer development in approximately 80% of subjects. Lynch, Li-Fraumeni, hereditary breast and ovarian cancer (BRCA), familial adenomatous polyposis, and Peutz-Jeghers syndromes represent other cancer types having a considerably lower risk (Joshi and Badgwell, 2021; Hansford et al., 2021; Lott and Carvajal, 2018).

Table 1. Risk factors for intestinal and diffuse-type gastric cancers

Intestinal-Type Risk Factors	*Diffuse-Type Risk Factors*
Helicobacter pylori-chronic superficial gastritis	Salty food/food stored in salt
Hypochlorhydria/ achlorhydria-gastric atrophy	Nitric acid components
Chronic inflammation-atrophic gastritis, intestinal metaplasia and dysplasia	Helicobacter pylori
	Epstein-Barr Virus
	Socioeconomic status

Etiology and Pathogenesis

It is possible to histogenetically divide gastric cancer into histological subtypes with varied prognostic and epidemiological characteristics, called intestinal and diffuse types, with the Lauren classification. There is a more close association of the intestinal type with dietary and environmental risk factors. There is a tendency for the intestinal type to dominate in areas with high gastric cancer incidence, whereas its incidence worldwide is decreasing. The glandular structure is absent in the diffuse type of cancer, which is comprised of poorly cohesive cells infiltrating the stomach wall. An important characteristic of diffuse-type cancers is special mucin-filled cells named signet-ring cells, which are not present in intestinal-type adenocarcinomas. The frequency of this type of cancer worldwide is the same, it emerges at a younger age and is related to a poorer prognosis compared to the intestinal form (Quante and Bornschein, 2019; Joshi and Badgwell, 2021; Abakay, 2019). Table 1 summarizes the risk factors for diffuse and intestinal-type gastric cancers.

Table 2 presents the classification of risk factors as definite, genetic, and probable risk factors.

Table 2. Classification of gastric cancer risk factors by definite, genetic, and probable

	Risk Factors	
Definite	*Genetic*	*Probable*
Adenomatous gastric polyps	Family history of gastric cancer (1st degree)	High salt consumption
Chronic atrophic gastritis	Familial adenomatous polyposis (with fundus gland polyps)	History of gastric ulcer
Smoking	Hereditary non-polyposis colorectal cancer	Obesity (Cardia adenocarcinoma)
Dysplasia	Juvenile polyposis	Pernicious anemia
EBV	Peutz-Jeghers Syndrome	Snuff tobacco use
Gastric surgery (Billroth II)		
Helicobacter pylori infection		
Intestinal metaplasia		

Quante and Bornschein, 2019.

Helicobacter Pylori (Hp)

Hp represents a Gram-negative microaerophilic bacterium infecting almost half of the population in the world and is considered the main etiologic agent of gastric cancer. Hp is transmitted by the fecal-oral and oral-oral routes. The International Agency for Research on Cancer (IARC), which is a branch of the WHO, classifies it as a class I (Definite) carcinogen. Infection with Hp has been detected in each studied population; however, its prevalence is found to be higher in developing countries and most parts of East Asia (Abakay, 2019; Ford et al., 2014).

Bacterial virulence factors take part in developing ulcers or cancer. Nevertheless, there are not sufficient data on its timing. The natural course of chronic Hp infection involves three potential outcomes: (1) simple gastritis, when subjects frequently remain asymptomatic; (2) duodenal ulcer phenotype that emerges in 10% to 15% of infected individuals, and (3) gastric ulcer/gastric cancer phenotype (Amieva and El-Omar, 2008).

Chronic inflammation triggers atrophy and intestinal metaplasia in the gastric mucosa over time. Due to molecular events induced by chronic inflammation, many important pathways, including normal cellular functions, may change, thus, the development of inflammation-induced carcinogenesis can accelerate (Nakajima et al., 2006). As is known, pathogenic agents can cause mutations in the cell genome structure through the genotoxins and oncoproteins they secrete, and they can also cause changes in the DNA repair pathways of the related proteins. Studies on the subject have revealed that chronic Hp infection leads to the formation of reactive oxygen species (ROS) or reactive nitrogen derivatives (RND), and accordingly, it takes an essential part in the formation of oxidative/nitrosative DNA damage, which leads to the development of gastric cancer. It has been indicated that the severity of inflammation in the stomach, the genetic properties of the host and the immune response, environmental factors, primarily diet, and bacteria-specific factors are all effective in gastric cancer development as a whole (Oral, D., Yirün, A., Erkekoğlu, P. 2019).

The virulence factors of *Helicobacter pylori* are shown also to take an essential part in gastric cancer development. Furthermore, there are findings indicating that *Helicobacter pylori* causes genotoxic effects independent of virulence factors and ROS formation (Oral et al., 2019; Mager, 2006).

Different environmental factors, involving nutrition and *Helicobacter pylori* infection, and irregularities in epigenetic and genetic mechanisms take part in the formation of gastric cancer. Whereas genetic changes lead to loss of function or protein expression in metabolic pathways in different ways, epigenetic alterations cause differentiation in the expression of tumor suppressor genes and oncogenes (Zhou et al., 2018).

Dietary Risk Factors

An increase in the consumption of fresh vegetables and fruits with the common use of cooling devices and the decreased consumption of pickled and salty foods in comparison with the past have led to decreased rates of gastric cancer. A decrease in temperature reduces the rates of bacteria and fungi in fresh food. The consumption of highly processed foods, excessive salt intake, and foods with nitrate and polycyclic aromatic amine contents may be related to elevated gastric cancer rates. Studies have also concentrated on the impacts of high nitrate intake. When bacteria or macrophages reduce nitrates to nitrite, it is possible for them to react with other nitrogenous substances and forming N-nitroso compounds, which are known as carcinogens and mitogens (Quante and Bornschein, 2019; Larsson et al., 2006).

The risk of gastric cancer increases with foods having a high salt content (soy sauce, pickled foods, dried and salted meat and fish). High salt intake has been linked to a higher prevalence of atrophic gastritis in animals and humans in the Hp infection medium and has been determined to increase the mutagenicity of nitrosated foods in animal models (Quante and Bornschein, 2019; Correa et al., 1990).

Smoking/Alcohol Consumption

It has been a known fact for long years that tobacco is carcinogenic, and a lot of epidemiological research has indicated a relationship between gastric cancer and smoking.

In general, the risk of gastric cancer increases moderately with alcohol consumption and is impacted by multiple factors (such as physical activity and tobacco consumption). Interestingly, it has been argued that alcohol consumption can increase the risk of gastric cancer in subjects having particular polymorphisms of the alcohol dehydrogenase gene (Duell et al., 2012).

Obesity

Obesity is recognized as a risk factor for different gastrointestinal tract malignancies. An increased body mass index is linked to a slightly to moderately elevated risk of gastric cardia cancer; however, it is not associated with noncardia cancer risk (MacInnis et al., 2006). The possible correlation between obesity and cardia cancer risk probably occurs through proinflammatory cytokines and adipokines generated by intra-abdominal visceral fat (MacInnis et al., 2006; Kant and Hull, 2011).

EBV (Epstein-Barr Virus)

It is thought that 10-15% of gastric cancers are linked to EBV. EBV-associated gastric cancers are situated in the stomach's cardia region and have a better prognosis with fewer lymph node metastases. It is often seen in diffuse-type histologies (Abakay, C. 2019; Lee et al., 2000).

Socioeconomic Status

It has been demonstrated to be related to proximal gastric cancer in individuals with high socioeconomic status and distal gastric cancer in people with low socioeconomic status (Powell et al., 1990).

Previous gastric surgery also increases the risk of gastric cancer. It is considered to be associated with the back leakage of alkaline bile and pancreatic fluid, especially after the Billroth II operation (Akeno et al., 2014).

Genetic Factors

In general, while intestinal-type gastric cancer is thought to be primarily due to environmental causes (especially Hp infection), diffuse gastric cancer is primarily accepted as a genetic malignancy.

As a result of environmental, genetic, and epigenetic changes, the pathways that control growth in normal tissue lose their functions with the deterioration of molecular mechanisms in the gastric tissue. Diet and Hp infection, the main environmental factors, can cause chronic superficial gastritis, intestinal metaplasia, chronic atrophic gastritis, and dysplasia in the gastric tissue.

Of gastric cancers, 1-3% are of hereditary origin. Gastric cancer syndromes are divided into three major groups: 1-Hereditary Diffuse Stomach Cancer, 2-Proximal Polyposis, and 3-Familial Intestinal Gastric Cancer. Hereditary gastric cancers are also related to Familial

Adenomatous Polyposis (FAP), Hereditary Non-Polyposis Colorectal Cancer (HNPCC), and Li-Fraumeni syndrome (Oliveira et al., 2015).

Chronic inflammation damages epithelial cells and reduces luminal ascorbic acid levels. This event increases cell turnover. In atrophic gastritis development, the loss of the exocrine glands causes hypochlorhydria and thus an increase in gastric pH, facilitating bacterial colonization. The risk is increased for both cardia and non-cardia tumors (Enta, 1998).

Intestinal metaplasia is a precursor lesion for intestinal-type gastric cancer. The rate of transformation of dysplasia to gastric cancer is 21%, 33%, and 57% according to a mild, moderate, and severe condition, respectively (Rugge et al., 1994).

Epigenetic Factors

Epigenetics is the science that examines differences in gene expression not resulting from genotypic alterations.

Epigenetic events are processes regulating gene expression without leading to any change in DNA sequence. These changes take a crucial part in tumor development and spread by causing irregularities in tumor suppressor genes and oncogenes. Epigenetic mechanisms may cause tumor formation with a sequence of events, such as DNA or RNA-based DNA promoter methylation, histone modification, chromatin rearrangement, and post-transcriptional gene expression regulation. Figure 1 shows the pathways of gastric cancer formation by Hp through the epigenetic mechanism.

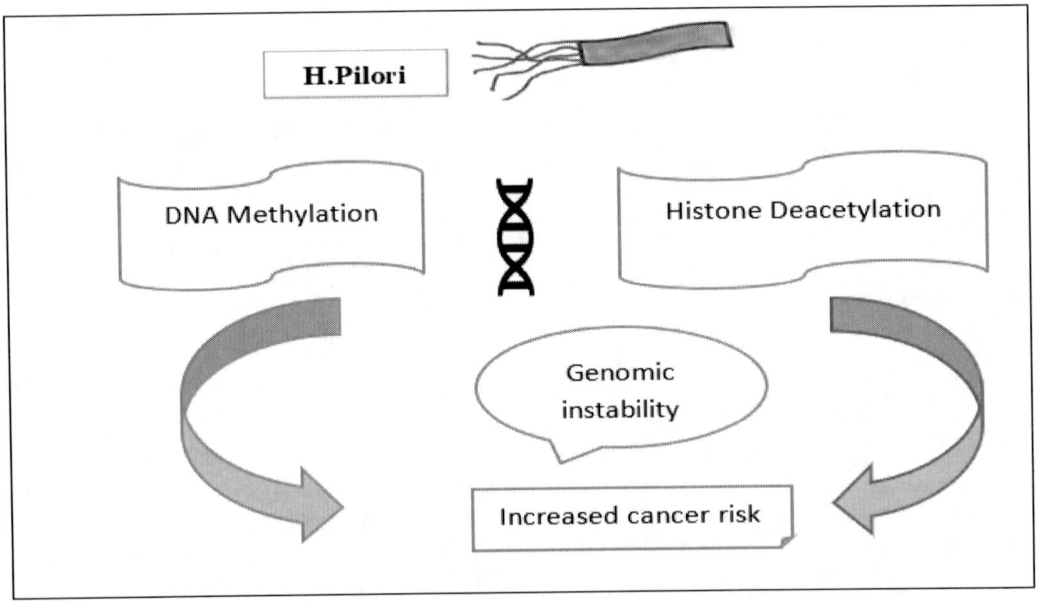

Figure 1. Pathways of gastric cancer formation by Hp through the epigenetic mechanism

Epigenetic mechanisms are separated into two groups as DNA or RNA-based (Figure 2). Molecular mechanisms involved in DNA-based epigenetic regulation are DNA promoter region methylation, histone modification, and chromatin rearrangement (Canale et al., 2020).

The two most important functional RNA groups, which are addressed in RNA-based epigenetic regulation in tumor biology analyses, are microRNA (miRNA) and non-coding long RNA (LncRNA) molecules (Samadani et al., 2019).

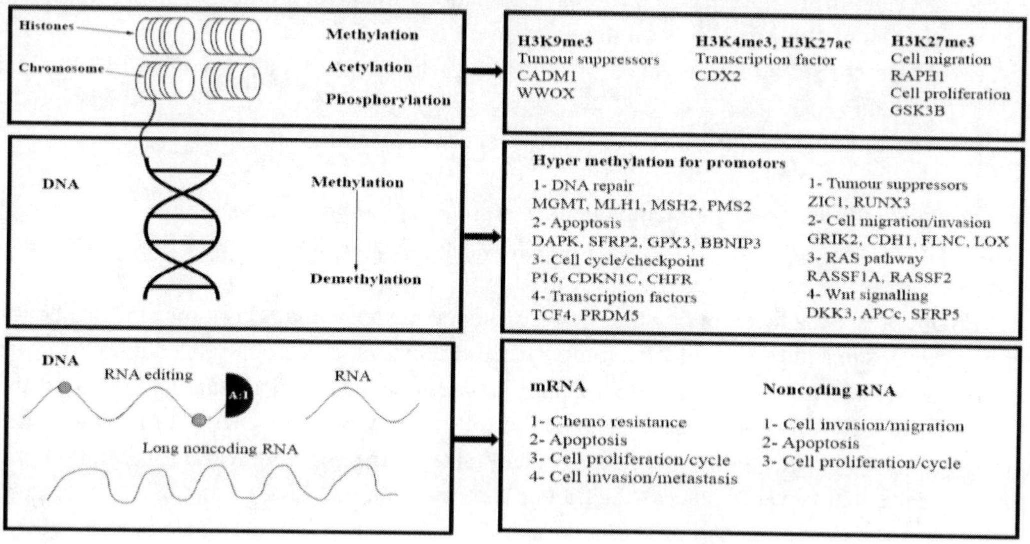

Figure 2. DNA and RNA-based epigenetic regulations supporting the development of gastric cancer (Samadani et al., 2019).

Surgery in Gastric Cancer

The treatment method for gastric cancer varies depending on the tumor stage and localization. Early gastric cancer (EGC) is described as a tumor limited to the mucosa and submucosa, independent of lymph node involvement (T1). Some studies report that the life expectancy of old and young subjects having early-stage gastric cancer is similar and that the life expectancy of young patients, including advanced gastric cancer, does not differ from that of old patients (Eguchi et al., 1999). The best life expectancy in gastric cancer is obtained in patients undergoing curative surgery.

To be able to perform endoscopic mucosal resection (EMR) in early gastric cancers, the tumor should be limited to the mucosa (T1a), without ulceration, well-differentiated and smaller than 2 cm in diameter. Additionally, it is also possible to apply endoscopic submucosal dissection (ESD) to EGC patients who have certain criteria (Japanese Gastric Cancer Association, 2014). In pathological findings after resection, all margins should be negative, and there should be no lymphatic and/or vascular invasion.

The EMR technique is commonly used for intestinal-type gastric cancers in South Korea and Japan, and research has demonstrated that only 3.5% of EGC subjects having lesions smaller than 2 to 3 cm have lymph node involvement, which makes the said lesions suitable for local treatment.

The following criteria have been recommended for EMR in gastric cancer:

(1) Cancer must be present in the mucosa, and the lymph nodes should not be affected, as shown by the EUS examination,
(2) The largest size of the tumor should be below 2 cm in case of the lesion being slightly elevated from the surface (type iia) and under 1 cm without ulcer scarring in case of the flat or slightly depressed tumor (type iib or iic),
(3) There should be no evidence of multiple gastric cancers or concomitant abdominal cancers,
(4) There should be intestinal-type gastric cancer (Soetikno et al., 2005).

In spite of the above-mentioned guidelines, it is usually impossible to remove lesions larger than 1.5 to 2.0 cm in the form of block with EMR, and piecemeal removal of EGC is linked to reduced curative resection rates (Lee et al., 2010).

ESD represents a technique, which was developed in Japan and allows for block resection of larger EGCs in addition to selected tumors with submucosal invasion. En bloc resection with ESD is suggested to provide the best chance of accurate histological staging and potential treatment for EGC. The Japanese developed the following expanded criteria for ESD for early gastric cancer: (1) intestinal-type cancer of any size in the mucosa without ulceration, (2) mucosal intestinal-type cancer less than 3 cm with ulceration, and (3) submucosal intestinal-type cancer less than 3 cm and its submucosal invasion less than 500 μm (Gotoda et al., 2000).

Bleeding (6-7%) and perforation (0.1-2%) are the two most common symptoms in endoscopic treatment. It is possible to treat both complications with endoscopic (endoclip, etc.) and conservative approaches (Quante and Bornschein, 2019).

Surgical resection is still the main curative treatment for gastric cancer. Nevertheless, survival after surgery alone is poor (20% to 50% in 5 years), and efforts should be made to improve outcomes for this patient group using perioperative chemotherapy or postoperative (adjuvant) chemoradiotherapy. Additionally, it also provides relief from symptoms in cases of obstruction (Quante and Bornschein, 2019).

Resection in gastric cancers is total or subtotal gastrectomy depending on the tumor stage and localization. Function-preserving surgeries (cases without lymph node involvement and outside the indication for endoscopic resection) are local resections together with pylorus-preserving gastrectomy, vagus-preserving proximal gastrectomy, or sentinel lymph node navigation.

Surgery, and especially laparoscopy, may be beneficial in cancer staging. Laparoscopy may assist in determining peritoneal deposits, primary tumor resectability, and suitable candidates for neoadjuvant therapy. According to Western guidelines, it should be performed in stage T3-4 tumors.

Total gastrectomy is generally conducted for proximal gastric tumors and diffuse gastric cancer, while partial gastrectomy is performed for distal gastric tumors. Large, randomized multicenter studies, which compared subtotal and total gastrectomy for antrum adenocarcinoma in France and Italy, revealed no difference in 5-year survival rates or operative mortality (Gouzi et al., 1989; Bozzetti, 1999).

The scope of lymphadenectomy accompanying gastrectomy has been debated for long years. The Japanese support a broader lymph node dissection (D2 resection) in comparison with their Western colleagues (D1 resection) and have higher published survival rates. D2 resection requires the resection of the celiac axis nodes and hepatoduodenal ligament besides the perigastric lymph nodes removed in the D1 procedure. In a 15-year follow-up of the said subjects, the researchers stated that there were no considerable differences in overall survival despite a significant reduction in gastric cancer-related mortality in the D2 resection arm (48% versus 37% in the D1 arm) (Songun I, Putter H, Kranenbarg EM, et al., 2010). The current recommendation to avoid "understaging" is a minimum D1 lymphadenectomy with the removal of at least 15 nodes (Songun et al., 2010). Table 3 presents the "D" classification according to the resection sites.

Table 3. "D" classification: Surgical resection width and lymphadenectomy

Definition	Resected Regions
D1	Removing all lymph nodes at a 3 cm distance from the primary tumor (1-6)
D2	In addition to D1, hepatic, splenic, celiac, and left gastric lymph nodes (7-11)
D3	In addition to D2, hepatoduodenal, retropancreatic, mesenteric root, diaphragm (12-14)

Sayek Basic Surgery, 2004.

There are numerous studies arguing that the surgical and oncological outcomes of laparoscopic and robotic operations are similar when compared to open surgery. Moreover, it has been suggested that combined chemoradiotherapy after surgical resection may be effective in improving overall survival in gastric cancers.

Conclusion

Gastric cancer still preserves its place among cancers with a poor prognosis. Opportunities for tumor behavior and the development of new treatment methods will increase through molecular pathways. Genetic changes in gastric cancers can be detected and subclassified. It is especially emphasized that epigenetic changes (miRNA, non-regular expressions of LncRNAs) together with genetic changes can help in dividing the tumor into molecular subclasses. There is a need for patient-based studies on these issues. As a result of the studies, it is considered that RNA molecules can be used in new treatment options. Furthermore, in surgical processes, the only curative method in localized gastric cancers is the complete resection of regional lymph nodes and tumors. Functional surgical methods can be preferred in suitable patients. Pancreas and spleen-preserving D2 dissection is preferred as a standard approach in serosa-positive and/or lymph node-positive cases.

References

Abakay, C. (2019). *Etiology, Risk Factors, Prevention and Early Diagnosis in Stomach Cancer: Current Approaches in Gastric Cancer Treatment. Turkiye clinics*, (1),1-6, https://www.turkiyeklinikleri.com/article/tr-mide-kanserinde-etiyoloji-risk-faktorleri-korunma-ve-erken-tani-85850.html.

Amieva, M. R., & El-Omar, E. M. (2008). Host-bacterial interactions in Helicobacter pylori infection. *Gastroenterology*, *134*(1), 306–323. https://doi.org/10.1053/j.gastro.2007.11.009.

Bozzetti, F., Marubini, E., Bonfanti, G., Miceli, R., Piano, C., & Gennari, L. (1999). Subtotal versus total gastrectomy for gastric cancer: five-year survival rates in a multicenter randomized Italian trial. Italian

Gastrointestinal Tumor Study Group. *Annals of Surgery*, *230*(2), 170–178. https://doi.org/10.1097/ 000 00658-199908000-00006.

Canale, M., Casadei-Gardini, A., Ulivi, P., Arechederra, M., Berasain, C., Lollini, P. L., Fernández-Barrena, M. G., & Avila, M. A. (2020). Epigenetic Mechanisms in Gastric Cancer: Potential New Therapeutic Opportunities. *International Journal of Molecular Sciences*, *21*(15), 5500. https://doi.org/10.3390/ijms2 1155500.

Correa, P., Haenszel, W., Cuello, C., Zavala, D., Fontham, E., Zarama, G., Tannenbaum, S., Collazos, T., & Ruiz, B. (1990). Gastric precancerous process in a high risk population: cohort follow-up. *Cancer Research*, *50*(15), 4737–4740.

Duell, E. J., Sala, N., Travier, N., Muñoz, X., Boutron-Ruault, M. C., Clavel-Chapelon, F., Barricarte, A., Arriola, L., Navarro, C., Sánchez-Cantalejo, E., Quirós, J. R., Krogh, V., Vineis, P., Mattiello, A., Tumino, R., Khaw, K. T., Wareham, N., Allen, N. E., Peeters, P. H., Numans, M. E., Bueno-de-Mesquita, H.B., van Oijen, M. G. H., Bamia, C., Benetou, V., Trichopoulos, D., Canzian F., Kaaks, R., Boeing, H., Bergmann, M. M., Lund, E., Ehrnström, R., Johansen, D., Hallmans, G., Stenling, R., Tjønneland, A., Overvad, K., Ostergaard, J. N., Ferrari, P., Fedirko, V., Jenab, M., Nesi, G., Riboli, E., González, C. A. (2012). Genetic variation in alcohol dehydrogenase (ADH1A, ADH1B, ADH1C, ADH7) and aldehyde dehydrogenase (ALDH2), alcohol consumption and gastric cancer risk in the European Prospective Investigation into Cancer and Nutrition (EPIC) cohort. *Carcinogenesis*, *33*(2), 361–367. https://doi. org/10.1093/carcin/bgr285.

Eguchi, T., Takahashi, Y., Yamagata, M., Kasahara, M., & Fujii, M. (1999). Gastric cancer in young patients. *Journal of the American College of Surgeons*, *188*(1), 22–26. https://doi.org/10.1016/s1072-7515(98) 00268-3.

Feldman, M., Friedman, L.S. & Brandt, L.J. *Sleisenger and Fordtran's Gastrointestinal and Liver Disease-* 2 Volume Set, 11th Edition. Elsevier. https://www.eu.elsevierhealth.com/sleisenger-and-fordtrans-gastro intestinal-and-liver-disease-2-volume-set-9780323609623.html.

Ford, A. C., Forman, D., Hunt, R. H., Yuan, Y., & Moayyedi, P. (2014). Helicobacter pylori eradication therapy to prevent gastric cancer in healthy asymptomatic infected individuals: systematic review and meta-analysis of randomised controlled trials. *BMJ (Clinical Research Ed.)*, *348*, g3174. https://doi.org/ 10.1136/ bmj.g3174.

Genta R. M. (1998). Acid suppression and gastric atrophy: sifting fact from fiction. *Gut*, *43 Suppl 1*(Suppl 1), S35–S38. https://doi.org/10.1136/gut.43.2008.s35.

Gotoda, T., Yanagisawa, A., Sasako, M., Ono, H., Nakanishi, Y., Shimoda, T., & Kato, Y. (2000). Incidence of lymph node metastasis from early gastric cancer: estimation with a large number of cases at two large centers..*Gastric Cancer: Official Journal of the International Gastric Cancer Association and the Japanese Gastric Cancer Association*, *3*(4), 219–225. https://doi.org/10.1007/pl00011720.

Gouzi, J. L., Huguier, M., Fagniez, P. L., Launois, B., Flamant, Y., Lacaine, F., Paquet, J. C., & Hay, J. M. (1989). Total versus subtotal gastrectomy for adenocarcinoma of the gastric antrum. A French prospective controlled study. *Annals of Surgery*, *209*(2), 162–166. https://doi.org/10.1097/00000658-198902000-00005.

Hansford, S., Kaurah, P., Li-Chang, H., Woo, M., Senz, J., Pinheiro, H., Schrader, K. A., Schaeffer, D. F., Shumansky, K., Zogopoulos, G., Santos, T. A., Claro, I., Carvalho, J., Nielsen, C., Padilla, S., Lum, A., Talhouk, A., Baker-Lange, K., Richardson, S., Lewis, I., Lindor, N. M., Pennell, E., MacMillan, A., Fernandez, B., Keller, G.,https://pubmed.ncbi.nlm.nih.gov/26182300/ Lynch, H., Shah, S. P., Guilford, P., Gallinger, S., Corso, G., Roviello, F., Caldas, C., Oliveira, C., Pharoah, P. D. P., Huntsman, D. G. (2015). Hereditary Diffuse Gastric Cancer Syndrome: CDH1 Mutations and Beyond. *JAMA Oncology*, 1(1), 23–32. https://doi.org/10.1001/ jamaoncol.2014.168.

Japanese Gastric Cancer Association (2017). Japanese gastric cancer treatment guidelines 2014 (ver. 4). *Gastric cancer: official journal of the International Gastric Cancer Association and the Japanese Gastric Cancer Association*, *20*(1), 1–19. https://doi.org/10.1007/s10120-016-0622-4.

Joshi, S. S., & Badgwell, B. D. (2021). Current treatment and recent progress in gastric cancer. *CA: A Cancer Journal for Clinicians*, *71*(3), 264–279. https://doi.org/10.3322/caac.21657.

Kant, P., & Hull, M. A. (2011). Excess body weight and obesity--the link with gastrointestinal and hepatobiliary cancer. *Nature Reviews. Gastroenterology & Hepatology*, *8*(4), 224–238. https://doi.org/10.1038/nrgastro.2011.23.

Larsson, S. C., Bergkvist, L., & Wolk, A. (2006). Processed meat consumption, dietary nitrosamines and stomach cancer risk in a cohort of Swedish women. *International Journal of Cancer*, *119*(4), 915–919. https://doi.org/10.1002/ijc.21925.

Lee, J. H., Kim, S. H., Han, S. H., An, J. S., Lee, E. S., & Kim, Y. S. (2009). Clinicopathological and molecular characteristics of Epstein-Barr virus-associated gastric carcinoma: a meta-analysis. *Journal of Gastroenterology and Hepatology*, *24*(3), 354–365. https://doi.org/10.1111/j.1440-1746.2009.05775.x.

Lee, T. H., Cho, J. Y., Chang, Y. W., Kim, J. O., Lee, J. S., Cho, W. Y., Kim, H. G., Kim, W. J., Park, Y. S., & Jin, S. Y. (2010). Appropriate indications for endoscopic submucosal dissection of early gastric cancer according to tumor size and histologic type. *Gastrointestinal Endoscopy*, *71*(6), 920–926. https://doi.org/10.1016/j.gie.2009.12.005.

Lott, P. C., & Carvajal-Carmona, L. G. (2018). Resolving gastric cancer aetiology: an update in genetic predisposition. *The Lancet. Gastroenterology & Hepatology*, *3*(12), 874–883. https://doi.org/10.1016/S2468-1253(18)30237-1.

MacInnis, R. J., English, D. R., Hopper, J. L., & Giles, G. G. (2006). Body size and composition and the risk of gastric and oesophageal adenocarcinoma. *International Journal of Cancer*, *118*(10), 2628–2631. https://doi.org/10.1002/ijc.21638.

Mager D. L. (2006). Bacteria and cancer: cause, coincidence or cure? A review. *Journal of Translational Medicine*, *4*, 14. https://doi.org/10.1186/1479-5876-4-14.

Ministry of Health of Turkey. *Health Statistics Yearbook 2019*. https://sbsgm.saglik.gov.tr/Eklenti/40566/0/health-statistics-yearbook-2019pdf.pdf.

Nakajima, T., Maekita, T., Oda, I., Gotoda, T., Yamamoto, S., Umemura, S., Ichinose, M., Sugimura, T., Ushijima, T., & Saito, D. (2006). Higher methylation levels in gastric mucosae significantly correlate with higher risk of gastric cancers. *Cancer Epidemiology, Biomarkers & Prevention: A Publication of the American Association for Cancer Research, Cosponsored by the American Society of Preventive Oncology*, *15*(11), 2317–2321. https://doi.org/10.1158/1055-9965.EPI-06-0436.

Oliveira, C., Pinheiro, H., Figueiredo, J., Seruca, R., & Carneiro, F. (2015). Familial gastric cancer: genetic susceptibility, pathology, and implications for management. *The Lancet. Oncology*, *16*(2), e60–e70. https://doi.org/10.1016/S1470-2045(14)71016-2.

Oral, D., Yirün, A., Erkekoğlu, P. (2019). Epigenetic and genetic changes caused by Helicobacter Pylori and their roles in gastric carcinogenesis. *J. Fac. Pharm.* Ankara. 43(3), 285-308, https://avesis. hacettepe.edu.tr/yayin/a40d14de-29f4-4a26-a621-c315f647b271/epigenetic-and-genetic-changes-caused-by-helicobacter-pylori-and-their-roles-in-gastric-carcinogenesis-helicobacter-pylori-nin-neden-olduu-epigenetik-ve-genetik-deisiklikler-ve-gastrik-karsinojenez-gelisimi.

Powell, J., & McConkey, C. C. (1990). Increasing incidence of adenocarcinoma of the gastric cardia and adjacent sites. *British Journal of Cancer*, *62*(3), 440–443. https://doi.org/10.1038/bjc.1990.314.

Quante, M., Bornschein, J. (2021). Adenocarcinoma of the stomach and other gastric tumors. In: Feldman M, Friedman L S, Brandt L J, eds. *Sleisenger and Fordtran's Gastrointestinal and Liver Disease*. 11th ed. Philadelphia, PA: Elsevier; chap 54, 820-841. https://www.eu.elsevierhealth.com/sleisenger-and-fordtrans-gastrointestinal-and-liver-disease-2-volume-set-9780323609623.html.

Rugge, M., Farinati, F., Baffa, R., Sonego, F., Di Mario, F., Leandro, G., & Valiante, F. (1994). Gastric epithelial dysplasia in the natural history of gastric cancer: a multicenter prospective follow-up study. Interdisciplinary Group on Gastric Epithelial Dysplasia. *Gastroenterology*, *107*(5), 1288–1296. https://doi.org/10.1016/0016-5085(94)90529-0.

Samadani, A. A., Noroollahi, S. E., Mansour-Ghanaei, F., Rashidy-Pour, A., Joukar, F., & Bandegi, A. R. (2019). Fluctuations of epigenetic regulations in human gastric Adenocarcinoma: How does it affect?. *Biomedicine & Pharmacotherapy = Biomedecine & Pharmacotherapie*, *109*, 144–156. https://doi.org/10.1016/j.biopha.2018.10.094.

Soetikno, R., Kaltenbach, T., Yeh, R., & Gotoda, T. (2005). Endoscopic mucosal resection for early cancers of the upper gastrointestinal tract. *Journal of Clinical Oncology: Official Journal of the American Society of Clinical Oncology*, *23*(20), 4490–4498. https://doi.org/10.1200/JCO.2005.19.935.

Songun, I., Putter, H., Kranenbarg, E. M., Sasako, M., & van de Velde, C. J. (2010). Surgical treatment of gastric cancer: 15-year follow-up results of the randomised nationwide Dutch D1D2 trial. *The Lancet. Oncology*, *11*(5), 439–449. https://doi.org/10.1016/S1470-2045(10)70070-X.

Sung, H., Ferlay, J., Siegel, R. L., Laversanne, M., Soerjomataram, I., Jemal, A., & Bray, F. (2021). Global Cancer Statistics 2020: GLOBOCAN Estimates of Incidence and Mortality Worldwide for 36 Cancers in 185 Countries. *CA: A Cancer Journal for Clinicians*, *71*(3), 209–249. https://doi.org/10.3322/caac.21660.

Takeno, S., Hashimoto, T., Maki, K., Shibata, R., Shiwaku, H., Yamana, I., Yamashita, R., & Yamashita, Y. (2014). Gastric cancer arising from the remnant stomach after distal gastrectomy: a review. *World Journal of Gastroenterology*, *20*(38), 13734–13740. https://doi.org/10.3748/wjg.v20.i38.13734.

Torre, L. A., Bray, F., Siegel, R. L., Ferlay, J., Lortet-Tieulent, J., & Jemal, A. (2015). Global cancer statistics, 2012. *CA: A Cancer Journal for Clinicians*, *65*(2), 87–108. https://doi.org/10.3322/caac.21262.

Van Cutsem, E., Van de Velde, C., Roth, A., Lordick, F., Köhne, C. H., Cascinu, S., Aapro, M., & European Organisation for Research and Treatment of Cancer (EORTC)-gastrointestinal cancer group (2008). Expert opinion on management of gastric and gastro-oesophageal junction adenocarcinoma on behalf of the European Organisation for Research and Treatment of Cancer (EORTC)-gastrointestinal cancer group. *European Journal of Cancer (Oxford, England: 1990)*, *44*(2), 182–194. https://doi.org/10.1016/j.ejca.2007.11.001.

Zhou, Z., Lin, Z., Pang, X., Tariq, M. A., Ao, X., Li, P., & Wang, J. (2017). Epigenetic regulation of long non-coding RNAs in gastric cancer. *Oncotarget*, *9*(27), 19443–19458. https://doi.org/10.18632/oncotarget.23821.

Editors' Contact Information

Sevgi Durna Daştan
Associate Professor
Faculty of Science, Department of Biology, Division of Molecular Biology
Sivas Cumhuriyet University
58140, Sivas, Turkey
sevgidurna@gmail.com

Nazan Yurtcu
Assistant Professor
Faculty of Medicine, Department of Obstetrics and Gynecology
Sivas Cumhuriyet University
58153, Sivas, Turkey
nazanyurtcu@cumhuriyet.edu.tr

Index

B

C

D

E

F

G

H

I

J

K

L

M

N

Q

R

T

U

V

W

X

Z